Advance Praise for *Lawless*

"Clear, rigorous, and deeply grounded in both scholarship and practice, *Lawless* is an essential resource for anyone working to make abortion access real. Drawing on her brilliance as a teacher and researcher, Paynter demystifies the different layers — legal, clinical, political, and social — that shape abortion care in Canada. This book is not only a must-read for scholars and activists in Canada, but also a powerful guide for global advocates seeking to understand what it takes to move from legal frameworks to meaningful access."

—**DIANA MORENO**, Advocacy Director, Profamilia

"Dr. Paynter has delivered a comprehensively researched and clearly written user guide for understanding the Canadian legal context for abortion and how this impacts upon delivery and access. Valuable for clinicians, researchers, and activists, in Canada and worldwide. As an international reader, I was fascinated by the history of Canada's abortion law reform and the continued struggle to ensure access to affordable, compassionate, and timely care. Understanding the Canadian journey is critical to countries like the UK, teetering on the brink of law reform and decriminalization, and *Lawless* guides the reader through the successes and challenges in that journey so far."

—**DR. JOHN REYNOLDS-WRIGHT**, University of Edinburgh

"*Lawless* is a compelling exploration of what full decriminalization of abortion can achieve—and what it cannot. As we in the UK confront the persistent criminalization of abortion and a troubling rise in prosecutions, this book serves as both an inspiration and a warning. Drawing from Canada's unique legal landscape as the only country to have fully decriminalized abortion, Martha Paynter's insights make clear that removing abortion from criminal law is essential, but ensuring equitable access demands systemic change across healthcare, education, and society. She makes clear how access to abortion protects health, dignity, and equality — and how denial deepens poverty and injustice. *Lawless* is an essential read for clinicians, policymakers, and advocates committed to advancing reproductive autonomy."

—**DR. PATRICIA A. LOHR**, Director of Research and Innovation, British Pregnancy Advisory Service

"This book brings into focus a vibrant picture of the past, present and future of abortion access in Canada. The scope of this book is amazing — each chapter is so well referenced and clearly written. Paynter expertly articulates how access to abortion and reproductive justice can be denied or limited, despite the removal of abortion from the criminal code in 1988. She describes the significant challenges overcome by the diverse reproductive justice movement, and lays out the next battles required to remove the remaining barriers to true reproductive justice for all Canadians."

—LIANNE YOSHIDA, MD, Reproductive Options and Services (ROSE) Clinic Halifax

"Dr. Martha Paynter cuts sharply through the shroud of secrecy and misinformation surrounding abortion in Canada. An invaluable resource detailing a path of resiliency, imperfection, victories, and struggles, this book is a clear map that leaves the reader informed, invigorated, and hopeful of change yet to come."

—NATASHA HINES, Chair, Wellness Within

"*Lawless* is a bold, timely, and essential exploration of what it truly means to provide abortion services free from the constraints of criminal law. With clarity, passion, and lived expertise, Dr. Martha Paynter exemplifies Canada's unique position as the only country in the world with complete decriminalization—while revealing the ongoing barriers, disinformation, and political resistance that persist. This book is a vital resource for women and gender activists, clinicians, educators and students of law, political scientists, historians, policymakers, and anyone interested in and seeking honest, accessible, and justice-driven insights into abortion care today. This book doesn't just inform—it empowers, calling readers to action in pursuit of a more equitable reproductive future."

—ABDUL-FATAWU ABDULAI, University of British Columbia

"Dr. Paynter is one of the few people in Canada whose combined experience as a frontline health care provider, researcher, teacher, and activist gives her a rare, birds-eye view of the legal, policy, and access dimensions of abortion. This book is a vital resource for anyone seeking to understand abortion not just as a medical procedure but as a political flashpoint and a cornerstone of gender justice. Accessible, grounded, and deeply informed, this book will reshape how we think and talk about reproductive rights in Canada."

—FRÉDÉRIQUE CHABOT, Executive Director, Action Canada for Sexual Health and Rights

"Dr. Martha Paynter's book, *Lawless*, offers a careful and rigorous analysis of abortion in Canada, illuminating the complexities of reproductive justice in a manner that is clear and conscientious. By centring patients over policy hurdles and offering a robust examination of inter-jurisdictional health care, Dr. Paynter's book also stands as a vital case study for anyone engaged in public health or service delivery. I especially appreciate how her scholarship situates abortion alongside the ongoing realities of forced, coercive, and involuntary sterilization of Indigenous Peoples, offering an essential lens of analysis for reproductive justice in this country."

—**KAREN LAWFORD, PHD**, Anishinaabe Midwife, Lac Seul First Nation

"*Lawless* is a bold, necessary, and deeply informed call to action. As a midwife and leader in reproductive and sexual health, I urge everyone working in health policy and care delivery to read this book. *Lawless* shows us how Canada can move from legal freedom to true, equitable access to abortion care for all."

—**CJ BLENNERHASSETT**, President, Canadian Association of Midwives

"Martha Paynter's book is a tour de force examination of the abortion situation in Canada today. She makes a strong case that decriminalized abortion in Canada has been a huge win for Canadians. It's helped enable ongoing improvements to abortion access, free care for almost everyone, higher quality services, and more providers — especially after the introduction of the abortion pill in 2017. While we still have gaps to work on and threats to fight against, Paynter's book reminds us to be proud of our accomplishments and gives us confidence to achieve even more."

—**JOYCE ARTHUR**, Executive Director, Abortion Rights Coalition of Canada (ARCC)

"Dr. Paynter's writing style is engaging, encouraging rapid page turning as Canada's story of abortion regulation within the context of complete decriminalization effortlessly unfolds. She has included all aspects I wanted to understand, and explained complex legal terms and processes in accessible and very readable prose. This is set to become a handbook for legislators and advocates in countries where abortion remains in criminal law, and it will undoubtedly be required reading for health care law courses across Canada."

—**WENDY V. NORMAN**, University of British Columbia

LAWLESS

LAWLESS

ABORTION UNDER COMPLETE DECRIMINALIZATION

MARTHA PAYNTER

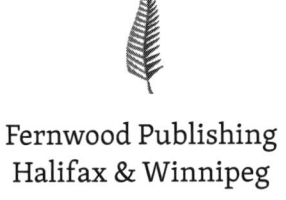

Fernwood Publishing
Halifax & Winnipeg

Copyright 2025 © Martha Paynter

All rights reserved. No part of this book may be reproduced or transmitted in any form by any means without permission in writing from the publisher, except by a reviewer, who may quote brief passages in a review. The publisher expressly prohibits the use of this work in connection with the development of any software program, including, without limitation, training a machine learning or generative artificial intelligence (AI) system.

Development editor: Fazeela Jiwa
Copyediting: Jenn Harris
Text design: Brenda Conroy
Cover design: Evan Marnoch
Printed and bound in the UK

Published by Fernwood Publishing
Halifax and Winnipeg
2970 Oxford Street, Halifax, Nova Scotia, B3L 2W4
www.fernwoodpublishing.ca

Fernwood Publishing Company Limited gratefully acknowledges the financial support of the Government of Canada through the Canada Book Fund and the Canada Council for the Arts. We acknowledge the Province of Manitoba for support through the Manitoba Publishers Marketing Assistance Program and the Book Publishing Tax Credit. We acknowledge the Nova Scotia Department of Communities, Culture and Heritage for support through the Publishers Assistance Fund. We also acknowledge the Urban Studies Foundation for publishing support.

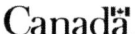 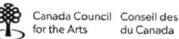 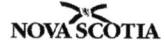 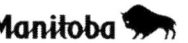

Library and Archives Canada Cataloguing in Publication
Title: Lawless : abortion under complete decriminalization / Martha Paynter.
Names: Paynter, Martha, author.
Description: Includes bibliographical references and index.
Identifiers: Canadiana 20250224917 | ISBN 9781773637501 (softcover)
Subjects: LCSH: Abortion—Canada—History. | LCSH: Abortion—Government policy—Canada. | LCSH: Abortion—Law and legislation—Canada. | LCSH: Abortion—Political aspects—Canada. | LCSH: Reproductive rights—Canada. | LCSH: Women—Health and hygiene—Canada.
Classification: LCC HQ767.5.C2 P39 2025 | DDC 362.1988/80971—dc23

For my parents, Beth and Jacques

CONTENTS

INTRODUCTION	Decriminalized Abortion	1
CHAPTER 1	What Is Abortion?	12
CHAPTER 2	With Laws Come Limits	24
CHAPTER 3	Defining Miscarriage, Stillbirth, and Infant Death	49
CHAPTER 4	The Mifepristone Revolution	59
CHAPTER 5	Belief-Based Denial of Care	85
CHAPTER 6	Crisis Pregnancy Centres	100
CHAPTER 7	Freedom of Expression and Assembly	113
CHAPTER 8	Expansion of Care	130
CHAPTER 9	Children and Youth	149
CHAPTER 10	Contraception	161
CHAPTER 11	International Law	169
CONCLUSION	Onward	177
ACKNOWLEDGEMENTS		181
ENDNOTES		183
INDEX		223

INTRODUCTION

DECRIMINALIZED ABORTION

Canada is the only country in the world in which abortion is completely decriminalized. This fact is remarkable, powerful, and enduring. In recent years, many countries have made significant progress towards partial and even widespread decriminalization. In 2024, France incorporated into its federal constitution the right to abortion to sixteen weeks gestational duration. In 2022, Columbia decriminalized to twenty-five weeks. In 2020, New Zealand decriminalized to twenty. There are many other examples. Meanwhile, the United States has notoriously lost ground in reproductive rights after the June 2022 Supreme Court ruled in *Dobbs v. Jackson Women's Health Organization* that the US Constitution does not protect the right to abortion and states can individually legislate abortion. In the tumult of these changes worldwide, public conversations about and understanding of abortion have changed. As a clinician and researcher in this area, I see how the public is increasingly curious about what abortion really is, brazen about asking for answers, and determined to see removed the remaining obstacles blocking access to care. Even after thirty-seven sustained years of complete decriminalization, the on-the-ground reality of abortion in Canada is uneven and unclear. The anti-choice lobby is robust, well-funded, and persistent — its members produce reams of disinformation to swell the results of any Google search. They poster and billboard, protest and march, and set up booths in schools and on sidewalks. Competing with this industry is laborious, and I often feel like factual publications are the needle in a haystack. This book is a needle, then, but hopefully a big one.

This book is intended for readers with an interest in clear, matter-of-fact, approachable information about how abortion works in a contemporary context of complete decriminalization, as well as guidance on important focal areas to improve access. Activists and champions for abortion may come away with stronger convictions and precise targets for new dimensions of advocacy. Community organization workers will recognize persistent barriers to care for clients and learn practical navigation strategies. Educators and students of law, women's and gender studies, political science, history, and sociology can use this book to develop different perspectives on the complexity of a topic significant to each discipline. Health professionals can learn about an under-taught, stigmatized, and yet essential service in ways that may change their practices and enhance their patient advocacy. Policy decision makers should read this book to see what matters most now and where they can be most impactful. Journalists should read this book to get the facts and disseminate them widely. Youth readers will learn what abortion is and the extent to which their privacy and autonomy are protected when seeking care. Parents, likewise, can read it to understand the regulatory and service landscape youth face when seeking sexual and reproductive health services — including gender affirming care — and to empower them to speak knowledgeably and compassionately with their children about options. My intention with this book is to introduce abortion to wide audiences in language and approaches that are pragmatic and positive.

My interest in abortion began as a child. My parents have always been deeply supportive of bodily autonomy and identify strongly as feminists. My mother worked as the executive director of Planned Parenthood New Brunswick. Reproduction was not kept secret. I remember when, at age six or seven, our neighbour miscarried and needed my mom's support. She explained to me what happened and said pregnancy loss was not shameful or uncommon. A classmate was sexually assaulted in my classroom when I was in elementary school, prompting my mother and I to demand thorough and early formal education about sex and consent. There was a nursery at my high school, and when two people in my homeroom class had babies one year, my mother encouraged me to visit them in hospital. My parents' friends ran the downtown Morgentaler abortion clinic. Abortion struck me, as a teenager, as simply a necessary part of life.

Over the past two decades, my role in the abortion movement in Canada has shifted and multiplied: I have led campaigns to fund Dr. Henry Morgentaler's legal battle against New Brunswick, volunteered as a free-standing clinic escort, helped take the provincial government of Prince Edward Island to court until they opened a clinic, badgered policymakers about financing mifepristone, worked bedside as an abortion clinic nurse, taught health professional undergraduate students their first and only modules about abortion, and researched nationwide changes to access. Over these twenty years the movement has experienced massive successes, most notably the approval of medication abortion, its public funding, and the immense expansion of abortion providers made possible through its complete deregulation and implementation in primary care. I am fervently committed to my colleagues in critical community organizations like Wellness Within: An Organization for Health and Justice, Action Canada for Sexual Health and Rights, the Women's Legal Education and Action Fund (LEAF), and the National Abortion Federation Canada (now named Abortion Care Canada); those on the front lines of care such as the Reproductive Options and Services (ROSE) Clinic in Halifax, named after longtime physician Dr. Jacques Desrosiers, and the New Brunswick Abortion Care Network; and those engrossed in family planning science at the University of New Brunswick and the Contraception and Abortion Research Team headquartered at the University of British Columbia. I say yes to (nearly) every ask by news media to speak about abortion access issues because when they get it wrong, the ramifications are dangerous, but also because the terrain is changing so quickly in recent years that, I recognize, it can be hard to get it right.

I am extremely proud and protective of Canada's position on abortion and dedicated to its perpetual improvement. The aim of this book is to explain how far we have come in recent years, through the relentless efforts by activists and abortion providers, and where we need to go from here. The title, *Lawless*, honours the rebellious energy of Canada's extraordinary position as a lone country globally with complete decriminalization. But Canada is not actually "lawless" at all: layers of laws and regulations at the federal, provincial, and territorial levels impact abortion, even if there is no one abortion law per se. This book tells the story of that complexity, while also drawing attention to the ways in which abortion access can be improved outside of legal frameworks, through research evidence, health professional leadership, frontline ingenuity, and the banal act of talking about abortion as a norm.

Abortion Access Varies because Health Care Varies

I decided I wanted to write this book while sitting in the audience at a very small conference in fall 2023 in Lethbridge, Alberta, at the Galt Museum, on the edge of the coulees. I was invited by ProChoice YQL, a small non-profit, to speak about my 2022 book, *Abortion to Abolition: Reproductive Health and Justice in Canada*. I consider Alberta to be one of the most challenging and fascinating sites of abortion access in Canada. Everyone thinks of New Brunswick's access as so terrible, and many people commented, when I chose to move home to New Brunswick in summer 2022, that I would have my work cut out for me. Indeed, the province has a twisted history of reproductive rights exceptionalism: it was the first province, back in the nineteenth century, to criminalize abortion. But New Brunswick has made incredible strides in access in recent years: it was the first province to announce and implement public funding for mifepristone and one of the first to warmly welcome nurse practitioner prescribing. New Brunswick has a population less than one-fifth that of Alberta, and it is physically only one-ninth the size of Alberta. Yet, New Brunswick has *more* self-referral facilities performing procedural abortion (three) than Alberta (two). That surprising information is never given a press headline.

At a National Abortion Federation Canada annual meeting in fall 2023, I met most of the nursing staff from the Women's Health Options Clinic in Edmonton. They perform forty procedures a day, working overtime almost daily. The main abortion facility in Calgary, the Kensington Clinic, performs similar volumes. I found these numbers flabbergasting. In Nova Scotia's main abortion clinic in Halifax, ROSE, where I nursed for several years and continue to hold a research appointment, we did not perform that many procedures in a *week*. In New Brunswick, there are fewer than 410 procedural abortions every year.[1] However, Alberta's abortion care providers face extraordinary demand and meet it. While astonishing and admirable, this is inarguably problematic: a small, feminized nursing and physician workforce is routinely absorbing extra work to keep the wheels of reproductive autonomy rolling for Albertans.

Which brings me back to ProChoice YQL. This small non-profit, with one paid staff member and not a single clinician, runs a 24/7 abortion hotline. Every few years they send a survey out to the entire primary care workforce in the region asking who is willing to prescribe medication abortion, and then they pool the results into an active registry of reliable abortion prescribers in southern Alberta. Whenever a patient calls the hotline asking for information, if they are under nine to ten weeks' gestation, eligible, and interested, a responding ProChoice YQL member refers them to an appropriate medication abortion prescriber. If the caller is not interested in or ineligible for medication abortion, they are directed to one of the two procedural abortion clinics. ProChoice YQL keeps track of which southern Alberta prescribers are willing to do prescriptions over the phone or through an online virtual appointment; which ones will not charge fees to non-citizens; and which ones have recently left the province because they are horrified by the political climate. Alberta Health has a $25 billion budget, yet a small group of mostly volunteers are responsible for ensuring southern Alberta has pregnancy termination care. They do this because no one else does. The burden facing Alberta's abortion work and volunteer forces has nothing to do with an abortion law and everything to do with health system funding, abortion stigma, and obfuscation. Access in Alberta will be remedied through complex changes to regulations, attitudes, and activities that surround and impact abortion care, and strategies to get there need to be prioritized.

The *R. v. Morgentaler* Canadian Supreme Court decision of January 1988 declared the section of the Criminal Code that governed abortion — Section 251 — to be unconstitutional. It was incompatible with Section 7 of the Canadian Charter of Rights and Freedoms, which asserts the right to life, liberty, and security of the person. That security of the self, that self-governance, would be undermined by any law restricting abortion. This is different from the logic of the US Supreme Court 1973 *Roe v. Wade* decision, which was based on the federal constitutional right to equal protection and privacy, and was, notoriously, revoked in June of 2022. In Canada, *Morgentaler* affirms a constitutional right to autonomy over your own body.

Canada remains the only country in the world with complete decriminalization of abortion. There are no legal restrictions on gestational duration, no required waiting periods, no mandatory counselling, no parental consent requirements, or any other legal barriers erected solely to delay and diminish abortion access. Most abortion care providers report feeling safe and free from harassment.[2] Yet in this context of complete decriminalization, a tangle of barriers persists and activists, lawyers, health care providers, and community organizations like ProChoice YQL continue to cut through it.

While safety from prosecution is certainly essential for patients to seek care and providers to provide it, decriminalization is insufficient. It is not an abortion-restricting law that ProChoice YQL is up against — it is Premier Danielle Smith's zest for privatization of hospitals and health services;[3] providers' fear of being open about prescribing mifepristone; social shaming of premarital sex and religious curriculum in southern Alberta public schools;[4] and escalating poverty, food insecurity, and homelessness in the province.[5] These represent structural barriers to patient autonomy, even if the Charter supports it. These barriers make ProChoice YQL indispensable.

Atlantic Canada is often touted as having the worst access in the country because consistent elective care beyond eighteen weeks gestation is not routinely available. Again, this is not because of a law. It is a complex issue, dependent on a combination of systems factors: health professional training and experience, access to equipment and space, clinic administrative staffing, and interprovincial care coordination. Work is underway to make these adjustments to expand gestational duration capabilities, but it may yet be years until one or every province in the region achieves the gestational capacities of the other provinces (twenty weeks or more). In the interim, the limits in Atlantic Canada may cause patients to feel judged and stigmatized for being "late" and being obliged to travel out of the region for care. Ironically, they may have to travel to Alberta.

While the complex task of equalizing gestational limits is going to take time, we could immediately make changes to remedy the unequal costs patients face to travel out of the region for services. We would do this by improving public funding for health services, simplifying the forms and hastening approvals of Medicare coverage for out-of-province or even out-of-country care, and recognizing pregnancy is on a timer and abortion is an essential service. If health professionals did not have to navigate these time-consuming logistical and regulatory hurdles of ensuring care affordability for travellers, we could focus instead on providing and improving clinical care locally.

Indeed, without the very heavy cloak of fear that criminalization casts, providers and advocates focus on different kinds of issues. We can reflect on how calling our clinics "Women's This" and "Woman That" is exclusionary and essentialist. We can realize it is not enough to change clinic names to generate gender-inclusive care environments. We can reckon with how our clinic spaces and equipment are fatphobic and ableist. We could notice that security guards at the entrances to our facilities are frightening to Black, Brown, and Indigenous people, who are disproportionately likely to face state violence. We can admit our pregnancy termination practice is submerged in the colonial swamp of forced sterilization and genocide. These changes would make a considerable and concrete difference in the lives of our patients. These conversations peel abortion back from the rhetoric of the criminal justice system and insert it into the complex realm of reproductive justice.

My first book, *Abortion to Abolition: Reproductive Health and Justice in Canada*, was an effort to connect the liberatory philosophy of the abortion clinic to the abolition of the prison cell. The book criticized the overemphasis some feminist activists and health professionals place on abortion in lieu of attention to other issues in reproduction critical to health equity in Canada: gender-affirming care, sexual violence, queer parenting, forced sterilization, assisted reproductive technologies, toxic water supplies, contemporary foster care, and the carceral system. Our focus on overall reproductive health must remain in these areas even as we make progress in abortion care.

Abortion is a Public Good

Individuals have abortions and support abortion, but abortion is not just individual. Abortion is a public good and its protection and promotion is a matter of public interest.

As a nurse and an undergraduate educator, I see firsthand the consequences of persistent stigma, confusion, and misinformation about abortion in Canada. Patients assume it is illegal and tumble into despair. Or they believe they need their parents' permission and cannot face the potential fallout from that judgment. Or they call their family doctor, and the office administrator books them four weeks out — four weeks spent puking, exhausted, and scared — and it's only when they get to the appointment that they learn the family doctor "doesn't do that." Or they are one of the 6.5 million people in Canada who do not have a family doctor. If they search "what to do?" on the internet, the first thing that comes up is an ad for a religious organization's crisis pregnancy centre, where the "support" they provide is shame and misinformation, further delaying access to real care. Abortion may have been completely decriminalized almost four decades ago, but care is still out of reach for many because of a vacuum of information.

Furthermore, as a health service, abortion is subject to the same challenges as all health services with respect to supply: are there enough people from enough disciplines providing it in enough places in enough ways? And even if there are, do patients know how to find these people and what types of abortion they can have when they do?

Canada holds a unique position as the only country in the world with complete decriminalization of abortion, in a global context of shifting reproductive rights. The way we think and talk about abortion is changing — it is becoming normalized — but the dangers of misinformation persist. Stigma and logistical barriers continue to hinder access to abortion services, as do a web of legal stipulations that are not about abortion per se, but dictate how abortion happens nonetheless. Abortion is health care, and improving access will come with systemic enhancements to health care for all, along with broader recognition of reproductive justice issues beyond abortion.

Chapter Summaries

Each of us can chip away at the persistent challenges to abortion access: we can educate ourselves and share factual, compassionate, helpful information. Know our rights to make decisions about our own bodies. Know the number to call to self-refer for an appointment and the URL for a trusted website. Know what the procedure involves and what to expect from the experience of dilatation and aspiration. Know in advance what a medication abortion (a pill-induced miscarriage) will look like: cramping and bleeding experienced at home. Know how to prepare for medication abortion with ibuprofen, a hot water bottle, and jumbo menstrual pads. Don't shy away or avoid this topic; know about it and talk about it. All of this will make a dent.

To begin the book, therefore, in Chapter 1, I explain what abortion is and discuss the prevalence, safety, and effectiveness of abortion services, how to seek care, and what we know about who seeks abortion care. I aim to capture how abortion is a health service, but also make clear its important political significance.

In Chapter 2, I trace how Canada arrived at this unique position as the only country in the world with complete decriminalization of abortion and describe the persistent but unsuccessful efforts from anti-abortion activists to reintroduce legislation to limit access. I argue that despite Canada not having "an abortion law" per se, the Canadian Charter of Rights and Freedoms and the Canada Health Act are profoundly important laws shaping the availability of abortion services across the country. I also honour Dr. Henry Morgentaler's legacy in the clinic and the courtroom, fighting for free and accessible care for all.

The complex legal definitions of miscarriage, stillbirth and infant death in Canada have implications on reproductive health privacy and autonomy, as I will explain in Chapter 3. The content in this chapter may be distressing, particularly for people who have experienced pregnancy and infant loss.

In Chapter 4, I present the extraordinary impact of mifepristone for medication abortion on the landscape of abortion service delivery. The chapter includes descriptions of how medication abortion works and compelling evidence about its safety and effectiveness. I recount how, despite this, it was a protracted effort to win its approval from Health Canada, some thirty-plus years after availability in Europe. That said, once implemented, Health Canada followed through with a swift process of deregulation, making "mife" into a normal prescription. Primary care prescribing of abortion and telemedicine allow vast expansions of the abortion workforce, improve geographic distribution of services, and reduce travel and other barriers to care.

One of the most frustrating barriers to abortion is belief-based denial of care, the subject of Chapter 5. Formerly called "conscientious objection" to provision of abortion services, belief-based denial of care collides with professional codes of ethics and provincial/territorial regulations. I describe these conflicts and contrast the Charter-protected freedom of individuals to religious practice with the "right" of institutions to deny care.

In Chapter 6, I introduce the concept and argue the harm of crisis pregnancy centres (CPCs), which are non-clinical operations run by religious organizations. As registered charities, CPCs may fundraise highly successfully and advertise themselves widely. More bountiful than actual abortion clinics, CPC advertisements and conversations with patients may cause confusion and result in delays in accessing abortion care. Very recently, the federal government launched efforts to stem their negative impact with law that ties their charitable status to transparency about their activities.

Graphic images and public protests are often used by the anti-abortion movement as symbolic, persuasive tools, and these may be perceived to be protected by Charter rights to freedom of assembly and expression. In Chapter 7, I recount how several universities have dealt with conflicts involving anti-abortion student groups over protests and displays of graphic images on campus: are these in public space, or not? The jury remains out. Another tactic of anti-abortion campaigning is to send unsolicited images in the mail: increasingly, municipalities are challenging the logistics of these efforts by introducing bylaws that require, at minimum, the images be sent in a sealed envelope.

Simultaneous to the types of access challenges captured in Chapters 5, 6, and 7, initiatives were underway to expand care. In Chapter 8, I describe some of the successful legal and political strategies that pushed the envelope on abortion access: reducing logistical barriers like referral requirements; launching services on Prince Edward Island; expanding scope of practice so that nurse practitioners and midwives could prescribe medication abortion; improving training opportunities; extending gestational duration capacity; and responding to the fall of *Roe v. Wade*. I also name priorities to continue to make access gains by improving services for diverse communities, including people with disabilities, enhancing gender inclusivity, responding to the needs of Indigenous people, addressing the disproportionate barriers faced by prisoners, and ensuring coverage for newcomers and undocumented people.

Youth seeking abortion services may have intersecting experiences of discrimination that deepen their vulnerability and the important role controlling fertility has on their ability to thrive. As I describe in Chapter 9, there are unique legal and practical considerations with respect to abortion care if a patient is under eighteen years of age, including how they consent to health services and when and whether they consent to sex.

In Chapter 10, I argue that because the financial, social and physiological burdens of unintended pregnancy are disproportionately borne by women, girls, and people with uteruses, gender equity hinges on need for universal access to publicly funded prescription contraception. British Columbia and Manitoba have implemented pharmacare coverage for contraception already, to wide fanfare and enthusiastic uptake. A comprehensive no-cost approach, like that taken with mifepristone, is not only the right thing to do, but the fiscally prudent thing to generate health system savings.

Finally, in Chapter 11, I describe the potential influence of international law, like the International Covenant on Civil and Political Rights (ICCPR)[6] and the International Covenant on Economic, Social and Cultural Rights (ICESCR), on abortion in Canada. While signing international treaties is not the same as passing law that can be enforced domestically, it is nonetheless an important symbol of what we value and believe. It allows us to take stock of progress towards these goalposts and what we still need to achieve.

* * *

This book is about abortion history, policy, practice, and experience. It is about progress and the challenges that persist long after Canada became the most legally progressive jurisdiction for abortion in the world. And it is about what we can do next.

CHAPTER 1

WHAT IS ABORTION?

> This chapter explains what abortion is and discusses the prevalence, safety, and effectiveness of abortion as a health service. Misinformation about abortion is a barrier to access in itself.

Even though one in three women or people with a uterus in Canada will have an abortion in their lifetime[1] and 100,000 abortions occur in Canada each year,[2] making it one of the most common health services available, abortion remains shrouded in secrecy. Requests for care are whispered and clear explanations of pathways and practices hardly exist. But information is always currency in accessing health services: what you know will expedite receiving care. Lacking information or being misinformed can result in delays in care. Care delayed can become care denied, especially for a time-dependent service like pregnancy termination.

Television and movie depictions of abortion are often inaccurate and sensationalistic.[3] More aggressive than gaps in information, anti-abortion extremists circulate myths and fabrications to deliberately misinform and fearmonger. When there is so little trustworthy, public information available about this highly stigmatized experience, journalists, community advocates, and even health professionals can end up circulating and amplifying untruths. Patients feel they are stumbling around in the dark and fill with anxiety. Yet this care can be so straightforward, compassionate, and quick. When I worked as a staff nurse at the Reproductive Options and Services (ROSE) Clinic in Halifax, patients would often say at the end of an appointment, "Oh, this is not what I expected at all."

Conceptualizing information as a critical element to access recognizes how timeliness increases clinical safety and reduces the social burdens placed on patients. At later gestational durations, the care is more complicated and is available in fewer places. The travel to care may not be just more costly but also more conspicuous: it is much harder to keep abortion a private experience when it requires days away from family and work. Information *is* access.

There are two types of abortion: medication abortion and procedural abortion. Medication abortion is also known as abortion with pills or "medical" abortion. However, "medical" can be confusing, since some people think all abortion is somewhat medical in nature, and others think "medical" refers to when abortion is indicated due to medical concerns such as maternal illness or fetal anomaly. For this reason, the term "medication abortion" is preferred. Procedural abortion, or what used to be called "surgical" abortion, is sometimes called aspiration abortion, vacuum abortion, dilatation and curettage (D&C), and dilatation and evacuation (D&E). In French, the term used is *avortement par instruments*, abortion with instruments, because, as the former list implies, the techniques involve using medical instruments such as speculums, tenaculum forceps, dilators, vacuum aspirators, and curettes. Procedural abortion is considered the best current terminology.[4]

Medication Abortion

Medication abortion using a product with the brand name Mifegymiso was approved by Health Canada in 2015. Prior to "mife" approval, medication abortion in Canada relied on use of less effective drugs and was very rare. Mifegymiso comes in a white box with two smaller boxes inside: the green box contains mifepristone, a highly effective and safe prescription anti-progesterone drug, and the orange box contains misoprostol, a prostaglandin. Misoprostol ("miso") was developed in 1973.[5] Misoprostol works alone as an abortifacient, a drug that causes abortion; however, it works less effectively and quickly when taken alone. Mifepristone became available in France in 1988; paired with misoprostol, it makes for an effective, safe, and timely regimen. It was approved by the Food and Drug Administration in the US in 2000. As a result of the long delay from its development in the 1980s to its implementation in Canada in the last decade, and because there have been no public promotion efforts to help Canadians understand what the drug is, medication abortion with mife remains poorly understood.

Many people believe emergency contraception is the same thing as mife.[6] Taken within a few days of unprotected sex, emergency contraception can prevent a pregnancy from occurring; abortion, by contrast, terminates an *existing* pregnancy. Mifepristone *can* work as a type of emergency contraception;[7] it is a remarkably flexible and useful drug, but it is not approved for that use in Canada. The three approved types of emergency contraception include levonorgestrel, ulipristal acetate, and the copper intrauterine device. Commonly known by the brand name "Plan B," the most common form of emergency contraception is levonorgestrel; since 2008, consumers have been able to purchase it over the counter (OTC) in pharmacies.[8] In 2018, there were over 124,000 units of levonorgestrel sold in British Columbia alone.[9] Ulipristal acetate, known by the brand name Ella, is a more effective medication than levonorgestrel. It works well to 120 hours (almost five days after unprotected sex), and it works better than Plan B for patients at higher weights. But it is only available by prescription. A study found that in 2018, there were 389 units of Ella sold in BC.[10] The copper IUD is usually used as a regular type of long-acting, reversible contraception. Unlike most forms of prescription birth control, which may take a few weeks to realize therapeutic effect, the copper IUD works so fast it will reliably prevent a pregnancy if inserted in the first few days after unprotected sex. Emergency contraception is used at vastly higher rates than medication abortion, has been available longer, and is unsurprisingly better known than mife.

The mife medication abortion regimen involves first taking one single pill of mifepristone to terminate the pregnancy, and then in the next twenty-four to forty-eight hours taking four pills of misoprostol, a prostaglandin, which causes uterine cramping and expulsion of tissue. Most people feel very little after the mife and only start to experience cramping and bleeding one to four hours after taking the miso. Medication abortion takes a varying amount of time to "complete" and normal bleeding can last over a week.[11] It is very similar to spontaneous abortion (miscarriage). While some patients experience medication abortion like a bad period, for others it may be much more difficult, with heavy bleeding and significant pain. Patients may experience minor adverse effects, including nausea, vomiting, diarrhea, fever, chills, and headache. Prescribers often recommend OTC non-steroidal anti-inflammatory medications like ibuprofen, antiemetics (anti-nausea medications), and non-pharmacological supports like a hot water bottle and herbal teas. Up to one-fifth of medication abortion patients have used cannabis to manage pain in states where cannabis is legalized.[12]

Many patients prefer medication abortion over procedural abortion because it is discreet; perhaps they have had a spontaneous abortion in the past and have an idea of what they will experience. They may feel it is more convenient and comfortable than a procedure in a clinic or hospital. However, patients may also dislike that the timeframe for medication abortion to take effect is uncertain. It may simply not line up with their employment or personal life. For some, knowing that medication abortion resembles a miscarriage is helpful. Some may not feel safe to experience their abortion at home because of intimate partner violence, reproductive coercion, or parental judgment. Some may not want to deal with discomfort, blood, and expelled products of conception at home without clinical support. Deciding between medication and procedural abortion is personal. That said, there are external pressures on this decision. Health Canada approved mifepristone for use at home up to nine to ten weeks' gestation, because the evidence of effectiveness is strongest up to this point, although elsewhere in the world it is commonly prescribed until twelve weeks. Patients beyond nine to ten weeks may not be offered a choice.

Chapter 4, "The Mifepristone Revolution," is an in-depth exploration of the impact of implementing medication abortion in Canada.

Procedural Abortion

Until the approval of mifepristone in 2015, over 96 percent of abortion in Canada was through procedural abortion. This involves the insertion of instruments through the vagina and cervix, into the uterus, which are used to remove the pregnancy tissue. Medications are usually administered in advance, to soften and open the cervix. These include oral or vaginal misoprostol tablets, or insertion of laminaria, a product that looks like a small stick, made out of seaweed. When inserted in the cervix, a laminaria stick absorbs fluid from the body and expands, gently dilating (opening) the cervix. At the beginning of the procedure, a speculum is inserted into the vagina to make the cervix visible, like in a pap test. Metal dilators of increasing diameters are inserted into and removed from the cervix, one after another, to open the cervix further. Then a rigid plastic tube is inserted, and suction (vacuum aspiration) is used to remove the tissue. The suction can be achieved manually, using a device that resembles a large syringe, or by attaching the tubing to an electric suction machine. It is standard procedure to offer patients oral and/or intravenous medications for pain relief, relief of anxiety, and antibiotics.

The procedure itself only takes about ten minutes in the first trimester; at later gestational durations it can take longer, and forceps may be used in addition to or instead of aspiration to remove larger tissue. Sometimes ultrasound imaging is used during the procedure to help the provider "see" what they are doing and ensure they have removed all the tissue. The pregnancy tissue is often called the "products of conception" (POC).

The term "surgical" abortion is being phased out because there is no cutting or "surgery" involved in procedural abortion, and neither is an operating theatre or surgical specialization required. Much of procedural abortion in Canada occurs in treatment rooms and is performed by family doctors. In terms of anesthesia, most procedural abortion is offered with optional conscious sedation, which means the patient receives medication such as fentanyl through an intravenous injection to reduce pain and/or anxiety but is still awake. General anesthesia, where the patient is "put asleep" for abortion, is rare, only occurs in some hospitals, and typically requires an anesthesiologist.

Who Gets an Abortion?

One in three people with a uterus will have an abortion in their lives.[13] Abortion is very common, and all types of people have abortions. There are callous, uninformed ideas in circulation that abortion seekers are irresponsible, promiscuous teenagers who use abortion as a form of birth control. None of that is true.

People in Canada seek abortion throughout their reproductive years, with 26 percent of patients being between the ages of twenty-five and twenty-nine.[14] Almost half of patients (48 percent) are over age thirty, and only 2 percent of abortion occurs among patients under age eighteen.[15] Although no Canadian data regarding marital status is available, in the US, the Guttmacher Institute's research has found half of all abortion seekers are married or living with their partner.[16] Most have at least one child already, and most are seeking abortion for the first time. People of all religions seek abortion,[17] as do people in all income brackets.[18]

Not all abortion patients are women and girls. Trans men and non-binary people get pregnant and choose to terminate their pregnancies, making the gendered language around abortion anachronistic and inappropriate. This book endeavours to use inclusive terms for abortion seekers except when citing studies or papers that use gendered language.

Prevalence of Abortion

Abortion is very common: there are approximately 100,000 abortions in Canada every year,[19] compared to 350,000 live births,[20] so, one abortion for roughly every 3.5 deliveries. To put this in further perspective: birth is the most common reason for hospitalization in Canada, and c-section is the most common type of inpatient surgery.[21] Reproductive experience is a dominant health concern in Canada, and abortion is a key element of that umbrella of care.

Although the Canadian Institute for Health Information no longer collects this information, available research suggests 95 percent of abortion (procedural and medication) occurs in the first trimester (up to thirteen weeks), and less than 5 percent of abortion in Canada occurs in the second and third trimesters.[22] There is no gestational duration limitation in law in Canada. "Late term abortion," a term widely circulated in anti-abortion messaging and recirculated by news media, is not a real clinical term and stigmatizes patients seeking care later in pregnancy. The best practice is to describe gestational duration factually, by trimester, as in "first trimester, second trimester, or third trimester."

In the third trimester, what usually occurs is a different type of medication abortion. A physician will make an injection into the fetus, usually of potassium chloride, to stop fetal cardiac activity. Then, labour is induced using additional medications and the fetus is delivered still. Maternal-fetal medicine specialist physicians are often engaged in this process. There are few cities in the country where this care is offered, including Vancouver, Toronto, and Montreal. The labour can be managed the same way as it is for spontaneous intrauterine fetal demise and stillbirth, involving midwifery or labour and delivery nurse care and doula support. The process takes several days. Third trimester abortion is extremely uncommon, and patients seeking this care may experience multiple intersecting forms of marginalization including poverty, language barriers, violence, and very young age. As such, clinical social workers often are involved in coordination and support.

Safety and Effectiveness

Both medication and procedural abortion are very safe — safer than colonoscopy or wisdom teeth removal, for example. Most complications are minor. In a US study of 55,000 abortions, 0.8 percent were associated with an abortion-related emergency department visit[23] and 0.2 percent with a major complication associated with hospital admission, surgery, or blood transfusion. A recent 2022 study by Schummers et al.[24] examining almost 300,000 abortions in Canada found the rate of complications to be 0.7 percent and of major adverse events to be 0.03 percent. The alternative to seeking an abortion is to give birth, which is fourteen times more likely to result in maternal death than abortion.[25] Furthermore, the same types of complications may follow spontaneous abortion (miscarriage). Abortion is safest the earlier it is experienced and when providers are well trained, supported, and experienced.

Medication abortion is associated with slightly higher rates of "failure" than procedural abortion, which means the medication did not actually cause an abortion or not all of the tissue was expelled, and either more medication is required or a patient should receive procedural care.

Mischaracterizations of the risks of abortion are a tool of the anti-abortion movement to dissuade patients from seeking services. Patients often ask about it, but abortion does not reduce future fertility; birth has a much higher rate of complications that can result in infertility.[26] It does not cause breast cancer.[27] Being denied an abortion can increase the risk of physical illness, including pre-eclampsia, chronic pain, and gestational hypertension.[28] Abortion does not cause psychological distress; being *denied* an abortion is much more likely to cause anxiety and low self-esteem.[29] Studies have found that for 95 percent of abortion seekers, their most common feeling afterwards is relief.[30] By contrast, the most common complication of pregnancy is depression,[31] affecting about 15 percent of people postpartum.

Getting an Abortion

There are many myths and misperceptions about the non-clinical "how" of abortion: the administrative or bureaucratic steps involved in seeking care. Most importantly, abortion is not something requiring physician approval: so-called "therapeutic abortion committees" were done away with in 1988 across Canada, although New Brunswick retained a cumbersome two-doctor consultation process until 2015. At later gestational durations, where provision of care requires coordination between multiple care providers, there are often "case conferences" where a plan is developed for the patient; this is not a permission-granting process as much as a planning one.

Abortion patients are not "wait-listed" in the way surgical patients may be placed in a queue until a surgeon has available operating room time. Pregnancy is time dependent, and abortion cannot wait. That said, abortion providers may book a patient for a few weeks into the future for a variety of reasons, including the patient's social needs (e.g., to arrange childcare, time off work, or transportation), clinical reasons (e.g., some providers prefer to wait until the pregnancy is visible on ultrasound, usually by six weeks, or until they can review blood work results), or staffing/facility issues (e.g., the clinic only has enough volume to operate one day a week). Abortion is also not a walk-in service: for security and logistical planning purposes, abortion seekers must always make appointments.

Abortion does not usually require a referral from a primary care provider. Almost all first-trimester providers accept self-referral, and in all provinces there is at least one abortion clinic where abortion seekers themselves simply need to call and they will be booked. Some hospital providers do require a referral. In Saskatchewan, for example, patients can call the Regina Women's Health Centre to book an appointment on their own; however, the hospital in Saskatoon requires a referral.

Only physicians are authorized to perform procedural abortion in Canada, but both nurse practitioners and physicians are authorized to prescribe medication abortion, and Quebec has also authorized midwives to prescribe. A 2019 Canadian workforce survey found primary care physicians provided over 71 percent of first trimester abortions,[32] 73 percent of procedural abortion in the first trimester, and 48 percent of second-trimester abortion. Nurse practitioners provided 2 percent of first trimester abortion, all by medication abortion.

The abortion seeker is autonomous in their decision making: abortion does not require anyone else's permission. People who cause pregnancies, including spouses and casual sexual partners, do not have any decision-making power regarding the decision to terminate a pregnancy. Parental consent is not required for abortion specifically, and neither does Canada have a specific age of consent for health care generally.[33]

However, the "age of majority" differs from province to province, and some provinces have unique regulations about consenting to care. For example, in New Brunswick, the age of majority is nineteen, but the Medical Consent of Minors Act stipulates that youth from sixteen to eighteen years of age may consent to medical treatment just as they would if they were at the age of majority. Those younger than sixteen may consent if

> in the opinion of a legally qualified medical practitioner, dentist, nurse practitioner, midwife or nurse attending the minor, (a) the minor is capable of understanding the nature and consequences of the medical treatment, and (b) the medical treatment and the procedure to be used is in the best interests of the minor and his continuing health and well-being.[34]

Abortion providers typically ask patients whether the decision to terminate is autonomous or if they are experiencing any coercion because of the risk of interference in patient consent.

Procedural abortion is likely to be experienced largely alone. Out of concern for both staff and patient safety, most clinics do not permit companions to accompany patients inside facilities at all. If support people are allowed in, they are usually required to wait in a designated area and rarely permitted in the procedure room. This includes parents, partners, and abortion doulas.[35] Protections against COVID-19 caused many facilities to tighten companion rules to be more restrictive. The benefit of protecting staff and patients from anti-abortion violence, intimate partner violence and reproductive coercion is believed to outweigh the potential harms of excluding companions. That said, many procedural providers require patients arrange to have a post-procedure escort, as most procedural abortion patients have taken one or more medications that would impair their driving ability. In some clinics, staff may even meet that escort at the clinic door to confirm their presence. Escort policies are based on concern about patient safety. The requirement for escorts means that when patients travel to another area for care, they either need a companion for the trip or a local volunteer to take on that responsibility.

The vast geography of Canada is an enduring challenge to access, resulting in significant travel requirements. In 2007, a study by Sethna and Doull[36] found that three-quarters of abortion patients travelled more than an hour for care, and patients with lower incomes were more likely to have to travel over 200 kilometres. As will be discussed in future chapters, intra- and interprovincial and even transnational travel for abortion is a longstanding norm in Canadian abortion care.[37] In 2013, Sethna and Doull[38] published a critical study that mapped the abortion journeys of 1,186 patients to care, visibly capturing the acuity of spatial disparities in access, particularly for Atlantic, northern, coastal, and Indigenous women. After decriminalization, overcoming geography has perhaps been the most challenging part of getting an abortion in Canada.

Geography is in some ways a proxy for provider numbers: if there were more providers in more places, patients' travel distances would fall. Mifepristone implementation inarguably ushered in waves of new prescribers, swelling the abortion workforce and reducing the need to travel to find someone able to provide care. Before mife, most abortion facilities were located close to the US-Canada border in major urban centres.[39] Now, mife is prescribed widely. But mife has an early gestational limit for approved use, and medication abortion is not clinically or socially appropriate for everyone even if they are earlier than nine to ten weeks.

Travel for abortion can be profoundly exhausting, humiliating, confusing, and expensive. The cost of flights, train or bus tickets, gas, meals, accommodations, childcare, and missed time from work adds up and is usually absorbed privately. Bringing a support person along can double those costs.

Abortion itself, whether procedural or with medication, does not usually require private payment. Provincial/territorial health insurance (using one's Medicare card) covers both, with few exceptions. However, if an abortion seeker does not have a Medicare card, the cost can be significant: from $350 for just the pills themselves, plus fees for physician time or blood work, to $3,000 for a procedure in a hospital. It can be cumbersome to present a Medicare card from one province in another province. For example, if a non-Quebecer seeks care in Quebec, they are required to pay upfront for services and then can seek reimbursement from their home province. While the abortion itself may be covered by one province for care in another, the associated costs, such as flights and hotel, may not: policies on this differ from one jurisdiction to another. Work to improve inclusiveness of public funding for abortion is discussed in Chapter 8.

Impact on Patients

Abortion does not negatively affect a person's life — quite the opposite. The harmful social and economic consequences of *not* having access to abortion and going on to give birth are very significant. A large and critically important US study called the "Turnaway Study" examined what happened to 1,000 people recruited through thirty abortion facilities who were "turned away" from abortion care, usually because they were past the gestational duration capacity in their state, compared to those who were not. Over the course of ten years, the research team followed up with participants. They found that the people who were turned away were more likely to live in poverty, less likely to be able to afford basic necessities like food and housing, and more likely to experience bankruptcy and eviction.[40] They were more likely to experience an abusive partner, and to parent alone. Their children were more likely to live in poverty and to experience worse child development outcomes. Abortion supports patients' quality of life and their families' prosperity.

Abortion is health care. But abortion is also much more than health care: it is a requirement for bodily autonomy, for women and people with a uterus to forge our own paths. It is not a women's issue or only relevant to people with uteruses: men and people who cause pregnancies benefit from the liberation abortion affords. Research has found young men who caused pregnancies that result in abortion are more likely to graduate from high school than when the pregnancy resulted in live birth.[41]

Abortion is health care, but abortion is political, too. While politicians should have no say in what a person chooses to do with their own pregnancy, the political ramifications of restrictions to abortion, and the political power generated through access to abortion, are enormously important. It is foundational to economic security, civic participation, personal safety, and self-actualization.

Abortion is foundational, not fringe. It is normal, not special. And it is power, not shame.

*   *   *

Despite both types of abortion — medication abortion (using mifepristone and misoprostol) and procedural abortion — being common health services, abortion in Canada remains shrouded in misinformation and stigma, which contribute to delays and unnecessary hardship in accessing care and which cannot be easily remedied through legal levers. Abortion is a fundamental aspect of health care and bodily autonomy for individuals of all genders, and there are social and economic implications of not having access to abortion care.

CHAPTER 2

WITH LAWS COME LIMITS

> This chapter explains how Canada came to be the only country in the world with complete decriminalization of abortion, the important roles of the Canadian Charter of Rights and Freedoms and the Canada Health Act in supporting access, and why we would not want an abortion law.

Canada is the only country in the world with complete decriminalization of abortion: no aspect of abortion services is restricted by criminal law. Canada also has no laws specifically asserting the right to abortion. The expectation of the US Supreme Court *Dobbs v. Jackson* decision, leaked by Washington-based digital newspaper *Politico* on May 2, 2022, and officially released on June 24, 2022, prompted a swell of discussion in Canada about whether or not we would be safe from a similar regressive trajectory; to protect ourselves, did we need an abortion law?[1] Canadian politicians even mused about the potential place for one.[2] The *Dobbs* ruling did prompt *other* countries to enact abortion law: in March 2024, France made history as the "only country" to enshrine the right to abortion specifically into its constitution.[3] The "only" aspect was debated as other jurisdictions have made similar constitutional strides: Yugoslavia's 1974 constitution included the right to decide on the birth of a child,[4] and Section 12 of the 1996 Constitution of South Africa states, "Everyone has the right to bodily and psychological integrity, which includes the right to make decisions concerning reproduction."[5]

Activists in Canada quelled the brief interest in law creation, which would be protracted and fraught due to the complexity and broad consensus any such change would require.[6] We can be happier with what we have than what was created in France, because with laws come limits. Most countries in the former Yugoslavia limit abortion to ten to twelve weeks,[7] and the South African Choice in Pregnancy Termination Act specifies abortion may be requested to twelve weeks or provided up to twenty weeks for maternal-fetal health reasons.[8] Although gestational duration capacities differ from province to province in Canada, these differences are not stipulated by law. Gestational capacity is a matter of policy, training, demand, experience, equipment, and how later gestational care — which takes longer than abortion in the first trimester — fits into clinic staffing and schedules.

While France's action was conceptualized as a huge win for "feminism and democracy,"[9] what remains to be seen is how this legislative manoeuvre will affect frontline care. In France, while abortion is 100 percent publicly insured, the law stipulates it is only available to fourteen weeks after conception, or roughly sixteen weeks since last menstrual period; it also requires two medical consultations.[10] When France first partially decriminalized abortion in 1975 under what was called the Loi Veil, after then–health minister Simone Veil, the limit was to ten weeks of pregnancy or twelve weeks of amenorrhea (the absence of menstruation).[11] It was extended to twelve weeks (fourteen weeks of amenorrhea) in 2001,[12] and fourteen weeks (sixteen weeks of amenorrhea) in 2022. Until 2015, a punitive and humiliating seven-day "reflection period" was required.[13] While people in France now have a constitutional right to abortion, it is the right to abortion provided according to current French law. This is a significantly more restrictive regulatory regime than in contemporary Canada. Canadian law went through a stepwise progression similar to France, but it did so earlier and more broadly, eventually resulting in no criminal-legal restrictions on gestational duration, no waiting periods, and no age limitations or requirements for parental consent, outside of any such requirements that apply to health services generally.

In 2018, Ireland voted to repeal the country's Eighth Amendment of the Constitution, a notoriously restrictive law banning abortion, and replace it with the Health (Regulation of Termination of Pregnancy) Act.[14] The Act legalized abortion under a set of heavy limitations: it is only legal until the eighty-fourth day of pregnancy (twelve weeks); a doctor must *certify* the patient is under twelve weeks; and the patient must receive that certification at minimum three days before the abortion.[15] If abortion is provided outside of these parameters, physicians can face up to fourteen years of imprisonment. Patients are not criminalized. The Irish Health Service Executive launched a 24/7 MyOptions hotline to facilitate access to care, and abortion services began on January 1, 2019. In the first year, 6,666 patients obtained abortion.[16] While these conditions are indisputably an improvement on the prior ban — which had egregious consequences for Irish people and caused the recent death of at least one woman, Dr. Savita Halappanavar[17] — they are taxing on clinicians. The mandatory requirement that patients endure a three-day wait between certification of gestational duration and receiving the abortion is particularly burdensome.[18] Clinicians become the face of a political compromise and are stuck justifying to patients something for which there is no clinical justification.

Just as it is argued that lawyers and judges should not be making our health care decisions for us, health care professionals are likely to argue against becoming agents of the law. Clinicians are unlikely to want to have to explain to every patient the legal limitations of care they might receive, and neither do we want to have to navigate those limitations. As a health care provider, I would have to say to an abortion-seeking patient one day beyond twelve weeks that they are not eligible for care — not because it's clinically inappropriate or because no one has the skills to perform it, but because *the law says so*. Health professionals do not prefer to work at the edges of legality, vulnerable to imprisonment. We want to provide evidence-based, clinically safe care. Activists, recognizing the burdens legal parameters to abortion would create, do not want a law either.

Who Wants a Law?

Canada's "lawlessness" is often used as a rallying cry in the anti-abortion movement. In fact, "We Need a Law" is the name of a national anti-abortion organization. In August 2018 it launched a Pattison billboard advertising campaign across thirty Canadian cities with "Canada Has No Abortion Law" in all caps. Sarah Baddeley, then-chair of Women's Legal Education and Action Fund (LEAF) Halifax, expressed that the point of these billboards was to "Foster stigma and create barriers to access by creating shame about abortion and shame about whether or not abortion is safe."[19] In response to the ads, the Abortion Rights Coalition of Canada (ARCC), under the longstanding leadership of Joyce Arthur, issued a formal complaint to the Ad Standards of Canada (ASC),[20] the self-regulatory body for advertisers. The very first provision of the ASC Code[21] is "accuracy and clarity" based on several principles, including "Advertisements must not contain, or directly or by implication make, inaccurate, deceptive or otherwise misleading claims, statements, illustrations or representations" and "Advertisements must not omit relevant information if the omission results in an advertisement that is deceptive or misleading." In its complaint about the "We Need a Law" campaign, ARCC argued,

> On its face, the ad statement that "Canada has no abortion laws" is accurate. However, that is not enough.... Ads must also not omit relevant information that results in a deceptive or misleading ad. The perceived misleading messages the ad sends are that abortion is completely unregulated, there's something wrong with abortion, and there should be laws restricting abortion. Further, the ad omits to say that abortion is in fact regulated by the Canada Health Act, the Canadian Medical Association, the provincial Colleges of Physicians & Surgeons, medical discretion, best practices, and clinical protocols. Just like any other healthcare. In fact, no healthcare treatment has criminal or civil laws governing it, as that is unnecessary, including for abortion.[22]

While Ad Standards Canada agreed the billboards violated the Canadian Code of Advertising Standards, their reasoning differed: "Coupled with regulations imposed by Canadian authorities on the conduct of abortions in Canada, the Supreme Court's decision in *R. v. Morgentaler* makes it clear that, contrary to the advertising claim, binding Canadian law that permits abortion in Canada does, in fact, currently exist."[23] The *Morgentaler* decision,[24] the critical juncture in Canada's abortion history, hinged on Charter law provisions protecting life, liberty, and security of the person.

Unlike a legal dispute such as *Canada v. Bedford* 2013 SCC 72,[25] when the Supreme Court decided existing criminal law governing sex work was unconstitutional and called for the creation of *new* criminal law, the *Morgentaler* decision determined existing criminal law governing abortion, Section 251-4 of the Criminal Code, was unconstitutional — and stopped there. Section 251-4 was "repealed," and that section of the current Criminal Code[26] is now empty. No new laws were created in its place. While the *Morgentaler* decision determined the constitutional rights of people in Canada were violated by the criminalization of abortion, it did not result in a *positive* right *to* abortion.

In 2020, having fought the ASC decision on the grounds that it violated Charter rights to freedom of expression, "We Need a Law" was allowed to repost its ads on London, Ontario, city buses.[27] But anti-abortion campaigns like "We Need a Law" serve to confuse the public. In 2014, in response to the "Canada Has No Abortion Law" billboards, activist Allison Sparling, in collaboration with South House, a student gender justice centre at Dalhousie University, launched a crowdsourcing campaign[28] to fund counter-content[29] billboards to promote abortion access. In effect, this is exactly what the abortion movement is most lacking: public relations and advertising. "We Need a Law" fundraised $80,000 for its billboard campaign. Unlike crisis pregnancy centres funded by religious organizations (discussed in Chapter 6, "Crisis Pregnancy Centres"), abortion clinics focus on providing abortion care, are almost entirely publicly funded for their services, and use these funds for salaries and to keep the lights on. There are no extra funds for self-promotion.

While the underlying goal was undoubtedly to affect public opinion, the stated intention of "We Need a Law" is to push the Canadian federal government into adopting supposed "International Standards Abortion Law"[30] with gestational duration limits. However, the only actual international standard for abortion services, the Abortion Care Guideline issued by the World Health Organization in 2022,[31] recommends complete decriminalization, recommends against any "grounds based" limitations (such as banning abortion for sex selection or only allowing it in cases of sexual assault/incest), and recommends against any gestational duration limitations.

Health care providers, advocates, and lawyers agree: an abortion law is not necessary because abortion is health care,[32] and health services are not crimes. There are no criminal laws governing knee replacements, but orthopaedic surgery is not provided in circumstances of chaos. Only orthopaedic surgeons can perform knee replacements. They are only indicated in certain clinical circumstances: arthroplasty is an option when a patient has osteoarthritis, not a muscle strain, and the surgery is not advisable if the patient has multiple co-morbidities and is unlikely to rehabilitate after surgery. Diagnostic imaging and other tests are required beforehand, to be performed by licensed, trained technicians. Operating room time is scarce, and there may be wait times and patients triaged on the waiting list according to acuity and need. Medically necessary health services provided by surgeons and in hospitals are publicly funded. These things are stipulated in all kinds of laws, policies, guidelines, and standards of practice. There are indeed laws outside of the federal Criminal Code that impact abortion — this book aims to illustrate this legal architecture. But first, this chapter will recount how we got here.

Prosecuting Abortion

As described in *Abortion to Abolition: Reproductive Health and Justice in Canada*, abortion criminalization in Canada was inherited from colonial Britain in the early nineteenth century. Great Britain had passed the (Lord) Ellenborough Act in 1803, which made providing abortion punishable by death if it occurred after "quickening" (around sixteen weeks, when fetal movement is first detectable). British laws were applicable in British North America. In 1837, the British Parliament made two changes to the Act, both removing the death penalty and the distinction between pre- and post-quickening legality, prohibiting provision of abortion at any gestational duration. When Britain passed the Offences Against the Person Act in 1861, it included criminalization of women seeking abortion:

> Every woman, being with child, who, with intent to procure her own miscarriage, shall unlawfully administer to herself any poison or other noxious thing, or shall unlawfully use any instrument or other means whatsoever with the like intent, and whosoever, with intent to procure the miscarriage of any woman, whether she be or be not with child, shall unlawfully administer to her or cause to be taken by her any poison or other noxious thing, or shall unlawfully use any instrument or other means whatsoever with the like intent, shall be guilty of felony, and being convicted thereof shall be liable … to be kept in penal servitude for life.[33]

The Act included vague provisions that abortion could be acceptable if a woman's life was in danger, but how that danger could be interpreted was highly subjective. As de Costa[34] describes, in the years following the Offences Against the Person Act, prosecutions and convictions for providing abortion in Britain were common and were concentrated among "backstreet abortionist" laywomen who charged very low fees, as "women have to help each other."

The harshness of the 1861 Act and ambiguous meaning of "life preserving" abortion motivated a prominent London gynecologist, Dr. Aleck Bourne, to challenge it outright. He openly provided an abortion at St. Mary's Hospital for a fourteen-year-old victim of rape who was referred to him for care by the girl's school and with her parents' consent.[35] He had provided abortion before, in more clearly therapeutic (life-preserving) contexts, but in this case, the girl was characterized "as normal and healthy, in medical terms there is nothing to be said."[36] (Davies, 1938). Bourne is quoted as stating,

> I ... decided to bring forward a test case, in which there would be no real danger to life ... but in which one might strongly suspect great danger to health. I was also concerned to establish in the eyes of the Law that mental health was just as important as physical health, and in certain cases perhaps even more so.[37]

In a summary of the case, in which Bourne was acquitted, presiding judge MacNaghten[38] explained,

> The surgeon had not got to wait until the patient was in peril of immediate death, but it was his duty to perform the operation if, on reasonable grounds and with adequate knowledge, he was of opinion that the probable consequence of the continuance of the pregnancy would be to make the patient a physical and mental wreck.

From then on, British physicians had the authority to determine whether an abortion was therapeutic or necessary for health.

Returning to the west side of the Atlantic and back to the nineteenth century, in 1867, the first four provinces of Canada (Ontario, Quebec, New Brunswick, and Nova Scotia) federated into their own territory. Swift on the heels of Confederation, the first Canadian law prohibiting abortion was passed in 1869, potentially resulting in sentences for life if convicted. Canada's first federal Criminal Code arrived in 1892, including a swath of legislation criminalizing sex work, contraception, and abortion. The penalty for a physician or person found guilty of providing an abortion could be life imprisonment; for women themselves procuring the service, up to two years. The law persisted until 1969. In the years between 1900 and 1972, almost 1,800 people were charged with procuring or receiving an abortion, of whom two-thirds were convicted.[39]

On March 8, 2023, International Women's Day, the federal minister of public safety, Marco Mendocino, announced that the abortion-related offences would be added to Canada's list of historically unjust offences.[40] Anyone ever convicted of crimes on this list is eligible to have their record expunged. The list includes many "crimes" related to sex and sexuality, including operating a bawdy house and homosexual sex. Although there were sixty-seven RCMP records of abortion-related convictions in 2023, it is not known how many people, if any, have applied to the Parole Board to have their records cleared.

Therapeutic Abortion Committees

The Pierre Trudeau federal government's Omnibus Bill of 1969, first introduced in 1967 when Trudeau was minister of justice and reintroduced two years later as Bill C-150 by then–minister of justice John Turner, decriminalized homosexuality and the sale of contraception, and it partially decriminalized abortion. It was the prompt for Trudeau's possibly most-famous quotation, "There's no place for the state in the bedrooms of the nation." The Omnibus Bill is a clear example of how progress in queer rights is deeply tied to reproductive freedom for people who can get pregnant.

The partial decriminalization of abortion in 1969 amounted to the creation of a new abortion law, Section 251 of the Criminal Code. It allowed for legal abortion on the basis of a stipulation, much like the result of the *Bourne* decision in Great Britain: the requirement of physician determination of therapeutic need. And not just from one physician, but three. Thus began the two-decade era of the therapeutic abortion committee (TAC) in Canada, from 1969 to 1988. In addition to the three-person TAC panel of physicians determining the procedure to be necessary, legal abortion had to be performed in a hospital and by a physician. Keep in mind that in 1957, the Hospital Insurance Act had introduced 50/50 cost-sharing between the federal government and the provinces/territories for acute hospital stays, and the 1966 Medical Care Act expanded that foundation of Medicare to include physician services. The 1985 Canada Health Act later solidified the standards and principles of Medicare, which, as it relates to abortion access, will be discussed below.

While a seemingly powerful compromise between lobbies for reproductive rights and for religious opposition to abortion, the 1969 law was dangerously and insultingly inadequate for patients on the ground.

Hospitals were not required to strike TACs. Even where they formed, patients were routinely turned away by TACs or turned off by the process of supplicating to their approval. Delay and rejection resulted in elevated clinical risks, social and economic ruin, and despair. Grassroots guerila feminism exploded. The revolutionary Abortion Caravan, started by the Vancouver Women's Caucus on the west coast, travelled across the country in 1970, gathering supporters as they went and trumpeting three demands:[41] (1) the repeal of all abortion laws; (2) the provision of free and safe birth control to all; and (3) the construction of community-controlled women's health clinics. Caravan members were subjected to RCMP surveillance. When the Caravan reached Ottawa, over thirty women secretly entered the House of Commons, chained themselves to their seats, and shouted until they shut Parliament down.

Amid the robust protest efforts, pragmatic frontline services emerged to help pregnant people navigate the TAC red tape within Canada and beyond. The Calgary Birth Control Association (CBCA), also formed in 1970, focused on dissemination of newly legal information about birth control and referrals for abortion care.[42] When legal abortion services from Alberta's hospitals with TACs became overburdened and the *Roe v. Wade* decision improved US access, CBCA stuck to its mandate of legal activities and started directing women over the border, to US services.

The *Roe v. Wade District Attorney of Dallas County*[43] decision in 1973, affirming the constitutional right to equal protection and privacy, and thus to abortion in the US, introduced a regimen for access that depended on the gestational week of pregnancy. In the first trimester, the mortality risks of abortion were understood as equal or less to those of a continued pregnancy, and the decision to terminate was left to the physician. In the second trimester, the state could regulate abortion in the interest of maternal health, but not ban it. In the third trimester, after fetal viability, the state could regulate or ban abortion, except when necessary to preserve the life or health of the pregnant person.

While individual states legislated protection for that right in different ways, several states were more hospitable than Canadian provinces, even if transnational patients were paying out of pocket. Between 1970 and 1975, a reported 50,000 women left Canada for US abortions,[44] with 9,627 in 1975 alone.[45] The red tape of TACs also allowed for opportunism and exploitation. Commercial abortion referral agencies emerged that deliberately misinformed patients about the legality and costs of abortion in Canada, encouraging them to seek services across the border.[46]

So evident was the resulting inequality in access to abortion post-1969 that in 1975, the federal government struck a committee, chaired by Robin Badgley and including Marion Cowell and Denyse Fortin Caron, with the task of conducting "a study to determine whether the procedure provided in the Criminal Code for obtaining therapeutic abortions is operating equitably across Canada."[47] The committee, and its nearly twenty-person staff, pursued an expansive and rigorous analysis of abortions, patients, and providers across the country. On top of the nearly three weeks between when a woman first suspected pregnancy to her first visit with a physician,[48] the committee found an average eight-week delay between when a patient first consulted with a physician about the abortion procedure to when it was performed.[49] The report authors describe this period as the "merry-go-round treatment," a consequence of physicians' lack of forthrightness and/or obstructiveness in facilitating TAC approval.

The Badgley committee found a lack of medical standards governing abortion services, inconsistent interpretation of the meaning of "therapeutic" or "necessary for health," and, despite partial decriminalization, profound and persistent ignorance among patients, the public, health professionals and hospital leadership about what the 1969 abortion law entailed, resulting in many continuing to believe it was outright banned. The committee's report also concluded insufficient public effort and investment was dedicated to factual education about and support for accessing contraception, and as a result, "more money is spent paying for the treatment and the care of women who have induced abortions than on ways of seeking a reduction in their numbers and on providing more effective programs of family planning and sex education."[50] As will be discussed in Chapter 10, "Contraception," contraception remains under-supported by public health funding today.

In the Badgley committee's interrogation of whether and why the 1969 abortion law caused inequality, one key element under scrutiny was the presence of TACs: if a TAC was required for legal abortion, legal abortion would be concentrated in areas with functional TACs. Of 1,348 civilian hospitals in the country, the Badgley committee found only 20 percent had a TAC. Further, a TAC, by definition, included three physicians who would approve abortions. The committee found that 40 percent of people in Canada lived in communities where the hospital was ineligible to form a TAC, simply because it had fewer than four physicians on staff. Further, in a national physician survey, they found half of all physicians believed abortion "lowered the value of human life," and physicians of this view "worked in virtually every hospital in Canada."[51]

The presence of a TAC was not enough to ensure services, as TAC operations varied from hospital to hospital. Two-thirds of the hospitals that *did* have TACs required the consent of the "father" of the pregnancy to approve the abortion.[52] The definition of "health" to be preserved through the abortion was subjective, and TACs were found to have on average four requirements on which their approval would rest — for example, only if the patient were under a certain gestational duration.

Although damning, the Badgley report did not prompt an urgent change to the law, although it was brought into evidence in the critical *R. v. Morgentaler* Supreme Court lawsuit in 1988. First, the enactment of the Canadian Charter of Rights and Freedoms in 1982, and then the Canada Health Act in 1984, would prove to be foundational for Canada's path to abortion "lawlessness."

Federal Legislation vis-à-vis Provincial Legislation

The Canadian Charter of Rights and Freedoms, the first part of Canada's Constitution, was enacted in 1982 and would come to play a critical role in improving abortion access. It is the supreme law in Canada, and any government (provincial, territorial, or federal) rule, regulation, or law in violation of the Charter is invalid. Many parts arguably have some bearing on abortion and activism around abortion access. Shortly on the heels of the Charter, the Canada Health Act (CHA) aimed to generate equity among Canadians by ensuring financial costs would not exclude people from access to care. Fred Chabot, executive director of Action Canada for Sexual Health and Rights, asserts that the CHA[53] is the only "abortion law" Canadians need[54] — it is the reason the mantra "abortion is health care" is actually, and only, true in Canada. It governs the icon of Canadiana that is "Medicare," public insurance policy for health services.

Introduced by then–health minister Monique Begin in 1984 at the tail end of Pierre Trudeau's tenure as prime minister, every single federal member of Parliament voted in favour of the CHA. It sets out national standards for receipt of the Canada Health Transfer; if provinces and territories fail to adhere to these standards, they face deductions in federal support for their health system costs. Although in effect it is voluntary, compliance is financially incentivized.

The CHA supplanted two prior federal Acts, the Hospital Insurance and Diagnostic Services Act (HIDSA) (1957), the first iteration of federal-provincial-territorial cost-sharing for hospital services, and the Medical Care Act (1966), which did the same for physician services. At that point in time, the federal share of these health system costs was about 50 percent;[55] in recent years it has dropped to about 22 percent, although overall costs have grown unabated, and Canada is one of the highest-spending countries in the world when it comes to health services,[56] at almost $9,000 per year per Canadian, a total of over $330 billion.

The Canada Health Act has five principles. "Medically necessary" care provided in hospitals and by physicians must be *publicly administered* and financed. It must be *universally available* to everyone who is eligible for publicly insured health care. This excludes people who are not citizens, without residency status, or a provincial health card. The coverage must be *comprehensive*, in that it includes blood work, nursing care, housekeeping, meals, and the medications that are administered in a hospital or health centre, as well as the costs of the clinical supplies, equipment, and physician fees. The coverage is *portable* from jurisdiction to jurisdiction: a New Brunswicker can receive their artificial knee in Ontario, and an Albertan can receive their appendectomy in Nova Scotia. The provincial governments, not the patients, will sort out responsibility for payment through a process called reciprocal billing. Finally, care must be reasonably financially *accessible*, provided without subjecting the patient to extra billing or user fees. Each province and territory generate their own policies and regulations to keep care delivery compatible with the CHA; if one violates the Act, they face a threat of the federal government withholding transfer payments.

The CHA causes a lot of confusion. Public administration does not mean public delivery: private companies, which family physician offices often constitute, are paid by the government for medically necessary services rather than physicians being paid as public servants. Nurses in hospitals, however, are paid as public servants. The drugs that are required during a hospital stay are always funded, but the same drugs as an outpatient, once care is located out from under the hospital roof, are unlikely to be. Portability refers to Canadians receiving care in the province in which they are not normally resident. Sometimes this is because more specialized and rarely required care only exists in certain specialized hospitals under the leadership of specially trained physicians: if a rural Nova Scotian child needs advanced pediatric neurosurgery, she may travel to SickKids hospital in downtown Toronto. SickKids bills Ontario, and Nova Scotia ensures Ontario receives appropriate payment through the reciprocal billing process. However, services outside of hospital and physician services covered by the CHA may not apply. For example, ambulance services are, perhaps shockingly, not in the so-called Medicare "basket." Many provinces subsidize the costs of ambulance services for their own residents, but not for visitors. So, if a visiting teen breaks their leg on a ski vacation in BC, the ambulance ride may cost their family $1,000 out of pocket, while the care in hospital for surgery and casting would be 100 percent covered.

Medication abortion, which will be discussed in much greater detail in Chapter 4, "The Mifepristone Revolution," is an example of how a service may have "sticky" portability. First implemented in Canada in 2017, mifepristone for medication abortion at home *is* publicly funded in Canada, an unusual exception to the only "drugs in hospital" norm. The patient simply presents their prescription and Medicare card at the community pharmacy and receives the medication free of charge. However, most provinces will not accept another provincial health card; they will not "reciprocally bill" for this "exceptional" case. And this can be problematic because of the type of patients who often need mifepristone: young people experiencing unintended pregnancy. Young people travel across the country in search of employment opportunities and to pursue their education. But because of the mifepristone exception, a young Ontario resident, studying for her Bachelor of Science in Halifax, will have to pay approximately $350 out of pocket for mifepristone, while her classmate who is a Nova Scotian resident will pay nothing. Ontario will reimburse the Ontarian student if she later submits receipts, but that is a lot of paperwork and a lot of money to have available up front.

Legal abortion in 1985 fit into the CHA basket: a medically necessary service always performed by physicians in hospitals with TACs. But abortion does not need to be performed in a hospital or hospital-based clinic. Dr. Henry Morgentaler, discussed much more below, started a revolution with his free-standing clinic in Montreal, and free-standing clinics remain an important element of care provision. But they have not always fit easily with interpretations of the CHA.

Morgentaler opened a clinic in St. John's, NL, in 1990. At the time, the provincial government did not provide funding for clinic abortions, and patients paid between $400 to $750 for procedures.[57] In 1993, the Newfoundland government agreed, as per the Canada Health Act, to cover the physicians' fees associated with abortion care, which reduced patients' out-of-pocket costs somewhat, but physicians remained responsible for financing equipment, supplies, and clerical and nursing staff. In 1995, then–federal minister of health Diane Marleau issued a letter[58] to all provinces and territories, now referred to as the Marleau Letter, ordering them to provide public funding for all medically necessary costs at clinics. A total of $280,430 was deducted from Newfoundland and Labrador's cash contribution from the Canada Health Transfer in 1995 because of the fees in place at the Morgentaler clinic. These annual deductions only ceased in 1998, when the province assumed responsibility for covering all medically necessary services.[59]

Comprehensive public funding of Newfoundland's free-standing abortion clinic ensured sustainability of a critical source of abortion access; at the time, the clinic provided close to 100 percent of abortion care province-wide, and it still does today. The Morgentaler clinic changed hands over the years and is now called Athena. It is located within a family practice office dedicated to providing abortion procedures one day a week. The public protections put in place in response to the first wave of COVID-19 — closing workplaces, bars, and recreation facilities — were associated with a drop in demand for abortion services. The current owner, Rolanda Ryan, found that per-patient funding from the province, at such reduced patient volumes, was insufficient. Recognizing the critical role the clinic played, the province agreed to fund Athena $1 million[60] every year, regardless of patient volumes.

New Brunswick was notoriously known for its exception to the Canada Health Act: Section 84-20 Section 2.a.1 of the provincial Medical Services Payment Act,[61] enacted in 1984,[62] precluded public funding for abortion in free-standing clinics. The Act long predated mifepristone implementation and was understood to only refer to procedural abortion; medication abortion prescribed by providers based in free-standing clinics was publicly funded. In fact, New Brunswick was the first province to agree to public funding for medication abortion, in 2017. When Dr. Morgentaler opened his clinic in Fredericton, NB, in the spring of 1994,[63] he did so without any access to public financing. The Marleau Letter (1995) insisted there be mandatory penalties if any clinic was found to be charging patients for services covered by the CHA (e.g., medical necessary hospital and physician services, including abortion). Yet no immediate action was taken against New Brunswick.

Although many patients were offered sliding scale and even free services, most patients at the Fredericton Morgentaler clinic paid out of pocket for care, about $750 each. This continued until Dr. Morgentaler died in 2013 and the clinic closed. Reopened in 2015 as part of a family practice office known as Clinic 554, the shadow of 84-20 persisted. Operational costs for an abortion clinic are not minor, and despite income through fee-for-service care through the family practice, the clinic faced challenges to financial sustainability. The family practice part of the business shuttered in 2020, and in early 2024, Clinic 554 permanently closed. Many headlines declared "New Brunswick's only abortion clinic closed!"[64] but since 2015, New Brunswick's two health authorities, Vitalité and Horizon, have operated abortion clinics within the walls of three hospitals: the Chaleur Hospital in Bathurst, and, in Moncton, the Georges Dumont Hospital and Moncton City Hospital, the latter of which runs five days a week. Procedural abortion services at these clinics are publicly funded.

Regulation 84-20 was a clear violation of the CHA and, as it did in Newfoundland, the federal government eventually took NB to task for failing to uphold Medicare principles. In 2020, approximately $140,000 was deducted from federal health transfers to New Brunswick, and approximately $65,000 in 2021, 2022, and 2023. These penalties represented costs reported by Clinic 554. The impact on the province was largely chastising and symbolic, as the deduction represented little compared to the province's annual health budget of $3.8 billion.[65] The province responded to the federal government's clawbacks with assertions that access was adequate, because of its three procedural clinics mentioned above, and availability of mifepristone in primary care. The Canadian Civil Liberties Association (CCLA) launched a lawsuit against NB in 2021, demanding NB abandon 84-20.[66] In November 2024, as her first act as the first female premier of New Brunswick, Susan Holt did just that, and CCLA discontinued its fight.[67]

Although the New Brunswick case has received abundant media attention, lesser known is how multiple free-standing abortion clinics in Ontario charge "booking fees"[68] likely disallowed by the CHA. From 2021 to 2023, $53,000 was withheld from Ontario each year for these types of fees.[69] Beyond CHT deductions, there have been other attempts to reproach provinces for private abortion clinic fees. In 2001, two women, both identified as Jane Doe,[70] filed a class-action lawsuit against the government of Manitoba because they were forced to pay out of pocket for abortion services at the Winnipeg Morgentaler Clinic. At the time, like New Brunswick, Manitoba had a regulation on the books, 46/93 of the Health Insurances Act, that denied funding for abortions outside of hospitals. When she discovered her pregnancy in September 1994, at about seven weeks' gestation, Jane Doe 1 made an appointment with the Health Sciences Centre hospital in Winnipeg. There she was told she would have to wait six to eight weeks to receive the abortion, pushing her into the second trimester. Instead, she paid $375 out of pocket to receive care from the Morgentaler Clinic, on September 29, 1994. Jane Doe 2 sought care in 2001. Like Jane Doe 1, she first tried the Health Sciences Centre and was informed the wait would be four to six weeks. Jane Doe 2 was on social assistance, and her case worker told her about the Morgentaler Clinic, where she received timely care. Because she was on social assistance, most of Jane Doe's fees were paid for by the province, despite the rule against public funding for clinic abortions. Jane Doe 1 and Jane Doe 2 were successful in their lawsuit, with Judge Oliphant declaring that Regulation 46/93 violated Sections 2, 7, and 15 of the Charter. In 2004 the regulation barring public funding for clinic abortions was removed. The Morgentaler Clinic closed and was reopened under community ownership as The Jane Clinic. Services were amalgamated with the Women's Health Clinic,[71] which is still in operation in downtown Winnipeg today.

On the heels of the Jane decision, in 2006 the Quebec Superior Court ruled the province was required to reimburse nearly 45,000 patients who had paid supplementary costs for abortions in free-standing clinics across the province between 1999 and 2005. At the time, approximately 44 percent of abortion in the province took place in free-standing clinics. The Association pour l'accès à l'avortement brought the lawsuit forward on behalf of the patients, and the total bill for the Quebec government was projected to be $13 million.[72] In her ruling, Judge Benard insisted not only on the restitution costs, but that the government make the necessary changes to ensure services be provided freely in future. The government did not appeal.[73]

As of this writing in 2025, there are no free-standing abortion clinics in PEI, Nova Scotia, Saskatchewan, Nunavut, the Northwest Territories, or New Brunswick. Where they do continue to exist, they can operate either as community health centre not-for-profits, like the Women's Health Clinic in Winnipeg, or be owned individually by health professionals, like the Cabbagetown clinic in Toronto, or be situated within family practices, like the Athena Centre in St. John's. Free-standing clinics can be another source of stickiness for portability because they do not as easily participate in reciprocal billing structures as clinics set inside hospitals. Hospitals have the routines and resources to ensure invoices for out-of-province patient care get sorted; independent clinics, less so. As a result, if a patient from Newfoundland needs care at twenty-two weeks, far beyond Athena's capacity of fifteen weeks, they may need to travel to Toronto for care at the Cabbagetown clinic, where services are available into the second trimester, but out-of-province patients need to pay for the service out of pocket and up front.

While worthy of much criticism, especially for what fell at the outset and continues to fall out of the "basket," the Canada Health Act has endured for forty years. Procedural abortion was always in the basket, and the pragmatism of home abortion has ensured mifepristone prescriptions are also included. The basket evolves: since 2017, nurse practitioners (NP) have been authorized to prescribe mifepristone, but NP care was not a specifically insured service. Most NPs work in hospitals and clinics that receive public funding for their salaries, but technically, NPs could have charged fees for their care. In January 2025, Minister of Health Mark Holland announced the Canada Health Act Services Policy would come into effect in April 2026, and include "physician-equivalent" services, such as NPs. However, post–COVID-19, virtual appointments make up over 30 percent of primary care, and virtual care is not necessarily in Medicare. Most glaringly, even if procedural and medication abortion are covered, prescriptions for post-abortion birth control are not. Chapter 8, "Expansion of Care," will discuss the need for and progress towards truly universal pharmacare, the inclusion of prescription drugs within our public health insurance model.

Dr. Henry Morgentaler

If the Canada Health Act is, as Chabot suggests, Canada's current "abortion law," it is only because Dr. Henry Morgentaler put criminal abortion law to bed. The Omnibus Bill of 1969 decriminalized abortion only when and if it was approved by a therapeutic abortion committee (TAC) and performed in an approved hospital. Recognizing this was an anemic compromise, that same year, Morgentaler opened a private abortion clinic in the east end of Montreal and began providing abortions on demand, no TAC approval required. He is often quoted for having explained to his biographer, Catherine Dunphy, "I decided to break the law to provide a necessary medical service because women were dying at the hands of butchers and incompetent quacks, and there was no one there to help them. The law was barbarous, cruel and unjust."[74]

Dr. Morgentaler came to Canada in 1950, twenty-seven years old, having survived years of deprivation in the Jewish ghetto of Łódź, Poland, the murders of his parents by the Nazis, and forced labour in the Dachau and Auschwitz concentration camps. He completed a medical degree in French in Montreal and opened a family practice in 1955. Profoundly affected by the injustices he experienced as a young adult, Morgentaler was drawn to humanism and action to advance human well-being and autonomy. Representing the Humanist Fellowship of Montreal,[75] he argued against the laws criminalizing abortion to the House of Commons in 1967, although at the time he was not providing abortion care. His presentation prompted a large volume of requests, however, and he is said to have performed his first abortion in 1968. He closed his general practice and came to focus entirely on family planning. He was not secretive about defying the Section 251 restrictions. On June 1, 1970, Montreal police raided his clinic and arrested him for illegal provision of abortion.

It was not until 1973 that he was tried, receiving a jury acquittal. The Quebec Court of Appeal overturned the verdict and handed down a sentence of eighteen months, ten of which Morgentaler served behind bars until he was granted release after a heart attack. By this point he was over fifty years old. In response to Morgentaler's experience, the federal government under then–prime minister Pierre Trudeau introduced a change to the Criminal Code that prohibited higher courts from reversing a jury acquittal, even when the jury ignored the law; instead, the court could only order a new trial. This was known as the "Morgentaler

Amendment."[76] This represented a powerful new standard. When tried a second time, Morgentaler was again acquitted. Quebec stopped efforts to prosecute him, and in 1976 the provincial government granted immunity to physicians performing abortions.[77]

In 1973, Morgentaler published a study[78] in the *Canadian Medical Association Journal* affirming the safety of 5,641 vacuum aspiration abortions he had performed by that point in his Montreal clinic and the superiority of this method to the usual dilatation and curettage performed in hospitals. Morgentaler would go on to open sixteen free-standing abortion clinics in his lifetime.

In 1983, Morgentaler opened a clinic in Toronto, on Harbord Street in the University of Toronto neighbourhood known as the Annex. The Ontario Coalition for Abortion Clinics had convinced him to set up shop in a new province and try to push the law again. On the day of the clinic's grand opening, Morgentaler was attacked by a man wielding garden shears, and feminist icon Judy Rebick[79] put herself between the attacker and Dr. Morgentaler, who credited her with saving his life. Predictably, Morgentaler was soon arrested, tried by the Ontario courts, and acquitted for performing abortions at the clinic. As per the Morgentaler Amendment, all the Ontario Court of Appeal could do was order a new trial, which it did. This is the trial that Morgentaler appealed to the Supreme Court of Canada.

On January 28, 1988, the Supreme Court ruled Canada's abortion law unconstitutional. The decision reads:[80]

> Liberty in a free and democratic society does not require the state to approve such decisions but it does require the state to respect them. A woman's decision to terminate her pregnancy falls within this class of protected decisions. It is one that will have profound psychological, economic and social consequences for her. It is a decision that deeply reflects the way the woman thinks about herself and her relationship to others and to society at large. It is not just a medical decision; it is a profound social and ethical one as well. Section 251 of the Criminal Code takes a personal and private decision away from the woman and gives it to a committee which bases its decision on "criteria entirely unrelated to [the pregnant woman's] own priorities and aspirations." Section 251 also

deprives a pregnant woman of her right to security of the person under s. 7 of the Charter. This right protects both the physical and psychological integrity of the individual. Section 251 is more deeply flawed than just subjecting women to considerable emotional stress and unnecessary physical risk. It asserts that the woman's capacity to reproduce is to be subject, not to her own control, but to that of the state. This is a direct interference with the woman's physical "person."

Justice Bertha Wilson concurred with the majority decision and went further, proposing criminalization of abortion also violated the Section 7 right to liberty. She defined liberty as the right to "individual decision-making in matters of fundamental personal importance" without interference from the state. Section 251 was struck from the Criminal Code.

Post-1988

The legal void left by the 1988 *Morgentaler* decision apparently "bewildered" the federal Conservative government of the time, led by Prime Minister Brian Mulroney.[81] Just doing nothing was objectionable, but there was also worry an overly restrictive response would be thrown out by the court or found unacceptable by the public. Conservative senator Lowell Murray was appointed chair of an ad-hoc abortion committee tasked with creating a new law.[82] Cabinet vigorously debated various proposals, with most early support leaning towards a three-stage model for greater access early in pregnancy with greater restrictions at later gestational durations, a similar compromise to that on which the US had landed in *Roe v. Wade*. Harder-lined anti-abortion MPs, led by then-health minister Jake Epp, pushed for a single, restrictive approach across all pregnancy stages. The final Tory proposal, Bill C-43, introduced in May 1990, did just that. It criminalized abortion at any gestational week, unless performed by a physician who considered the women's life or mental or physical health to be threatened. Convictions would be punishable by two years in prison. In a free vote in Parliament, 140 MPs favoured the bill, while 131 voted against. On January 31, 1991, the bill progressed to the Senate, where the vote tied at 43–43. According to Senate rules, a clear majority is required to pass a bill.[83] The bill was a very narrow failure, and there was appetite to revisit and reframe.

Barbara MacDougall, then minister for the status of women, commented that "It is best to let sleeping dogs lie. It is a personal moral decision for each woman."[84] The House of Commons made no further action to reintroduce the bill.

Even after the monumental win of the 1988 *R. v. Morgentaler* decision, Dr. Morgentaler would persist to the end of his ninety-year life with legal battles to make abortion ever more accessible. In 1989, the province of Nova Scotia sought and received a court injunction to prevent Morgentaler from performing abortions at his clinic on Halifax's McCully Street.[85] Nova Scotia had introduced provincial legislation, Section 4 of the Medical Services Act, prohibiting abortion outside of hospitals. Morgentaler appealed to the Supreme Court of Canada,[86] which ruled the Nova Scotia regulation against free-standing clinics was effectively a provincial effort to make criminal law outside of its jurisdiction. However, a requirement for out-of-pocket payment for clinic abortion care remained.

The problem of private fees became moot when the Halifax Morgentaler Clinic closed in 2003. Morgentaler determined adequate access was available through the Termination of Pregnancy Unit (TPU) at the city's Victoria General Hospital,[87] where all care was publicly funded. He moved on to other battles. The TPU is now known as the Reproductive Options and Services (ROSE) Clinic,[88] named to honour Dr. Jacques Desrosiers who worked there for thirty years. Desrosiers trained under Morgentaler, as did current medical co-director of the clinic, Dr. Lianne Yoshida.

New Brunswick had its own version of the Nova Scotia ban on abortion clinics, Bill 92, passed by the Richard Hatfield provincial government in 1985.[89] The bill amended the NB Medical Services Act to place in jeopardy the medical licence of any physician performing abortion in a free-standing clinic. After his win in Nova Scotia, Dr. Morgentaler sought to have Bill 92 declared invalid and won. However, New Brunswick would continue to refuse to publicly fund abortions provided in clinics, a regulation that continued until 2024, with Morgentaler fighting it steadfastly until his death." As described previously, the Fredericton Morgentaler Clinic opened in 1994, closed after his death in 2013, reopened as the rebranded Clinic 554 in 2015, and closed permanently in 2024. Abortions at the clinic were never publicly funded. As her first act in office, Premier Susan Holt removed the restriction on public funding for abortion in free-standing clinics.

Prince Edward Island fiercely resisted Morgentaler's January 1988 victory and took a series of steps to ensure the island remained abortion-free. Later in 1988, the province introduced a resolution opposing abortion except to save the life of a pregnant woman, and then, in 1994, enacted a policy against public funding for abortions performed outside of hospital and/or without a finding to be medically necessary. Morgentaler fought back in court but lost on appeal.[90] It was not until a feminist coalition launched a fresh lawsuit in 2016 that PEI would capitulate and welcome abortion services on the island. More on that case in Chapter 5.

Legal Status of the Fetus

Despite the layers of laws governing health service provision, location, and funding that provinces and territories in Canada have navigated through, abortion's "lawlessness" serves as a bottomless source of fuel for individual anti-abortion activists and organizations. They lobby relentlessly for the introduction of laws to directly or indirectly restrict abortion, often framing them as rights protective. Beyond prosecution of physicians for providing care, and penalties for funding restrictions, a swath of legal disputes in Canada have addressed the autonomy of pregnant people vis-à-vis the fetus and the question of fetal personhood. Several key cases serve as a strong foothold for the longstanding recognition in Canada of the fetus as embodied within the pregnant person, not a person in itself.

In the late 1970s Joseph Borowski, formerly an NDP member of the Legislative Assembly (MLA) in Manitoba, brought a case forward challenging the constitutionality of Section 251 of the 1969 Criminal Code, arguing it was too permissive and violated fetal rights. By this time, Borowski's political career had imploded, and he was well-known for anti-abortion extremism, including a protracted hunger strike. His legal case took years to progress, well into the late 1980s. After the 1988 *Morgentaler* decision struck down Section 251, the Supreme Court of Canada determined Borowski's case, based on the 1969 law, to be moot. It was dismissed in 1989.[91]

In 1989, Chantal Daigle's[92] abusive ex-boyfriend, Jean-Guy Tremblay, sought and received an injunction from the Supreme Court of Quebec to prevent her from seeking abortion care, arguing he was protecting fetal right to life, and he had rights to decide the fate of the pregnancy as a father. Upheld by the Quebec Court of Appeal, Daigle appealed the injunction to the Supreme Court of Canada and won. On the question of fathers' rights, the judgment explained,

> There does not appear to be any jurisprudential basis for this argument. No court in Quebec or elsewhere has ever accepted the argument that a father's interest in a foetus which he helped create could support a right to veto a woman's decisions in respect of the foetus she is carrying.[93]

Further, the decision clarified the fetus is not considered a person and does not have the substantive rights of a person.

The *Dobson (Litigation guardian of) v. Dobson* 1999 case[94] examined whether Cynthia Dobson should have been held liable for the mental and physical disabilities her son Ryan Dobson experienced after a car accident that occurred when Cynthia was twenty-seven weeks pregnant. Again, the judges found that the pregnant person is inseparable from the fetus and cannot be required to have a duty of care to that fetus as if it were a unique person. Cynthia won. These cases have effectively eliminated the possibility of any successful litigation to limit abortion access on the grounds of "fetal rights."

"Women-Centred" Attacks on Abortion

Facing routine failure with fetal rights arguments as in these cases, anti-choice activists have shifted to frame their efforts to limit abortion as women-centred. In 2012, Mark Warawa, the late Conservative MP for Langley, BC, introduced a motion (M-408) in the House of Commons calling for condemnation of "discrimination against females occurring through sex-selective pregnancy termination."[95] The House Affairs Committee determined the motion was out of order[96] and it did not proceed to debate or vote.[97] Again in 2016, Warawa attempted to introduce a similar motion, which also failed. In 2020, Conservative MP for Yorkton-Melville, SK, Cathay Wagantall introduced Private Members' Bill C-233, "An Act to amend the Criminal Code (sex-selective abortion)," which sought to criminalize medical practitioners who performed abortion based on sex selection with a prison term of five years. The bill was defeated.[98]

The Society of Obstetricians and Gynaecologists of Canada (SOGC) strongly opposes sex-selective abortion, as it is without clinical benefit; however, patients are not required to share any rationale for seeking abortion. To ascertain who was seeking abortion for sex selection could introduce grounds-based limitations to abortion care. Notably, in 2012, SOGC spokesperson and IWK Health maternal fetal medicine specialist Dr. Michiel Van den Hof called for a ban on "entertainment" ultrasounds, which are accessed outside of the public health care system and may reveal fetal sex.[99] These private ultrasound businesses now abound; there has been no associated increase in abortion but there are issues staffing publicly financed ultrasound departments.[100] This is one of the insidious ways abortion access can be lost irrespective of legislation or regulation about abortion itself: when private, for-profit, health service or health service–like operations multiply, they remove human resources from the publicly funded system where abortion and its required adjuvant services, like blood work and diagnostic imaging, are located.

Anti-abortion efforts to insert fetal protections into law — and in so doing, interfere in the legality of abortion — are persistent and deceptive. In January 2023, Wagantall changed course from a focus on sex selection, introducing Private Members' Bill C-311,[101] "An Act to amend the Criminal Code (violence against pregnant women)," which would introduce knowledge of a victim's pregnancy as an aggravating factor in sentencing their assailant. In the context of epidemic violence against women in Canada, the bill hovers under the pretense of support for survivors, but its intentions are to muddy the definition of who is a victim and who is a human being under Canadian law. Criminal Code[102] Section 223 states, "A child becomes a human being within the meaning of this Act when it has completely proceeded, in a living state, from the body of its mother." It is already a crime to assault a pregnant person, because it is a crime to assault a person, period. Bill C-311 was defeated.[103]

With Bill C-311, Wagantall argued for extra criminalization of those who harm pregnant people and that a victim's pregnancy ought to be considered an aggravating factor in sentencing decisions. The principles of sentencing in Canada do not highlight pregnancy as a potentially mitigating factor, and pregnant people are not routinely prioritized for non-custodial consequences. Yet incarceration arguably has a direct and harmful impact on maternal and fetal health, as pregnancy while incarcerated in Canada is associated with lack of access to obstetrician-gynecologist care,[104] elevated risk of inadequate prenatal care,[105] and premature birth,[106] the leading cause of neonatal death. There have been several criminal prosecutions related to negligence in the context of neonatal death and stillbirth that have intersected with understanding the status of the fetus in Canada. These potentially triggering topics are discussed in the next chapter.

*　*　*

No criminal laws restrict abortion services in Canada. The loss of constitutional protection of abortion from criminalization in the US because of the *Dobbs v. Jackson* Supreme Court decision has raised concerns in Canada about potential legal threats here, along with the need for a dedicated abortion law. Yet even those countries, like France, that have enacted constitutional protections for abortion still impose limitations, such as gestational duration caps. In the absence of criminal law, abortion is health care governed by the Canada Health Act, subject to access variations that result from provincial/territorial policies, regulations, and health system operations.

While anti-abortion protestors zealously insist Canada's lawlessness requires urgent intervention, abortion care in Canada is hardly unruly: it is provided within layers of institutional, professional, clinical, and legal parameters; it is publicly funded under the Canada Health Act; and it remains resiliently identified by the courts as a necessity for fundamental rights and freedoms.

CHAPTER 3

DEFINING MISCARRIAGE, STILLBIRTH, AND INFANT DEATH

CONTENT WARNING: This small chapter addresses a few aspects of Canadian legislation relevant to abortion that may be triggering for some readers as they relate to miscarriage, stillbirth and infant loss.

> Although legal cases have clarified that the fetus in Canadian law does not have personhood, this chapter explains the legal conceptualizations of miscarriage, stillbirth and infant death and how they can have implications for abortion.

Legal Definition of Stillbirth

By law, stillbirths, as a type of death, must be registered with Vital Statistics. "Stillbirth is currently defined as the complete expulsion or extraction from its mother of a product of conception, which did not at any time after birth breathe or show other sign of life."[1] This definition applies when the fetus has reached twenty weeks or more gestation, and/or when it has a weight at or equal to 500 grams. At this gestation duration and/or weight, all fetal demise is classified as a stillbirth, whether it occurred spontaneously, for fetal reduction in the case of multiples, stemming from a diagnosis of fetal anomaly, or as an abortion. All abortions after twenty weeks' gestation are registered with Vital Statistics as stillbirths.

Stillbirths have not always been defined this way, and over the past hundred years Canadian data about stillbirths has shifted. There were no reliable data prior to 1921. In the first half of the twentieth century, stillbirth was limited to loss after twenty-eight weeks, and the rate was about thirty to thirty-five per 1,000 pregnancies. By comparison, in

2017, the rate of stillbirth at or after twenty-eight weeks had decreased to 2.8 per 1,000.²

However, in 1959, Canada shifted the definition of stillbirth from twenty-eight to twenty weeks. In Quebec, the dual criteria of gestational duration and/or weight is still not used; rather, the province uses the World Health Organization (WHO) recommendation of a single criterion of 500 grams or more.³ New Brunswick and Saskatchewan used the single criterion until 1996 and 2001, respectively,⁴ but now use the dual criteria. The dual criteria increase the size of the number of stillbirths included in the statistic. The definitions are somewhat arbitrary: in Australia, the cutoff is twenty weeks and/or 400 grams, not 500, and in the United Kingdom, it is twenty-four weeks,⁵ regardless of weight.

As a result of the inclusive Canadian definition, and because it encompasses both spontaneous stillbirths and abortion, the rate of stillbirth in the country has increased in recent years: in 2002 it was six per 1,000, and in 2017 it was eight per 1,000.⁶ This makes it seem like pregnancy in Canada is becoming less healthy and more likely to result in stillbirth. But as prenatal testing has improved, assisted reproduction has expanded, and maternity care has become more sophisticated,⁷ there are more terminations for fetal anomaly and fetal reduction, such as from triplets to twins,⁸ and fewer spontaneous stillbirths, particularly at later gestations. The current rate of stillbirth (0.8 percent, or eight in 1,000 pregnancies) is higher among multiple pregnancies like twins and triplets (13.5 per 1,000) than single pregnancies (4.8 per 1,000).⁹ The inclusive definition of stillbirth makes stillbirth seem like a greater risk in Canada now than it did previously and when compared to other countries, including the US,¹⁰ where the rate is 0.57 percent, or fewer than six per 1,000.¹¹

In the current system, when a loss at twenty weeks or 500 grams or more occurs, parents must register the stillbirth with their local, provincial, or territorial Vital Statistics registrar, just as they must register a live birth. They must also include a medical certificate, completed by a physician or coroner, stating the cause of the stillbirth. The guidelines for investigations of fetal death stipulate that parents should be informed that half of all stillbirths are not explained, and parents must consent for an autopsy to be performed.¹² Research has found involvement of parents in reviews of spontaneous perinatal death to be valuable for improving patient safety and helping bereaved parents process grief.¹³ If the products of conception do not meet the definition of a stillbirth — that is to say, the fetus was not at least twenty weeks or 500 grams — a burial permit cannot be issued and stillbirth registration is not required, but parents can contact a funeral provider to handle disposition of the remains.[14] In BC, a burial permit is required for disposition of the stillbirth remains.[15]

The stillbirth registration form includes information[16] such as the deceased child's name,[17] as well as date and place of stillbirth; the sex, birth weight, and gestational age of the fetus; the parents' ages, marital status, and their birthplaces; the mother's place of residence; the type of birth (single or multiple); and the mother's parity (the number of live births to date).[18]

Pregnancy loss of all types is stigmatized; however, spontaneous stillbirth in an intended or wanted pregnancy, termination of pregnancy due to fetal anomaly, and abortion in an unintended or unwanted pregnancy are very different emotional and clinical experiences. The circumstances of loss have long been understood to impact how pregnant people and their partners may experience pregnancy loss.[19] When a wanted pregnancy is lost, families can experience profound and complex grief. This can be complicated by the conditions of stillbirth: families lack memories with the baby, mothers may feel a sense of biological failure, families may feel their grief is minimized by others, and they may feel confusion and uncertainty about future pregnancies and parenting.[20]

Because of the very different nature of spontaneous fetal death and abortion, experts in the field have described the current Canadian definition of stillbirth as "anachronistic."[21] They recommend making a distinction between fetal deaths that occur spontaneously and those occurring through abortion. They advocate spontaneous fetal deaths be reported and registered as vital events, while abortions after twenty weeks should be counted as abortions and not be entered into the vital registration system. And they recommend health care providers take responsibility for the registration of fetal death rather than require it from parents. If the parents wish to be involved, they could opt in, rather than face mandatory participation as is the current requirement. This may be particularly helpful for people who sought abortion care.

The definition of stillbirth has an impact on abortion service delivery. In Atlantic Canada, Manitoba, and Saskatchewan, elective abortion is only available up to sixteen to twenty weeks; each province has its own capabilities and related gestational duration caps.[22] None of these clinics or providers would be involved in registration of stillbirths. There are abortion services in Quebec, Ontario, Alberta, and British Columbia that offer care to twenty-four weeks and beyond; in these provinces, abortion care providers must be able to advise patients on the process.

The Alberta Health Services policy governing abortion, generally emphasizing compassion and patient-centredness, stresses that, save for in exceptional circumstances, abortion should occur before twenty-one weeks. After twenty-one weeks, abortion is available only in cases of maternal interests, fetal anomaly, and fetal reduction.[23] A second physician must be consulted prior to proceeding, and the physicians must have appropriate privileges at appropriate acute care hospital settings. Free-standing abortion clinics in Alberta are not approved to provide care beyond twenty weeks. This is not a criminal matter but one that relates to payment: for physicians to receive remuneration for services, they must proceed in the approved manner. This is also not to say that care beyond twenty weeks in free-standing clinics is not safe or not happening elsewhere. Indeed, clinics like the Cabbagetown Women's Clinic in downtown Toronto provide services to twenty-four weeks, fully covered for patients with OHIP (the Ontario health card/Medicare).[24]

How stillbirth is classified has employment repercussions as well. Federal employment insurance in Canada provides two types of support to families with new children: maternity benefits, up to fifteen weeks, which are only available to a person who has given birth and are related to the time needed for physical healing; and parental benefits, up to sixty-nine weeks, which all eligible parents, including fathers or adopting parents, can receive, and which can be shared between multiple parents. If a pregnancy ends before twenty weeks, the pregnant person may only be entitled to sick leave, whereas if the pregnancy ends after twenty weeks, they may be entitled to EI maternity benefits.[25] EI benefits only apply to people eligible for EI who have paid into the program for an adequate length of time. For example, most self-employed people are ineligible.

Alberta and Ontario each have provisions for sixteen weeks of unpaid leave for people experiencing pregnancy loss within sixteen weeks of their due date, which is to say at approximately twenty-four weeks gestation or later. Since 2021, PEI has granted one day of paid leave and two of unpaid leave for pregnancy loss, regardless of gestational age, just as it does for the death of an immediate family member.[26] In 2023,

Nova Scotia enacted a multi-part end-of-pregnancy leave policy, where employees receive five days unpaid leave before twenty weeks, and sixteen weeks if the pregnancy reaches twenty weeks or beyond.[27] The different provisions, types of leave, and variations across Canada are complicated. As Nova Scotia business professor Stephanie Gilbert explained, "Most bereavement leave policies do not state pregnancy loss, but only 'loss of a child' ... does pregnancy loss count as a loss of a child?"[28]

The confusion and slippage about defining stillbirth and "child" further intersects with elements of the Criminal Code and crimes related to the treatment of children or of the remains of children.

The Criminal Code

Section 223 of the Criminal Code of Canada defines "when a child becomes a human being" as "when it has completely proceeded, in a living state, from the body of its mother."[29] A child very clearly must be alive in 223 to be a child. Section 218 of the Criminal Code, unlawful abandonment of a child, explains,

> every one who unlawfully abandons or exposes a child who is under the age of ten years, so that its life is or is likely to be endangered of its health or is likely to be permanently injured, is guilty of an indictable offence and liable to imprisonment for a term not exceeding five years.

Again, in this section, the child must be alive. However, Section 243 of the Criminal Code, which addresses the crime of concealing the body of a child, does not distinguish between a stillbirth or a child born alive. In fact, it clearly includes both:

> Every person who in any manner disposes of the dead body of a child, with intent to conceal the fact that its mother has been delivered of it, whether the child died before, during or after birth, is guilty of (a) an indictable offence and liable to imprisonment for a term of not more than two years; or (b) an offence punishable on summary conviction.

The contemporary purpose of Section 243 is to facilitate investigations of possible newborn homicides. Criminalizing the disposal of the remains of a child deters offenders from disposing of the evidence required to determine if death occurred before or after birth.[30]

Section 243 does not define when a fetus becomes a child. It has been interpreted to not include abortions or miscarriages, terminations of pregnancy and pregnancy loss before twenty weeks, but it does not stipulate that. Using this interpretation, if a person miscarries at nine or nineteen weeks and disposes of the fetal tissue themselves, they have done nothing unlawful. If they do so at twenty-one weeks, however, they have committed a Section 243 offense and can be imprisoned for two years.

It is unrealistic to imagine all pregnant people know the exact gestational duration of their pregnancy. The definition of gestational duration is not well understood; many patients incorrectly think pregnancy starts the day they had sex, when weeks are actually counted from the first day of the last menstrual period, which is roughly two weeks before conception. Further, many people are not aware of their last menstrual period date, and even techniques such as fundal length (uterus size) assessment and ultrasound are imperfect measures of gestational duration.[31] Some patients do not realize they are pregnant at all, let alone have a precise understanding of gestational weeks.[32]

The consequences of this not-knowing can be complex. For example, in Halifax, there is an assortment of health care institutions patients are to turn to at different stages of pregnancy and for different pregnancy outcomes: If a patient is choosing abortion and the pregnancy is earlier than sixteen weeks, they seek care at the ROSE clinic in the Victoria General Hospital (VG). If they are miscarrying before twenty weeks, they are to go to the Emergency Department at the Halifax Infirmary (HI), an adult acute care hospital. If they are beyond twenty weeks and need either a termination for maternal-fetal indication, or experience spontaneous fetal demise (stillbirth), or go into labour for a live birth, they are cared for at the IWK Health Centre, a regional pediatric and maternity centre that is part of a separate health authority from the VG or the HI. All three health centres are within a three-block radius of each other. These different locations and instructions are perplexing to patients and problematic for clinicians in each site, because there is slippage between all these states and circumstances of pregnancy. Patients can arrive at the IWK with a threatened miscarriage only to learn that because they are nineteen weeks, not twenty, they must seek care elsewhere. Having different facilities for different outcomes becomes convoluted because reproductive experiences are not binary: a threatened miscarriage at nineteen weeks, managed at the HI, can become fetal demise at twenty-three, managed at the IWK. It is very challenging for patients to understand how so much about their care can change depending on the moment of pregnancy.

Patients' unfamiliarity with gestational timing and pregnancy viability is a backdrop to recent prosecutions for Section 218 and 243 offences. In 2007, a woman identified only as ADH,[33] then twenty years old and completely unaware that she was pregnant, went into precipitous labour in a Walmart washroom while shopping in Prince Albert, Saskatchewan.[34] She went into the bathroom, delivered the baby into the toilet, and, thinking the baby was not alive as it was not apparently breathing, she cleaned up as best she could and left. The baby was discovered in the toilet, revived, taken to hospital, and determined to be perfectly healthy. ADH was charged under Section 218 for child abandonment. ADH's case reached the Supreme Court of Canada in 2013, where the judges determined that while she did leave the baby, she did not intend to cause harm, as she genuinely thought the baby was stillborn. They determined that to convict her would require proof of intention.

Another case concerned Ivana Levkovic in Mississauga, Ontario.[35] In April 2006, the remains of a baby were found on a balcony by a building superintendent, who called police. A few days later, Levkovic went to the police station and stated that during a period of drug use, and having not known she was pregnant, she fell and delivered a stillborn baby girl, the body of which she wrapped in a bag and left on the balcony.[36] Levkovic was charged under Section 243 for unlawfully disposing of the body of a child. The forensic pathologist testified the fetus had a gestational age of thirty-six weeks but was unable to determine if the baby was born still or alive and if birth had occurred spontaneously or through a self-induced abortion.

Levkovic's lawyers argued that Section 243 was overly vague in its failure to distinguish between a miscarriage and a stillbirth and for its combining of the term "child" with the term "before birth," when a child only becomes a child once it is born. They argued that, effectually, Section 243 as written violated Charter rights to life, liberty, and security of the person by criminalizing women for choosing not to publicly reveal a failed pregnancy. In 2008, Levkovic was acquitted by trial judge Justice Casey Hill, who agreed. The acquittal was overturned by the Ontario Court of Appeal and the Supreme Court of Canada, which found that Section 243 was indeed constitutional because it was about birth and limited to cases where the fetus had reached a point of maturity where it was *likely* to have been born alive. Justice Fish wrote in the decision, "in its application to a *child that died before birth*, S. 243 applies only to stillbirths — not to miscarriages or abortions."[37] The Supreme Court chose not to specify an exact gestational duration where likelihood to be born alive began, which would have been fodder for anti-abortion extremists, and left Section 243 as it was. They ordered a new trial for Levkovic, and she was again acquitted in 2014.[38] In this case, Judge Skarica referred to the Supreme Court's clarification that Section 243 does not include abortion; because it could not be confirmed that Levkovic had not self-induced an abortion, she could not be convicted under Section 243.

These cases are disturbing, and there may always be unanswered questions about what really happened and what each woman knew. In a commentary on these cases, Stephanie Voudaris wrote,

> Perhaps it is difficult to talk about foetuses abandoned in toilets at Wal-Mart, or left on balconies of apartment buildings, because if we talk about this, then we also have to talk about broader issues regarding the ways in which society has failed women in the area of reproduction (i.e., the failure to provide free contraception), and the ways in which these failures influence decisions women make about reproduction.[39]

Importantly, the ultimate results of these cases confirm an understanding that Section 243 applies to the hiding of stillbirth and infant death, not to harm to children. Further, it cannot be applied to criminalize hiding miscarriage and abortion, regardless of the gestational duration at which the abortion occurs.

Another important case, known as *R. v. Sullivan and Lemay*, amplified the understanding of the status of the fetus in criminal law. It concerned the actions of two lay midwives, Mary Sullivan and Gloria Lemay, during a birth in Vancouver in 1985. At the time, "lay" midwives trained through informal apprenticeship and could be hired privately by patients for home births only. Lay midwives could not and did not practice in hospitals. In the spring of 1985, Ms. Jewel Voth hired Sullivan to attend her home birth, with Lemay serving as a backup. She went into labour late on the evening of May 7, with first Sullivan and then Lemay arriving in the morning of May 8. The baby's head was delivered at about 2 p.m., then contractions stopped, with the rest of the body not yet delivered. After twenty minutes, emergency health services were called. They transported Voth to nearby St. Paul's hospital, where a waiting intern facilitated "basic delivery" by way of traction (pulling). The baby was stillborn. Pathology determined the cause of death to be lack of oxygen.

The sections of the Criminal Code were numbered differently at the time, and Sullivan and Lemay were charged with criminal negligence causing death (then Section 203), and criminal negligence causing bodily harm (then Section 204). The latter applied to Voth, who was exhausted and experienced severe pain and volume depletion during the labour. At trial in fall 1986, Judge Godfrey found them guilty of the former and not guilty of the latter, summarizing the physical harm to Voth as "bruising."[40] Although the Criminal Code specified that a child becomes a human being when it has proceeded *completely,* in a living state, from the body of its mother, Godfrey relied on a 1979 case, *R. v. Marsh*, where the judge had determined "a full-term child in the process of being born is a person within the meaning of s. 203, notwithstanding that it would not be a human being for the purposes of s. 206" (now Section 223). She acknowledged that if she had not determined the fetus to be a person, she would have found Sullivan and Lemay guilty of causing bodily harm to Voth, because the fetus was part of Voth.

Sullivan and Lemay appealed their conviction, and the Crown did not appeal the acquittal for negligence causing bodily harm. The BC Court of Appeal substituted Sullivan and Lemay's conviction for criminal negligence causing death with a conviction instead for criminal negligence causing bodily harm. Sullivan and Lemay appealed again, as did the Crown, in objection to the substitution. The Women's Legal Education and Action Fund served as intervenors in the Supreme Court of Canada case, because of the implications the appeals had for definition of personhood, the status of the fetus, and access to abortion.[41] The majority of the Court agreed that "a foetus is not a 'human being' for the purposes of the Criminal Code"[42] and upheld the acquittal for negligence causing death. They also determined the Court of Appeal should not have substituted one conviction for another and acquitted both Sullivan and Lemay for the Section 204 offences. In short, the lay midwives were not convicted of either charge, and the case again clarified that a fetus is not a person in the eyes of Canadian law.

BC passed legislation in 1998 requiring anyone practising as a midwife to be registered with the BC College of Nurses and Midwives.[43] To use the label of "midwife" and not be registered is a crime. Registered midwives are publicly funded by the province and work in the formal health care system, which includes providing care for birthing parents at home. When it started in 1998, twenty-eight midwives registered with the BC College. Twenty-five years later, there are over 320 midwives in BC, and they attend nearly 25 percent of the province's 44,000 births.[44] In 2000, shortly after midwifery was legislated in BC, the Supreme Court of British Columbia issued an injunction against Lemay, prohibiting her from attending births in the province. She defied the injunction, attending at least ten births in the interim, and was sentenced to five months in jail in 2002. In response to the sentence, Lemay had stated, "I hope that until the day I die I fight for women's freedom that they can have who they want in their own bedroom to help them give birth to their baby."[45] In January 2025, Lemay was charged with manslaughter for her involvement in the birth process of a baby girl born in December 2023 in Nanaimo, and who died ten days later.[46]

Registered midwifery is legislated in all provinces and territories in Canada — the first being Ontario in 1991, and the most recent additions including New Brunswick and Newfoundland and Labrador, both in 2016,[47] the Yukon in 2022,[48] and lastly, PEI in 2024.[49] Lay midwifery is prohibited in all contexts with midwifery legislation. The emerging role for registered midwives in abortion care will be discussed in Chapter 4, "The Mifepristone Revolution."[50]

* * *

All pregnancy loss after twenty weeks, including abortion, is classified as stillbirth, requiring registration with Vital Statistics and resulting in an emotional toll on abortion seekers and potential misrepresentation of the physiological health of pregnancy. Experts have called for a distinction between spontaneous loss and that resulting from termination. While a fetus is not considered a person under the Canadian Criminal Code, hiding a stillbirth can be criminalized, as can negligence in birth care that may result in stillbirth and unlicensed work in regulated health professions providing care to pregnant people. Clarity is important to protect abortion seekers and destigmatize abortion care.

CHAPTER 4

THE MIFEPRISTONE REVOLUTION

> This chapter explains what medication abortion is, how it came to be approved and deregulated in Canada, and the important role it plays in expanding access to abortion.

The introduction of mifepristone to the Canadian health care system in 2015 was, without argument, the most impactful shift to the abortion movement since the *R. v. Morgentaler* Supreme Court of Canada decision in 1988. Finally, a safe and effective method for medication abortion at home could be available, offering not only discretion and convenience for patients *and* providers, but potentially alleviating the enormous travel burdens Canadian geography often presented to procedural care. While there were several hiccups in implementation, nothing has changed the abortion landscape more drastically than "mife."

Despite complete decriminalization of abortion, Canada went decades without *legal* access to the only medication specifically indicated for abortion: mifepristone. Without federal regulatory approval of the drug, it did not exist in Canada and could not be prescribed. When it did arrive, there was the question of who could or would be able to prescribe it. What falls within the scope of different types of health care providers is determined by provincial/territorial legislation, professional regulatory bodies, and tensions between professions for territory and remuneration. Compared to many other jurisdictions, including the US, and despite World Health Organization recommendations to widely broaden the pool of health workers in abortion care,[1] Canada's definition of "abortion provider" was tightly constrained only to physicians until 2017. The extension of mifepristone prescribing authority to nurse practitioners and midwives not only improves access but augments efforts to destigmatize and normalize abortion as a common and essential element of sexual and reproductive health care. Implementation of mifepristone has shed light on the critical roles of other health care professionals, including nurses, social workers, and pharmacists, as well as clerks and doulas, in the abortion care team.

What is Medication Abortion?

Medication abortion, or the "abortion pill," is actually a set of five pills: one 200-milligram tablet of mifepristone, swallowed, followed twenty-four to forty-eight hours later with four 200-microgram tablets of misoprostol, which dissolve in the cheeks (buccal administration) or inside the vagina. Mifepristone is an anti-progestin; it acts like a decoy, occupying hormone receptors expecting to bind with progesterone. A supply of progesterone is necessary to sustain a pregnancy; when it is cut off, the endometrium lining of the uterus starts to break away, the cervix softens, and the uterus begins to contract. The patient subsequently takes misoprostol, a prostaglandin, which stimulates strong contractions that release the contents of the uterus, the pregnancy tissue (products of conception).

In terms of the experience, a medication abortion is similar physiologically to a spontaneous abortion (miscarriage). While it is sometimes described as "a very bad period," patients can feel very significant cramping and pain and will experience heavy bleeding. They may also experience nausea, vomiting, and diarrhea. It is not "magic"; contrary to some expectations, the patient does not take a pill and suddenly become "unpregnant." Despite the expected side effects, satisfaction with medication abortion is very high. Having the ability to choose between types of abortion is empowering and increases patient satisfaction.[2] Medication abortion is a very safe and effective way to terminate a pregnancy. If the patient is housed and the home is safe, there are many benefits to being able to do so in the comfort and privacy of the patient's own home.

As described in Chapter 1, "What is Abortion?," while mifepristone technically could be used as effective emergency contraception, it is not what we generally mean when we say "emergency contraception" in Canada. Emergency contraception, if taken in the days immediately following unprotected sex, prevents pregnancy from occurring in the first place. Its efficacy to prevent pregnancy decreases the longer the time interval between the unprotected sex and ingestion of the pills. Plan B, the most known form of emergency contraception, contains levonorgestrel, a synthetic progesterone hormone, which is also used in hormonal intrauterine devices like the Mirena and Kyleena. To reduce delays to access, in 2008, Plan B was approved by Health Canada for out over-the-counter (OTC) non-prescription sale.[3] Unlike in the US, where proof of age over eighteen was required to purchase the medication until 2013,[4] Health Canada did not set a mandatory minimum age. Health Canada did, however, institute a requirement that consumers ask the pharmacist for the medication rather than simply take it from a store shelf themselves.

While OTC status for a medication removes the need to arrange an appointment with a primary care provider to get a prescription first, it also results in the drug being ineligible for coverage by most private health plans. And Plan B is not cheap: it is about $37 each time.[5] Further, Plan B is most effective for people under about 165 pounds or with a BMI under 25;[6] while less effective does not mean *not* effective, it is recommended that heavier patients take an alternative form of emergency contraception known as Ella. Ella contains ulipristal acetate, also a progestin, is effective for five days, but is only available by prescription. Notably, a third form of emergency contraception frequently used in Canada is the copper intrauterine device (IUD), which, if inserted in the seven days after unprotected sex, works quickly to prevent pregnancy.[7] The copper IUD is also only available by prescription, and requires a competent provider to insert it. If a patient is already pregnant, none of these methods will work to make them unpregnant, but mifepristone will.

Mifepristone Safety and Effectiveness

Mifepristone is on the World Health Organization list of essential medicines[8] — medications the global health advisory body has determined must be available to a population for basic well-being. It is safe and effective. Chen and Creinin[9] conducted a systematic review of twenty studies examining the mifepristone + misoprostol combination of medicines used before sixty-three days' (nine weeks') gestation and found it to be 96.7 percent effective, meaning that in ninety-seven times out of a hundred, the pills cause a successful termination of the pregnancy. The most common complications patients encounter with medication abortion are continued pregnancy (0.8 percent), excessive bleeding requiring blood transfusion (0.03–0.6 percent), and hospitalization (0.04–0.9 percent).

To check if medication abortion is effective and the termination "complete," measurements of a patient's pregnancy hormone (ßhCG) present in the blood can be taken before the abortion, and again one to two weeks later: although the hormone may not have totally disappeared, the level should fall by at least 80 percent. Another method is to wait a month after the medication abortion and confirm termination using a urine pregnancy test, which can be taken easily and inexpensively at home.

Like spontaneous abortion, medication abortion has a small risk of some tissue remaining inside the uterus. This is called "retained products of conception." Retained products can cause infection or prolonged bleeding and can be treated with an additional dose of misoprostol medication or through a procedural abortion. Because of the potential need for this follow up procedural care, some health care providers are reticent about prescribing medication abortion in environments where that procedural care is unavailable. Procedural care to complete an abortion is the same as would be required to complete a spontaneous miscarriage that resulted in retained products. Procedural care may be unavailable either because the setting is remote and such services are always unavailable or because of the beliefs of the physicians who would be asked to provide procedural follow up. This will be discussed further in Chapter 5, "Belief-based Denial of Care."

As with spontaneous abortion, medication abortion carries a risk of hemorrhage requiring emergent response. This is another reason why a prescriber might be reluctant to prescribe to patients in rural and remote locations: what if this patient is that one rare patient who requires emergent blood transfusion, and the resources are not available?[10] The science on the extent of the risk of hemorrhage after medication abortion is imprecise, and consequently, there is no clear clinical guideline about acceptable distance from emergency or blood transfusion services for prescribing medication abortion. Further, what exactly constitutes hemorrhage is debated: more than 250 millilitres of blood loss, or more than 500 millilitres, or blood loss requiring hospitalization, or even requiring transfusion?[11] Research on this aspect of medication abortion safety is ongoing. An international research team led by Dr. Wendy Norman received funding from the Canadian Institutes of Health Research in 2024 for a multi-year, multiple-methods study to examine the question of "How far is too far?"[12] Hemorrhage may also occur in the event of spontaneous abortion.

Another potential complication involves ectopic pregnancy — when a pregnancy occurs outside of the uterus, such as in a fallopian tube. This is not caused by the abortion; it was pre-existing, but mifepristone will not work to terminate an ectopic pregnancy. Ectopic pregnancies are non-viable and must be terminated on an urgent basis.[13] Failure to treat ectopic pregnancy through induced abortion is unethical. Receiving an injection of the medication methotrexate, a chemotherapy agent, may work by stopping the growth of cells and dissolving existing cells.[14] If methotrexate is contraindicated or the ectopic pregnancy has ruptured, surgery is required. The ectopic pregnancy can be removed through a dilatation and curettage procedure through either the cervix or a caesarean section.

Contraception and Abortion Research Team UBC epidemiologist Dr. Laura Schummers and colleagues examined the rate of complications observed among nearly 200,000 abortions before mife implementation in Canada (from 2012–2016) compared to over 80,000 afterwards (2017–2020). They found no significant difference between the periods with respect to the rate of complications, serious adverse events, or undetected ectopic pregnancy. There was a very small increase in the rate of incomplete abortion (ongoing pregnancy) by 0.08 percent.[15]

Other Medication Abortion Products

Before the approval, implementation, and deregulation of mifepristone in Canada, medication abortion occurred very infrequently and was estimated to constitute less than 4 percent of all abortion in 2012.[16] Dr. Ellen Wiebe, now likely best known for her activism to advance access to medical assistance in dying (MAiD), was an early medication abortion pioneer. Out of her Vancouver, BC, practice, the Willow Clinic[17] (formerly the Women's Willow Clinic), she studied the effectiveness and safety of a combination of the medications methotrexate followed by misoprostol. Methotrexate, discussed previously as a treatment for ectopic pregnancy, was approved for use in Canada in 1955. It is a chemotherapeutic drug used in cancer treatment and for autoimmune disorders.[18] Using it as an abortifacient is "off label," a use unapproved by Health Canada. Manufacturers cannot promote off-label uses, but prescribers may choose to use medicines for these purposes based on evidence of effectiveness.[19]

In 1996, Wiebe published findings from a study of one hundred patients from her clinic, all under eight weeks gestation, who were highly motivated to experience a non-surgical, medication abortion. Using the combination of methotrexate followed by the prostaglandin misoprostol, forty-eight study participants experienced an abortion within twenty-four hours of taking the misoprostol.[20] An additional dose of misoprostol was offered at day eight. By day ten, an additional twenty-one patients had completed an abortion, and a further twenty did by day forty-four. In total, 89 percent achieved a "non-surgical" abortion. Seventy-one stated they would choose the methotrexate-misoprostol approach again, which surprised the study author as high. While the study demonstrated reasonable success and adequate patient satisfaction, because of the number of continued pregnancies, Wiebe concluded this regimen was most appropriate only when follow up could be ensured. Methotrexate is a potent teratogen: it can cause severe birth defects,[21] and continued pregnancies after taking this medication would be very concerning. Notably, Wiebe's study of methotrexate took place eight years after France had approved the vastly more effective mifepristone in 1988; she was trying to figure out how to support patients who needed a non-surgical option within the limited list of Health Canada-approved medications at the time.

Because it causes such strong uterine contractions, misoprostol alone can also work as an abortifacient. It is used alone around the world for medication abortion where mifepristone is illegal, overly expensive, or otherwise unavailable. Indeed, with recent restrictions to abortion across the US, protocols for its use alone are increasingly in demand.[22] However, it was never commonly used as such in Canada, even prior to the approval of mifepristone, because of the much higher effectiveness of procedural abortion and because abortion was decriminalized in 1988.

These days, the Willow Clinic is one of several clinics in Canada that *only* offer medication abortion: other examples include the Vancouver Island Women's Clinic[23] and the SHORE Centre[24] in Ontario. They are ahead of the curve in that sense. Always innovative, Wiebe's clinic also offers non-scalpel vasectomy procedures, fully covered by BC Medicare. Wiebe has studied the value of cannabis in enhancing sexual experience[25] and is a key voice in MAiD advocacy and research.[26]

Wiebe has described her envelope-pushing approach to medicine as a reaction to the shooting of Dr. Gary Romalis,[27] a dedicated obstetrician-gynecologist who survived a sniper attack against him through a window into his home in November of 1994. At the time, Wiebe and Romalis were colleagues at Vancouver's longstanding Elizabeth Bagshaw[28] (abortion) Clinic. He rehabilitated and returned to work, continuing to provide abortion care until his death in 2014. Romalis attributed his drive to practise in the area of abortion care as stemming from learning about the sepsis death of a woman who had sought illegal abortion in 1962.[29] Wiebe and Romalis are two links on a labyrinthine chain of extremely dedicated care providers in Canada who have advanced abortion care, regardless of the legal climate.

The Long Road to Mife Approval

Mifepristone for medication abortion was only approved by Health Canada in 2015, a full thirty-five years after it was discovered by French researcher Etienne-Emile Baulieu in 1980. Born in 1926,[30] this revolutionary biochemist and endocrinologist continues, as of this writing, to work as a lab scientist. His father, Leon Blum, a physician, died when he was three years old, and he was raised in "*un environnement exclusivement féminin*" [an exclusively feminine environment] with his mother, Therese Lion, a feminist who worked with British suffragettes, as well as his grandmother and sisters.

Like Canada's icon of abortion activism, Dr. Henry Morgentaler, Baulieu is Jewish and a survivor of the Holocaust. He was a member of the French Resistance in World War II and devoted his long and much-decorated life to scientific advances that would reduce human suffering. Inspired by Dr. Gregory Pincus' work on the contraceptive pill in the 1960s,[31] and deeply affected by witnessing women harmed by unsafe abortion and unintended pregnancy, he was motivated to create what he described as an "unpregnancy pill."[32] He worked with chemist Dr. Georges Teustch from the pharmaceutical company then called Roussel-Uclaf. They synthesized mifepristone in 1980. The medication became known in France as "RU-486," the 38,486th compound synthesized by Roussel-Uclaf. Baulieu organized early human clinical trials in collaboration with an obstetrician-gynecologist friend, Dr. Walter Hermann. The trials found that the pill not only worked as intended but was 95 percent effective when combined with a prostaglandin. The method was described as preferable to a procedure because it avoids having to be touched by a health professional, seems more like a spontaneous or natural miscarriage, and avoids anesthesia and hospitalization.[33] Roussel-Uclaf's application for drug approval in France met with international anti-abortion resistance but was eventually successful in 1988.³⁴ Bowing to continued pressure, Roussel-Uclaf *renounced* the approval, prompting France's then–minister of health Claude Evin to threaten to award the medication to another company. He stated, "*RU-486 est la propriété morale des femmes*" [RU-486 is the moral property of women].³⁵

Mifepristone was approved in Great Britain and Sweden in 1991, and by the Food and Drug Administration in the United States in 2000 under the brand name Mifeprex. In 2005, it was added to the World Health Organization's list of essential medicines.³⁶ Yet it was not until October 2011 that pharmaceutical company Linepharma brought an application for approval to Health Canada.³⁷ Notably, at this point, mifepristone had been approved in sixty countries around the world and had accumulated decades of safety data.³⁸ Despite this, Health Canada requested additional documentation from Linepharma, requiring a refiling of the approval application in 2012. Dr. Joel Lexchin,³⁹ one of the most-cited researchers in the world for his critical examinations of drug approval, marketing, and pricing practices, remarked in 2014 that the protracted delay to approve mifepristone was "unusual."⁴⁰ Health Canada has a standard of 300 days at most from application to approval; the norm is nine months. Mifepristone took two and a half years.⁴¹ While that lengthy approval process is unarguably peculiar and was only ever explained by Health Canada's "requests for additional information" and "confidentiality policies,"⁴² perhaps the greater question is why it took so long to *start* the approval process in the first place.

In Canada, a new medication is only considered for approval when a pharmaceutical company applies to Health Canada for its approval. Advocacy groups or even health care professionals who recognize the value and importance of a clinical innovation cannot bring an application; otherwise, perhaps the Abortion Care Canada (formerly the National Abortion Federation Canada)⁴³ or mifepristone supporters like Dr. Wiebe and Dr. Norman may have done so themselves. Furthermore, Health Canada or any other government body itself cannot even respond to the WHO placing a medication on its list of essential drugs to spark an application. Health Canada must wait for the company to apply, and the makers of RU-486 were not in a hurry to penetrate the Canadian market. Studies have found that applications for approval of novel contraceptives take longer to be initiated in Canada than in the US or the UK, and the approval process itself also takes longer.⁴⁴

In the case of mifepristone, Erdman, Grenon, and Harrison-Wilson[45] attribute the delay to two causes. First, it was not anticipated to be highly profitable. The Health Canada application process is expensive, and mifepristone is not a lucrative drug. While abortion may be more common than people think, with one in three people with a uterus likely to have an abortion in their lifetime,[46] for a medication, this does not amount to frequent use. Compare that to a birth control pill taken daily for thirty-five years, the average reproductive lifespan.[47] There are also public agency pressures to keep costs low for a drug like mifepristone that is so critical to well-being. Second, Erdman and colleagues suggest there may be a political bias against reproductive health medicines. For example, "the requirements for approval of oral contraception in Canada as compared with the United States and Europe have been described as onerous."[48] Indeed, another example would be the extended delay to approve the single-rod contraceptive implant that uses the hormone etonogestrel, known by the brand name Nexplanon.[49] The size of a matchstick, this form of long acting contraception is inserted into the arm and is highly effective as birth control for three to five years. Nexplanon was approved by Health Canada in 2020 after already being available in the US for fourteen years, since 2006.[50]

Deregulation

When Health Canada finally *did* approve the combination product (mifepristone and misoprostol), sold under the brand name Mifegymiso by the company Linepharma, it did so with a peculiarly high number of regulatory requirements.[51] Only physicians could prescribe it, even though nurse practitioners routinely issue reproductive health-related prescriptions (for example, contraception). Physicians intending to prescribe mife first had to complete an educational course. They had to register with the manufacturer, Celopharma, stock and dispense the medication themselves, and witness the patient swallow the first pill in their office in front of them. They were required to review ultrasound imaging before seeing the patient, and patients thus needed multiple appointments: to the primary care physician for that referral, then to the diagnostic imaging department, and back to the physician for the subsequent prescription, not to mention follow-up care. Patients also had to sign a consent form. These requirements were unprecedented and made mifepristone seem dangerous, intimidating, and simply exhausting to become involved with, despite the international evidence of mifepristone safety and effectiveness. As a result, almost no one, besides those physicians already performing procedural abortion, was interested in taking up medication abortion prescribing. Moreover, some of the requirements contradicted other policies. For example, physicians do not generally dispense medications,[52] as this is out of their scope and squarely in that of pharmacists.

Recognizing these restrictions would likely inhibit most potential prescribers from adopting mife into their practice, the Contraception and Abortion Research Team (CART-GRAC), an interdisciplinary, cross-country team headquartered in the Faculty of Medicine at the University of British Columbia (UBC) and under the leadership of family physician Dr. Wendy Norman,[53] embarked on a study of barriers and facilitators to mife implementation. As they interviewed ninety care providers and stakeholders, they shared emergent findings with Health Canada, namely that the host of mifepristone restrictions made prescribing unnecessarily complicated and burdensome.[54] One by one, Health Canada repealed the restrictions:[55] dropping the requirement of observed ingestion, for patient consent, for prescriber training, physician dispensing, and eventually, making ultrasound optional[56] until, by 2019, the drug was completely deregulated. During this time, Health Canada also extended the approved gestational duration from the initial seven weeks (forty-nine days) to nine weeks (sixty-three days).

The combination of mifepristone and misoprostol medications is also clinically useful at any gestational duration for pregnancy termination care and treatment of miscarriage and stillbirth.[57] Some providers are willing to prescribe beyond nine weeks; such "off-label" prescribing is beyond what Health Canada has reviewed and authorized.[58]

The Changing Provider Workforce: Abortion Integration into Primary Care

The Contraception and Abortion Research Team (CART) first surveyed abortion providers in 2012 to understand the workforce and its workload.[59] At the time, ninety-four abortion facilities (hospitals, community-based clinics, and physician offices) were identified, nearly half of which were in Quebec and most of which were in large urban centres. The respondents to the national survey (from seventy-eight of the ninety-four facilities) reported providing 75,650 abortions in 2012, of which only 4 percent were described as medication abortion. More than half of the facilities provided fewer than 500 abortions per year. All abortions were provided by physicians, 60 percent of them identifying as general practitioners and family doctors in primary care. Two-thirds of respondents indicated no experiences of harassment or violence in the prior year; notably, 85 percent of respondents from Quebec experienced zero harassment, while only 14 percent of Ontario facilities responded the same. This survey would prove to be an important baseline to measure changes over time.

In 2019, CART sought to readminister the workforce survey to capture changes since the implementation of mife. Because the nature of abortion provision had changed so much, and mifepristone could be prescribed through primary care, the denominator in the survey changed from *facilities* providing abortion to *individuals* providing abortion. One of the sudden impacts of deregulatory changes was that abortion was no longer the purview of physicians alone: it could be prescribed by other primary care providers, including nurse practitioners. The 2019 survey included thirty nurse practitioners, constituting about 8 percent of all medication abortion providers, and providing about 2 percent of all medication abortions (about 327).[60] Half of all survey respondents had less than five years' experience providing abortion care, a clear indicator that mifepristone implementation had caused the numbers of abortion providers to skyrocket and changed the very nature of who was doing the work. Including family doctors and nurse practitioners, primary care professionals provided 71 percent of the nearly 50,000 abortions reported in the survey and constituted 83 percent of the total respondents providing medication abortion.

Quebec's College of Physicians (Collège des médecins du Québec) responded to Health Canada's mife deregulation by intervening with Quebec-specific requirements: prospective medication abortion prescribers must first be trained as procedural abortion providers. The special medication *and* procedural abortion training must take place in person.[61] Quebec's physician regulator is the only such regulator in the country with these powers. The College's rules effectively blocked the path for any nurse practitioner involvement, as only physicians are authorized to perform procedural abortions in Canada. It also excluded primary care physicians who were not performing procedural abortions in their offices. For all intents and purposes, only the physicians already working in abortion clinics as procedural abortion providers would be eligible and interested in prescribing medication abortion.

In the aftermath of the *Dobbs* decision in the US, over 300 Quebec physicians signed a petition against the College's restrictive requirements, which were subsequently removed in summer 2022.[62] The College stated, "It is up to the physician to ensure that he has the knowledge and skills necessary to prescribe this medication, as for any other care, medication or treatment, in accordance with his ethical obligations." In their 2019 survey of the Canadian abortion workforce, Renner et al.[63] found that of all the regions, Quebec had the lowest proportion of providers only providing first-trimester medication abortion, at 10 percent. Quebec also had the lowest proportion of first-trimester medication abortions, at only 12.5 percent of all abortions, compared to 28 percent in the sample as a whole.

Quebec is home to the country's first abortion clinic, which Dr. Henry Morgentaler opened in 1969 in Montreal, and it was for care he provided there that he was famously sent to provincial jail. Over the years, nearly fifty more clinics opened their doors in the province. Now there are more clinics in Quebec than in any other province, territory, or US state. By the often-used metric of "facilities per province," Quebec knocks abortion access out of the park. However, facilities-per-province is a very blunt measure, increasingly irrelevant as primary care prescribing expands.

Dr. Edith Guilbert, a founding member of CART and family physician with a long history of leadership in abortion care in the province, wanted to find out why medication abortion uptake was so much lower in Quebec. In 2021, she and co-author Dr. Geneviève Bois designed a "mystery shopping" experiment and had researchers call forty-seven clinics using fake patient profiles with pregnancies under sixty-three days.[64] Of the forty-seven clinics, medication abortion was only an option at thirty-nine. On average, the clinics required 2.9 clinic visits for medication abortion, compared with 2.3 for procedural abortion. No clinic offered medication abortion through telemedicine. Most tellingly, "Unfavorable comments about medication abortion were frequent" from the staff people who answered the calls, in that exaggerations were made about likelihood of complications or ineffectiveness. In a second part of this study, Guilbert and Bois analyzed the quality of the information clinic staff provided to the mystery patients and found it to be insufficient for informed decision making between medication and procedural abortion options.[65]

At the Unfinished Revolution,[66] a landmark abortion conference on Prince Edward Island in summer 2014, almost three years before the province finally opened an abortion clinic, one of the more controversial issues discussed in the hallways and coffee breaks was the potential "threat" posed by medication abortion, which at that point was under review by Health Canada. Those concerned felt that taking abortion out of the clinic and into community, into homes, could kill the clinic model, and the symbolic, even spiritual meaning of the clinics to the abortion movement. Procedural abortion at abortion clinics, and specifically Morgentaler clinics, had propelled access forward for four decades.

Today, ten years after the Unfinished Revolution conference, it is evident that primary care access to medication abortion is indeed decentring the clinic from abortion, with revolutionary consequences. Dedicated abortion clinics and procedural abortion services remain critical — not only because of the gestational duration limitations to mifepristone prescriptions, but because patients may be clinically ineligible for medication abortion for other reasons such as allergy or blood disorders, or they may simply prefer the experience of procedural abortion. But demand for procedural abortion is unarguably falling and falling fast: from 96 percent of all abortion in 2016 to 68 percent in 2020.[67] In the US, where Mifeprex launched in 2000, more than half of abortions are by medication. In Sweden, where mifepristone was approved in 1991, the rate of first trimester abortions by medication is 96.7 percent.[68] There is reason to believe free-standing, privately owned clinics that rely on procedural abortion revenue to stay open will need to make operational adjustments, such as expanding types of services or renegotiating funding arrangements with the provinces. It is possible some clinics may close. Ironically, these closures would be a result of *increased* access to services. In 2003, the Morgentaler clinic in Halifax closed when it became apparent that access through the hospital-based clinic was adequate to meet patient needs.[69]

Interestingly, although the majority of procedural abortion was provided by primary care providers in CART's 2012 national survey, that had shifted by 2019 to mostly obstetrician-gynecologist specialists.[70] Renner et al. comment that their survey did, however, illustrate "rejuvenation" of the procedural abortion workforce, which had been declining prior to mifepristone implementation. Although the number of procedural abortions provided in Canada each year appears to decline, increasing the number of providers willing and able to provide this service can improve patient options, equalize access across Canadian geography, and protect against loss of access when older physicians justifiably decide to retire. It also reassures medication abortion prescribers that backup is there when their patients may need it.

Nurse Practitioner Prescribing

The World Health Organization takes the position that "[a]bortion can be safely and effectively performed in a range of settings and by a variety of people, including different types of health workers, and in early pregnancy by the woman herself."[71] The evidence supports this: a 2015 meta-analysis by Barnard et al.[72] found no difference in the safety of medication abortion provided by physicians when compared to "mid-level providers" such as nurses and midwives, as well as no statistically significant difference in the risk of complications from first trimester procedural abortions.

In 2017, Health Canada removed the requirement that only physicians could prescribe mifepristone. In response, nursing regulatory bodies across Canada looked at the evidence of safety of mifepristone and the precedents for nurse practitioner (NP) prescribing and began authorizing their NP members to prescribe. With the notable exception of Quebec, all jurisdictions adopted NP prescribing within the year. However, work is needed to integrate appropriate content into NP training programs and to nourish the mentorship networks that support competence and confidence in these skills.[73] In 2024, the Canadian Association of Schools of Nursing (CASN)[74] launched entry-to-practice competencies in abortion care for graduates of all undergraduate (registered nurse) and graduate (nurse practitioner) nursing programs. In 2020, CART researchers studied the implementation of mifepristone among nurse practitioners in Canada,[75] interviewing forty-three people, including sixteen NPs who prescribed medication abortion. When asked about what supported the adoption of mife into their practices, the most important issue raised was having access to education and mentorship.

Medication abortion is usually very straightforward: confirm the patient is pregnant and below nine to ten weeks, advise them the sequence in which to take the pills and the difference between normal and concerning symptoms, and ask them to do follow-up blood or urine testing to confirm effective termination. But new or prospective prescribers worry about how to respond to patient questions: what should you say to make sure they know *this* much bleeding is appropriate, but *that* much bleeding is not? That *this* much pain — a completely subjective experience — is expected, but *that* much pain is cause for alarm? When should the patient be referred for ultrasound to check for retained products? When should they wait it out for a bit, see if the products pass on their own? These types of questions are easily answered by experienced providers, but the deep stigma that has long surrounded abortion prompts secrecy and isolation between providers and generated profound barriers for patients.

Safety from Violence and Harassment

As abortion permeates primary care, it becomes but one of a thousand routine prescriptions coming out of a general or family practice. It normalizes abortion for patients and providers, and the safety of the experience of abortion provision increases. In the CART 2019 survey, only 8 percent of low-volume providers, who provide fewer than thirty abortions per year, reported that they experienced harassment.[76] Among higher-volume providers, people providing more than thirty abortions per year, the rate was 21 percent.

Bringing abortion out of the clinic and into community reduces the vulnerability of clinics and clinic patients to harassment and violence. Anti-abortion extremism and terrorism is much more acute in the US than in Canada.[77] The Abortion Rights Coalition of Canada (ARCC)[78] reports that between 1977 and 2015, there were 7,200 acts of violence against US abortion providers, including "42 bombings, 185 arson attacks, and thousands of death threats, bioterrorism threats, and assaults. In addition, more than 234,300 acts of disruption were reported, including bomb threats, hate mail, and harassing calls."

There have been no acts of violence in Canada since the 1990s, but that decade saw the militarism evident in the US cross the border. In May 1992, Morgentaler's Toronto clinic was burned to the ground. No one was hurt in the fire, which happened overnight, but the arsonists were never found.[79] On November 8, 1994, Dr. Gary Romalis was shot in the thigh in a sniper attack at his home in Vancouver. Romalis saved his own life with a homemade tourniquet;[80] the case went unsolved. On November 10, 1995, Dr. Hugh Short was shot in his home in Ancaster, Ontario. James Kopp was initially charged with attempted murder, but Ontario police dropped the charges.[81] On November 11, 1997, Dr. Jack Fainman[82] was shot in the shoulder at his home in Winnipeg, and although Kopp was considered a "person of interest" in the case, he was not charged. Fainman was no longer able to work as an obstetrician-gynecologist after the shooting, although he too survived. Kopp, an American, later pled guilty for the 1998 murder of Dr. Barnett Slepian, an abortion provider in Buffalo, New York, and received a life sentence with no possibility of parole.

The escalation of anti-abortion violence of the 1990s, coupled with the discouraging actions of multiple provinces to stifle abortion access in clinics and the lack of abortion training opportunities in medical schools,[83] drove physicians away at the time. Abortion care became highly stigmatized beyond potential religious objection; it was considered dangerous. The fears and stigma have persisted: a 2018 study found most family medicine residents in Canada received no training in abortion at all.[84] Decades later, the privacy of medication abortion and its immersion in the ubiquity of primary care has helped remove stigma and encourage participation. While anti-abortion extremism continues with terrifying regularity in the US,[85] from assaults on clinic escorts to Molotov cocktail attacks and vandalism, it is unusual in Canada today.

Public Funding for Mifepristone

Even at the time of his discovery in France, Baulieu recognized that medication abortion represented a vastly more affordable approach to abortion than procedural care for both individuals and health systems.[86] At a hospital-based abortion clinic, a procedural abortion, including the associated services like ultrasound, blood work, nursing care, sterile processing of instruments, medications and administration costs, can amount to $2,000 or more if paid for out of pocket, which people without a Medicare card must do. Comparatively, a package of Mifegymiso costs about $350.

When mifepristone arrived on the market in Canada, activists and clinicians alike were swift to point out it only made sense for governments to foot the bill. Canada is the only country in the world with a "universal" health care system and yet no universal coverage for drugs.[87]

When first approved as a prescription medication, prescribed in primary care settings and dispensed by community pharmacies like any other prescription medication, the cost of mifepristone was expected to be borne by the patient. Organizations including National Abortion Federation (NAF) Canada and the Women's Legal Education and Action Fund (LEAF) lobbied persistently and successfully to include mifepristone under Medicare.[88] New Brunswick was the first province to agree, in 2017,[89] and every province and territory followed eventually, with Saskatchewan taking the longest to align.[90]

The one-by-one domino effect among the provinces/territories in this case was relatively quick, but variation in public funding for mifepristone is an example of how provincial/territorial jurisdiction for health services can result in significant inequalities between patients in different parts of the country. As of this writing in spring 2025, British Columbia, Manitoba, the Yukon and PEI have all signed agreements with the federal government to provide universal coverage to all residents for hormonal contraception. The newly elected Liberal premier of New Brunswick, Susan Holt, has announced plans for her province to offer coverage, as well. The cost of birth control is a driving factor in the choice to use it;[91] further, patients forced to pay out of pocket are more likely to choose the lower-cost options, even if they are less effective.[92] Irregular policies for prescription drug coverage, when the prescription drugs in question are for sexed and gendered experiences like pregnancy prevention and termination, are a problematic consequence of the Canadian model of care. The role of truly universal coverage for prescription contraception will be discussed further in Chapter 8, "Expansion of Care," and Chapter 10, "Contraception."

The cost of medication abortion is not, however, only the fee of the pills themselves. The pharmacists have dispensing fees; there may be blood work drawn by nurses and analyzed by lab technicians, ultrasounds conducted by radiation techs and reviewed by radiologists, clerks employed to book appointments for each step, and clinic and hospital administrators creating, compiling, and filing patient charts. Prescribers must take the time to talk with patients, make sure they are confident in the decision to choose medication abortion over procedural, explain how it works and what to expect, and to describe the expectations in terms of follow up: possibly more blood draws and even more visits. Providing medication abortion is not exactly like writing up a prescription for penicillin.

When provinces started publicly funding mifepristone prescription costs, they had not yet sorted out how to compensate prescribers for the comparatively more time-consuming work of a mifepristone prescription compared to penicillin. Most family physicians in Canada work on a fee-for-service basis, with each service they provide connected to a billing code for which they invoice the province. It takes longer to counsel a patient about medication abortion than it does about penicillin. Community and physician advocates engaged in a whole other round of efforts to prompt provincial/territorial governments to create new codes specific to the demands of medication abortion.[93] Again, there is inter-provincial variation to these codes and their values.[94] Alberta still, seven years after implementation, does not have billing codes for medication abortion prescribing.[95]

A shadow side of mifepristone's increased affordability through public funding is that it has caused abortion clinics to become vulnerable to significant revenue loss. Until 2016, 96 percent of abortion was procedural: family doctors and obstetrician-gynecologists performing the service in either free-standing clinics or within hospitals were billing the province accordingly. Free-standing clinics are private businesses: the province pays for the care, but the clinic owners must pay their bills. Staff salaries, electricity, mortgage or rent — these depend on bringing in enough revenue from services provided. If a provider used to bill $1,000 for every procedural abortion and can only bill $200 for prescribing mifepristone, and more and more patients are choosing medication abortion, and the abortion rate in a population stays the same or even decreases as access to contraception improves ... how do you keep the lights on?

Another concern is that despite the promise of access afforded by public funding for mifepristone, many already underserved patients in Canada are ineligible for this financial coverage. This includes people without a provincial health card in any province/territory, and often people with a health card for one province but living in another. As described in Chapter 2, "With Laws Come Limits," the Canada Health Act protects portability of care, but there are some hiccups: Many provinces require patients to pay up front for mifepristone if they arrive at the pharmacy counter with an out-of-province card. For example, a Torontonian studying at Dalhousie University in Halifax, Nova Scotia, cannot present their Ontario Health Insurance Plan (OHIP) card (provincial Medicare) and receive mifepristone free of charge: they first pay approximately $350 up front and then file paperwork with OHIP for reimbursement.

Some students will not even qualify for reimbursement. International students face delays from when they arrive in Canada to when they can apply for a provincial Medicare card, and often the emergency health coverage arranged through their university, meant to address emergencies in that interim period, fails to cover mifepristone. Nova Scotia[96] requires international students to wait thirteen months before applying for Medicare. Quebec requires newcomers to the province wait three months before applying for provincial insurance; however, the province makes an exception for pregnancy.[97] There were over 1 million international students registered in Canada in 2023.[98]

Telemedicine and Lower-Touch Care

Reducing use of potentially unnecessary corollary services in medication abortion — such as ultrasound, blood work, and in-person appointments with prescribers — reduces system costs and expedites access. Efforts to minimize travel and time devoted to the process of abortion seeking benefits patients by reducing direct and indirect costs. Very shortly after mife implementation, providers experienced a second wave of innovation coinciding with the COVID-19 pandemic: telemedicine. It became apparent early on that opportunities to reduce patients' physical contact with health facilities was optimal to protect everyone (patients, staff, and families at home) from illness. Keeping abortion patients, who are clinically well, out of health facilities was especially prudent. Being very new to abortion provision, many providers began to make the leap to prescribing it without ever sitting down with their patients.

There are several parts to a medication abortion that can be "telemedicinized." Instead of booking an appointment to consult with a prescriber, an initial intake can be done over the phone, by either the prescriber or a nurse or clerk. Blood work and ultrasound, if required at all, can be done as close to the patient's home as possible, and the results read online by the prescriber. The conversation about the process and medication can also be by phone or Zoom, as can follow-up calls to check on how the patient fared. The prescription itself can be faxed to the local pharmacy. Instead of follow-up blood work, a patient could use a urine test at their own home to confirm completeness of the abortion. Any or all steps could be made "lower touch" or even "no touch."

The Health Canada requirement for ultrasound for medication abortion was abandoned in 2019, before COVID-19. Health Canada's 2019 survey of abortion providers, also pre-pandemic, found 44 percent of first trimester medication abortion providers used some amount of telemedicine in their care, and 90 percent of patients received an ultrasound.[99] Of those providers using telemedicine, 86 percent used it for their initial consultation with the patient, 82 percent for issuing the prescription, and 92 percent for follow up.[100] Challenges to use of telemedicine included lack of ultrasound to confirm gestational duration and lack of blood testing to confirm beta-human chorionic gonadotropin (ßhCG), lack of an appropriate physician fee code for billing, and lack of emergency services in the event of complications.[101]

Guilbert et al.[102] created a clinical practice guideline for the Society of Obstetricians and Gynaecologists of Canada to support telemedicine prescribing. The guideline walks the prescriber through confirming patient identity, advising them to seek a high-quality urine test to confirm pregnancy, determining gestational duration by confirming date of last menstrual period (LMP), and discussing risks of ectopic pregnancy. These risk factors include previous ectopic pregnancy and current use of an IUD. If an ectopic pregnancy is present, the medication abortion medications will not cause harm; however, they will not resolve the issue, either. If there are ectopic risks, or if the LMP is uncertain, ultrasound and/or blood work will be required to confirm the pregnancy is not further along than nine to ten weeks, as well as the location of the pregnancy in the uterus.

The danger with unconfirmed gestation or location is that the pregnancy will be too far along for the mifepristone to work optimally, or that an ectopic pregnancy will go undetected and rupture — a serious obstetric emergency. Although research has found that there is poor understanding among the public of how to date pregnancies,[103] once patients learn that this is measured from the date of last menstrual period and not from the date of last sexual intercourse, they can be quite accurate in their self-assessment of gestational duration.[104]

Many studies have found telemedicine abortion to be very safe. A 2018–2019 US survey by Aiken et al.[105] found that among nearly 3,000 telemedicine medication abortion patients, 96 percent had a successful termination without surgical intervention, and 1 percent reported treatment for serious adverse events. In a much larger UK study, Aiken et al.[106] analyzed over 50,000 medication abortions provided in the winter and spring of 2020, comparing pre-COVID onset to post: 22,000 medication abortions were by the traditional pathway, 18,000 by telemedicine, and 11,000 by a telemedicine–in person hybrid. There was no difference in treatment success, serious complications, and ectopic pregnancy between the groups, but the telemedicine patients waited on average four days less from referral to treatment. Eighty percent of patients would choose telemedicine again.

There has yet to be a replication of the 2019 CART survey in the post-COVID Canadian reality to determine just how providers are adjusting their practices considering the Aiken et al. (2021) findings,[107] the Guilbert et al. guidelines, and the general routinization of virtual care experienced in the past few years. It is likely that providers with easiest access to ultrasonography, such as those in well-resourced clinics with their own ultrasound machines and trained techs, will continue to prefer patients receive imaging. Those without such easy access to ultrasound and technicians are likely more frequently prescribing without imaging. Confirmation of pregnancy and an approximation of gestational dating early in pregnancy can be achieved by tracking successive blood tests for the trend in ßhCG: generally speaking, the value doubles in the first ten weeks of pregnancy but then stops increasing and begins to fall,[108] but the sensitivity of this approach decreases after six weeks.[109]

Again, if a patient is very sure of their pregnancy and the date of their last menstrual period, determining ßhCG levels through blood analysis can be avoided. Blood work also shows complete blood count values, such as hemoglobin levels, which, if very low, would make medication abortion at home less acceptable. Patients must be informed of these risks, and providers must ultimately feel comfortable themselves that the likely benefit of "low-touch" care that avoids blood work and ultrasound outweighs any potential harm.

There are providers who resisted telemedicine medication abortion during COVID-19 and who remain uncomfortable and unconvinced by the practice. For many, one bad experience, such as a missed ectopic or a serious error in dating, is enough to dissuade them from the practice. But for many, familiarity with at least some level of lower-touch care is steadily increasing. For patients without a Medicare card, some prescribers may make profound efforts to avoid the costs of blood work and ultrasound, forego their own prescriber fees (basically donating their time), and arrange for Action Canada for Sexual Health and Rights,

Abortion Care Canada (formerly NAF Canada), or another charity to pay for the mifepristone prescription. The variations in practice are many and depend on patient clinical factors as well as geographical considerations and system organization and resources. Indisputably, however, increasing uptake of lower-touch care through medication abortion has improved convenience for patients and reduced costs.

Because of these variations, it can be a bit complicated to explain to abortion seekers exactly what they will encounter when they first call to arrange care. This may make medication abortion seem unwieldy and daunting, and much less efficient than a single clinic visit, where ultrasound, blood work, and procedure are completed all together in one appointment. What patients find optimal is individual, and the experience of abortion must balance what providers can comfortably offer and what patients find acceptable.

Telemedicine in family planning butts up against a hard limit when it comes to long-acting reversible contraception, the most effective type of birth control available. There is no way to insert an IUD or contraceptive implant online or by phone. Abortion patients are people who have already experienced unintended pregnancy: they are at elevated risk of future unintended pregnancy without effective contraception. A BC study of post-abortion contraception uptake before both the approval of mife in 2017 and of Nexplanon in 2020 found a quarter of patients chose IUDs, and these patients were less likely than those choosing oral contraception to undergo a subsequent abortion.[110] US researchers have found post-abortion IUD uptake is lower among medication abortion patients than procedural abortion patients.[111] Some providers value meeting patients in person for medication abortion prescriptions so that they build a relationship and can support patients with post-abortion family planning decisions and care. Efforts to enhance public funding of contraception in Canada will need to be matched with efforts to expand access to clinicians competent in insertion of long-acting contraception options.

Pharmacy Stocking

A prescription to pick up a medication in a community pharmacy is only useful if the pharmacy in question has the medication in stock. Since mifepristone was introduced in Canada, clinicians, patients, and advocates have shared concern about pharmacy stocking. There have been several efforts, such as the Canada Abortion Providers'[112] virtual community of practice, to identify and "map" participating pharmacies, however, these efforts are difficult to maintain with up-to-date information. Community pharmacies are privately owned and operated, and generally cannot be compelled to stock something if they find it morally or otherwise objectionable.

A 2019 survey of 433 pharmacists across the country reached encouraging conclusions: 93 percent were ready and willing to dispense mifepristone;[113] half of the respondents routinely kept mifepristone in stock, and 67 percent had dispensed the product an average of twenty-six times per year.[114] Mifepristone is a relatively expensive drug, at $350 or so retail; it has a shelf life of five years;[115] and, as described above, from a per-patient perspective, it is infrequently prescribed. Unsurprisingly, Zusman et al.[116] found that barriers to keeping mife in stock included low demand from consumers/patients, relatively short shelf life, and drug shortages. Almost 97 percent of pharmacist respondents reported their communities did not present resistance to their provision of medication abortion, and the authors concluded that mifepristone is well-supported by pharmacists in Canada. In 2022, the Canadian Pharmacists' Association (CPhA) released a statement in support of pharmacists' roles in medication abortion,[117] and in winter 2024, the CPhA published a collection of evidence-based professional development resources to support pharmacists in dispensing mife.[118]

Pharmacists are authorized to prescribe contraception in eight provinces in Canada;[119] the only exceptions are Ontario, Manitoba, and the three territories. The future of mifepristone may involve pharmacist prescribing as well.

Promoting Mifepristone

One of the lingering and perplexing challenges with the promise of mifepristone is how to let more people know about it. The Food and Drugs Act[120] governs the manufacture, distribution, and sale of medications in Canada. It also governs the advertising of prescription drug products. Direct-to-consumer advertising (DTCA) of prescription drugs is not permitted in Canada. As such, mifepristone has never had a manufacturer's marketing campaign to enhance public understanding of its existence and purpose. As Gardner, Mintzes, and Ostry[121] explain, advertising prescription drugs can threaten public safety: "Compared with OTC drugs, prescription-only products are generally more toxic and are used to treat conditions that are not easily self-diagnosed and self-managed." The authors describe how it is new drugs that are usually the most heavily promoted, when less information is available about potential benefits and harms.

While profoundly relevant to many products, DTCA restrictions on mifepristone are unsuitable in some ways. Mifepristone is *not* new to the market; it was first approved in France in 1988. It is not "generally more toxic": it is a very safe drug, associated with fewer than five deaths per million patients, a death rate of 0.0005 percent.[122] Its introduction into Canada was not associated with any increase in adverse events associated with abortion.[123] Finally, pregnancy *is* relatively easy to self-diagnose; urine pregnancy tests at home are highly acceptable to users and very effective.[124] Medication abortion is also called "self-managed abortion" because it is so autonomous. Perhaps at one point, mifepristone will be removed from prescription-only status, and the prohibition on promotion under the Food and Drugs Act would no longer apply. The future of mifepristone may be very dynamic.

The Future of Mifepristone

Dutch physician Rebecca Gomperts founded Women on Waves[125] in 1999, an anarchistic abortion ship service that sailed around the world for over a decade, offering abortion in the international waters off the coast of countries with restrictive abortion law. More recently, it has used drones to drop abortion pills into Poland, where abortion is severely restricted. Aid Access,[126] a splintering-off from Women on Waves, serves the United States specifically and in response to recent accelerations in abortion restrictions, delivered 85,000 packages of pills in 2023 alone. A sister organization, Women on Web,[127] emerged as a global abortion pill distribution service sending mifepristone and misoprostol packages by post to patients facing abortion bans. Beyond her innovations in medication abortion delivery through these organizations, Dr. Gomperts is a leading player in mifepristone research worldwide.

Research has long suggested that mifepristone could be used as a form of contraception.[128] Gomperts is spearheading current trials of a once-weekly oral mifepristone pill regimen that is anticipated to be both effective and without side effects associated with estrogen or progesterone-based birth control methods, such as weight gain, mood disorder, loss of libido, thrombosis, or breast cancer.[129]

There is interest in advanced, prophylactic prescription of mifepristone, so that when and if it is needed, there are no delays. Between 2021 and 2023, Aid Access received 50,000 such requests.[130] While these requests were made in the context of anticipating and then experiencing the fall of *Roe v. Wade* in the US, and widespread anxiety about the banning of abortion, advanced provision has applicability in areas where abortion is legal but cumbersome to access. Consider a rural area in Canada where, even if there is a prescriber, that one prescriber may go on vacation for a month a year. The relentless expansion of abortion bans across the US have generated significant discussion about the need for and value of advance prescribing in politically hostile contexts; this need and value also may be evident in low-service contexts.

Who can prescribe mifepristone will continue to expand. As mentioned previously, pharmacists, already prescribing birth control in most jurisdictions, could possibly start prescribing mife as well. In BC, registered nurses with advanced training are able to prescribe contraception; Ontario launched a similar program in January of 2024.[131] Eventually these programs could include all provinces and territories. Mifepristone has a higher safety profile than most prescribed forms of birth control; nurse and pharmacist prescribing of mifepristone is a sensible next step.

Joanna Erdman, an international legal scholar of abortion, urges regulatory bodies in Canada go even further than expansion of prescribing authority and telemedicine. Erdman wants to remove all gatekeeping and put pills in peoples' hands by allowing mifepristone to appear on shelves as an OTC product, available without a prescription.[132] In 2023, for the first time, the US Food and Drug Administration approved OTC sale of OPill, an oral contraception medication.[133] If this and emergency contraception are available without a prescription, there is a strong argument for mifepristone to be, as well.

Rather than courtroom battles, it is pragmatism and health evidence that has driven deregulation, resulting in ever-improving mifepristone availability in Canada.

* * *

The hard-won implementation of medication abortion (mifepristone) in Canada in 2017 was a transformative moment comparable to the *R. v. Morgentaler* decision. Safe and effective medication abortion in the privacy and comfort of home can improve patient satisfaction and decrease geographic barriers to care. Expanded prescribing authority, improved uptake of telemedicine, and increased public education and understanding are necessary to optimize use.

CHAPTER 5

BELIEF-BASED DENIAL OF CARE

> This chapter explains the limits of health professionals' "conscientious objection" to provision of abortion services in Canada.

Democratization of medication abortion throughout primary care has a potential shadow side: with any family doctor or nurse practitioner now a possible prescriber, patients may face more uncertainty about who might refuse to provide care or even refer them to other care providers. I have borrowed the term "belief-based denial of care" from Joyce Arthur, the longtime leader of the Abortion Rights Coalition of Canada (ARCC). I first heard her use this phrase in fall 2023 at the National Abortion Federation (NAF) Canada conference in Vancouver, BC. She has also called the practice "dishonourable disobedience."[1] This framing of the phenomenon, instead of "conscientious objection," takes away any neutrality. It captures the potential injuriousness of care withheld rather than the traditional, military understanding of conscientious objection as avoidance of participation in harm.

The Ethics of Conscientious Objection

The concept of conscientious objection gained currency in Canada early in the twentieth century. Refusal to participate in military service based on religious grounds has existed since at least Roman times.[2] Conscription into full-time military service was implemented in July 1917, three years into World War I, when Canada was facing vast casualties and declining voluntary enrolment. Widespread opposition to the US Vietnam draft in the 1960s served to push conscientious objection into the field of health services and spurred "draft dodgers" to seek safety in Canada. As Kessler[3] argues, "major religious organizations, the press, and the federal judiciary all came to embrace the individual conscientious objector as a legitimate and even laudable kind of citizen, enforcing the country's constitutional commitment to individual liberty in the face of a heedless war machine."[4] Further, he describes how it was "closely associated with a critique of government-authorized killing" and therefore "provided fertile ground for the anti-abortion and anti-contraceptive social movements that emerged during the later years of American involvement in Vietnam."[5]

Moving conscientious objection out of the domain of war into that of care had highly gendered consequences. The US anti-war movement coincided with the Food and Drug Administration's approval of the birth control pill in 1960,[6] its subsequent popularization, and of the *Roe v. Wade* Supreme Court Decision of 1973 legalizing abortion. In Canada, the discourse of conscientious objection in health services for years focused on medical professionals' non-participation in "women's health," although it later came to include medical assistance in dying (MAiD). In any context of health care, when each individual practitioner is bound by professional codes against patient abandonment, refusing to participate is ethically fraught; in the field of sexual and reproductive health, this refusal disproportionately affects women and people who can get pregnant. There are jurisdictions around the world, such as Sweden, where conscientious objection in medical care has no legal standing: health care professionals do not have the right to refuse to provide services based on religious or moral objections.[7] Being turned away due to health professionals' beliefs elevates the stigma of seeking abortions, a denial of which only women and people with a uterus can be subject. Belief-based denial drives delays and inequalities in access, and ultimately it may result in forced childbearing and gendered, highly inequitable clinical and socioeconomic consequences. Fiala and Arthur[8] argue against the translation of conscientious objection from military contexts to health services, insisting that "[t]he two have nothing in common (for example, objecting doctors are rarely disciplined, while the patient pays the price)." Indeed, dodging the US draft was punishable by five years in prison; in the context of abortion, a patient denied care is unlikely to even complain because of a combination of stigma and lack of understanding of even how to complain.

Conscientious objection in health care is generally understood as an individual's right to not do that care themselves, balanced with the health professional ethical requirement to ensure the patient is indeed cared for: a referral to an alternate provider is the lynchpin for this to function. For some objectors, however, the referral is itself interpreted as participation, and this compromise is untenable.[9] The referral makes the abortion possible, so, McLeod states, to impose the requirement to refer is to "defend the moral permissibility of abortion."[10]

Until 2017, when nurse practitioners were authorized everywhere but Quebec to prescribe medication abortion, abortion depended on physician involvement. But other health professionals certainly play critical roles in abortion care,[11] and physician-centred discussions of belief-based denial of care miss the team basis of much of abortion care. A registered nurse on a maternity unit could refuse an assignment with a patient who is terminating a pregnancy, regardless of whether the termination is for either fetal-maternal clinical reasons or patient's choice. While perhaps the physician will still provide the aspiration procedure, who is going to monitor the patient's vitals, administer medications, and provide comfort? Or perhaps an ultrasound technician will not see a patient who requires a dating ultrasound prior to an abortion. Or a phlebotomist may refuse to draw the blood work necessary to ascertain pregnancy hormone. Or a pharmacist who does not and will not stock mifepristone.

Adding to the interdisciplinary team of players, the Canadian environment for regulating belief-based denial of care is highly complex because there are many levels and types of ways health professional and ethical practice may be defined and governed. To begin with, each province/territory has its own unique laws governing the regulation of health professionals; in turn, each province/territory may have its own regulatory body for each regulated health profession. In some places there may be some collation, resulting in multiple health professionals being covered by one regulatory regime. This has been the case in Nova Scotia since November 2023, when the Conservative government passed Bill 323, the Regulated Health Professionals Act.[12] Meanwhile, Ontario has separate acts for nurses,[13] midwives,[14] and physicians.[15]

The provincial/territorial acts may define health professionals' scope of practice. The regulatory bodies then set standards that both inform professionals about their accountabilities and stipulate what the public should expect from their care.[16] As a result, what a certain type of professional can do depends on location. For example, nurse practitioners

(NPs), a profession that has grown substantially in recent years, may do different things with different levels of autonomy across the country. An example of how these manifest in practice: in every province except Quebec, NPs have the unrestricted ability to conduct advanced assessment and diagnosis of patients; they have full hospital privileges in four jurisdictions, none in Quebec, and restricted privileges in the others.[17] Rather than an abortion law, across Canada there are layers of regulations governing the practice of potential abortion providers.

The health professional regulator, often called a college, represents the interests of the public; it is the job of the regulator to respond to patient or peer complaints against a health professional for inappropriate conduct, which could include failure to provide adequate or appropriate care. Recall in Chapter 3, "Defining Miscarriage, Stillbirth, and Infant Death," how the BC College of Nurses and Midwives sought to protect members of the public from inadvertently hiring an unlicensed midwife after midwifery legislation in 1998.

Beyond provincial/territorial laws and the self-regulatory bodies that uphold them, there are national organizations that draw up health professional ethical codes. The Canadian Medical Association's (CMA) Code of Ethics and Professionalism[18] explains the "ethical and professional commitments and responsibilities" of every physician. The National Association of Pharmacy Regulatory Authorities[19] sets out ethical standards for pharmacists and pharmacy technicians. The Canadian Nursing Association (CNA)[20] does the same for all nurses and NPs in the CNA Code of Ethics, which stipulates, "if nursing care is requested that is in conflict with the nurse's moral beliefs and values but in keeping with professional practice, the nurse provides safe, compassionate, competent and ethical care until alternative care arrangements are in place to meet the patient's needs or desires."[21] Nurses are to place patient needs ahead of their own beliefs, at least until another nurse can step in. Health care is a needed service, not an optional add-on.

The CMA Code begins with a stipulation that each medical doctor must "Accept the patient without discrimination (such as on the basis of age, disability, gender identity or expression, genetic characteristics, language, marital and family status, medical condition, national or ethnic origin, political affiliation, race, religion, sex, sexual orientation, or socioeconomic status)." With specific respect to conscientious objection, it states physicians must follow their conscience, respect colleagues' values, while also meeting the duty of not abandoning the patient. Physicians are to inform the patient when they hold beliefs that may influence their recommendations about or actual provision of a medical intervention. While these elements could be interpreted as supportive of abortion access, they do not provide strict instruction that care must be provided or that an effective referral must be made.

In 1988, in response to the *R. v. Morgentaler* decision, the CMA published a policy on induced abortion,[22] which clearly stated acceptance of the removal of Section 251 from the Criminal Code. The contents of the policy begin with a definition of abortion as pregnancy termination before fetal viability — before the fetus could survive independent of the mother's body. The policy explains that viability depends on the weight of the fetus, its degree of development, and the gestational duration of the pregnancy; survival may be possible for a fetus weighing over 500 g or beyond twenty weeks' gestational duration. Beyond viability, the policy indicated abortion could occur only under exceptional circumstances.

The CMA positions acknowledge the health risks of abortion are lowest in early pregnancy, and so diagnosing pregnancy and determining the plan to manage the pregnancy (whether abortion or not) ought to occur as early as possible. While stating, "Induced abortion should be uniformly available to all women in Canada," the positions also include assertions that physicians cannot be compelled to participate in abortion and that physicians who do not provide abortion should not face discrimination. Furthermore, "the right of personal decision in this area must be stressed." This results in a conflict: how is abortion care to be uniformly available if individual physicians can pick and choose whether they will refer for it, let alone provide it? Why is the right of personal decision stressed over the safety of the patient who requires expedited care?

In a 2007 editorial in the *Canadian Medical Association Journal*, health law scholars Jocelyn Downie and Sanda Rodgers interpreted these policies to mean

> Physicians are not required to perform abortions (except in emergency circumstances); however, regardless of their personal beliefs, they should not prevent women from accessing abortion. Health care professionals who withhold a diagnosis, fail to provide appropriate referrals, delay access, misdirect

women or provide punitive treatment are committing malpractice and risk lawsuits and disciplinary proceedings. Physicians who prevent women from accessing abortion also breach the CMA's Code of Ethics, which prohibits discrimination on the basis of sex, marital status and medical condition. They also violate CMA policy and positions taken on abortion, including, for example, its positions taken on full and immediate counselling and access without delay.[23]

The CMAJ received a plethora of letters to the editor in sharp disagreement with this conclusion, prompting the editor, Jeff Blackmer, to subsequently publish a case example of a patient at seven weeks gestation who seeks a family physician's care for abortion. Appropriate conscientious objection, Blackmer explained, requires a physician to inform patients that they do not provide abortion services and will not provide a referral to another physician unless in an emergent scenario. The objecting physician may not impede the patient's right to obtain abortion care, and so, if asked by the patient, they must inform them as to how to obtain a referral.[24]

It is unclear how the "no delay" principle above could be accomplished without a physician providing immediate assistance with at least a referral. Conveniently, the patient in Blackmer's case was at seven weeks, and not 15.5 or beyond, when appropriately trained providers become fewer and farther between. Even the controversial compromise of simply offering a referral can be highly problematic in practice. What if the hospital is very short-staffed, as so many of them are in the post-COVID-19 era of protracted health human resource crisis, and the nurse asked to care for a patient booked for procedural abortion is the only nurse available, but she declines to provide care? What if the patient is eight weeks pregnant and the physician refers the patient to a colleague who usually prescribes mifepristone, but this month that colleague is on holiday? What if the pharmacist who will not stock mifepristone sends the patient to a pharmacy across the small town, but that pharmacy closed a half hour ago for the long weekend? What then?

The discourse that the decision to have an abortion "rests between a woman and her doctor" has reverberated for decades as a rallying cry to take abortion out of the courtroom or the legislature, to leave it to the halls of health services. Certainly, abortion is health care. But abortion is also more than health care, because without it, women and gender-diverse people face threats to participation in civil society — lack of abortion care access is a threat to democracy. Without it, women and gender-diverse people are subject to violence, poverty, and social subjugation. Placing access to abortion in the decision-making hands of physicians, when physicians can be so legitimately divested of responsibility to provide care, is troubling. Why does a physician decide if abortion is right? Even after the 1969 Omnibus Bill decriminalized abortion, it could only proceed with the approval of a therapeutic abortion committee (TAC), made up of physicians, and I have discussed the various reasons this was problematic in Chapter 2, "With Laws Come Limits." Physician authority over and participation in abortion is longstanding and taken for granted. In 2024, du Toit and Macleod[25] introduced the concept of "doctorability" to describe the required performance by abortion patients towards their abortion providers to present "their situation as worthy." The authors examined pre-abortion counselling conversations in South Africa, where abortion on demand is entirely legal in the first trimester.

In a review of the complexity of policies regarding physician conscientious objection, Downie, McLeod, and Shaw[26] found abundant variation that could cause confusion and result in differences in options and outcomes for patients, the costs faced by individuals and systems, interprofessional friction, and uncertainty about what services can be expected. Provincial/territorial health professional regulators refer to national documents like the CMA Code, and some supplement them with their own moral standards. Some affirm the need to provide referral, and some do not. Whether a patient can expect a timely referral depends on where they live. The Abortion Rights Coalition of Canada (ARCC), in their position paper entitled *The Refusal to Provide Health Care in Canada*, presents the example of the Yukon Medical Council's brief, *Moral or Religious Beliefs Affecting Medical Care*,[27] which requires the objecting physician to ensure their patient is offered timely access to another physician. By contrast, the College of Physicians and Surgeons of Nova Scotia's 2022 *Obligations for Services for Patients* asserts, "Physicians have the right to limit the health services they provide for legitimate reasons of conscience, religion, or scope of practice. When exercising this right, physicians must not discriminate against patients. The rights of patients are paramount, and their interests must prevail."[28] ARCC responds, "There is no such established right, and it is neither possible nor appropriate to determine whether someone's personal beliefs are "legitimate." [29]

In 2014, the *Ottawa Citizen* reported that a trio of Ontario family physicians based at the Care-Medics Medical Centre distributed a letter to patients extolling their right to refuse care based on freedom of conscience.[30] "[We] do not refer for vasectomies, abortions nor prescribe the morning after pill or any artificial contraception. If you are interested in the latter, please be aware that you may approach your own family doctor or request to be seen by another physician." The article included a quote from Planned Parenthood Ottawa encouraging patients needing contraception to call them instead. At the time, pre-mifepristone, abortion was only available as a procedure and often required a referral just to book an appointment. While not as bad ten years ago as in 2025, at the time of writing, the primary care provider shortage meant securing time with *any* family physician was challenging, let alone pursuing one after another in the hope of securing care.

Shortly thereafter, the College of Physicians and Surgeons of Ontario updated its policy[31] governing human rights in the provision of health care. From 2015 onward, it required doctors who object to providing care on religious grounds to make effective referrals to ensure patients receive timely care. Objectors took the College to court. Five individual physicians and the Christian Medical and Dental Society of Canada, the Canadian Federation of Catholic Physicians' Societies, and Canadian Physicians for Life[32] argued that the referral requirement violated Section 2 of the Canadian Charter of Rights and Freedoms, which protects freedom of religion, and Section 15, the so-called equality provision, which prohibits discrimination based on religion. It is worth noting that the Charter also prohibits discrimination based on sex.

The court ruled that while the policies do infringe on physician freedom of religion, that infringement is justified. Section 1 of the Charter[33] clarified, "The *Canadian Charter of Rights and Freedoms* guarantees the rights and freedoms set out in it subject only to such reasonable limits prescribed by law as can be demonstrably justified in a free and democratic society." In 2019, the Ontario Court of Appeal reiterated support for the referral requirement,[34] explaining that because of patient vulnerability and the time sensitivity of pregnancy care, the potential harm of a denied referral is significant. Patients should be able to trust their physicians to help them navigate the health system.

Institutions

What of providers with no personal objection to abortion who nonetheless find themselves working for institutions that claim conscientious objection to justify belief-based denial of care? This is a vexing problem in religious-affiliated hospitals across the country. The Charter protects *individual* freedom of religion, not institutional.

When new staff and physicians join St. Martha's Regional Hospital in Antigonish, Nova Scotia, they are reminded of their "legal obligation" to uphold the "Mission Agreement" in place at the facility, which requires the continuation of the "Catholic identity of the hospital." This Catholic identity would oppose participation in abortion, contraception, and MAiD, regardless of the moral or religious beliefs of practitioners working for the facility. Here, it is worth looking at some of the legislation around MAiD as it relates to belief-based denial of care and abortion.

First opened as a six-bed cottage hospital in 1906,[35] only ninety years later was ownership of St. Martha's Hospital transferred from the Sisters of St. Martha to what was then called the Eastern Regional Health Board. As a condition of this transition in leadership, the Health Board, the provincial Department of Health, and the Sisters signed a tripartite agreement, requiring the Catholic identity to be maintained. This agreement came under intense scrutiny in the late 2010s as a barrier to the provision of MAiD, first introduced into federal law in June 2016. Catholic opposition to suicide includes assistance with suicide.[36] "The Agreement" at St. Martha's would exclude the possibility of providing MAiD on site, even if it were legalized across Canada.

Canada's MAiD legislation is the product of many extraordinary women who pursued a series of legal battles. Unsuccessful in seeking an order from the BC court, Sue Rodriguez[37] was a forty-two-year-old mother living in British Columbia who had appealed to the Supreme Court of Canada in 1993 for the right to end her own life. Her case argued that Section 241b of the Canadian Criminal Code, the prohibition on assistance in suicide, violated Section 7 of the Canadian Charter of Rights and Freedoms, the right to life, liberty, and security of the person. Although there was agreement that the MAiD prohibition did impinge on Section 7 liberties, the justices ultimately applied Section 1 of the Charter to their ruling, which allows limitations on rights if such limitations are justified in a free and democratic society. They argued the blanket prohibition on MAiD was justified to "protect the vulnerable." Regardless of the ruling, Rodriguez sought the support of an unnamed physician and died in 1994.

The legal landscape did not shift again until 2012, when Gloria Taylor, supported by the BC Civil Liberties Association, looked to the British Columbia Supreme Court to determine that MAiD criminalization was unconstitutional. Justice Lynn Smith ruled that criminalizing physician assistance in suicide discriminates against people with disabilities who would require assistance to die by suicide, while able-bodied people might not require such assistance.[38] People with disabilities are protected from state discrimination under Section 15 of the Canadian Charter of Rights and Freedoms. At the time of the ruling, Justice Smith allowed lawmakers one year, until 2013, to make necessary changes. She granted Taylor, who also had amyotrophic lateral sclerosis (ALS), a progressive neurological disease, an exemption to allow her to seek MAiD care in the interim. However, Taylor died in October of 2012 from an infection.

A contemporary advocate of Taylor's, Kay Carter, who had spinal stenosis, travelled with her daughter, Lee Carter, to the Dignitas clinic in Switzerland in January 2010 for physician assistance in dying. Although she was the tenth Canadian to seek support in dying at the clinic, her death was the first to be publicly known.[39] The trip was planned in complete secrecy, for over six months, and cost the family over $35,000.

In 2015, Taylor and Carter's families joined together to sue the government of Canada for legally accessible MAiD in *Carter v. Canada* 2015.[40] This time, the justices agreed: the prohibition on assistance in suicide in Section 241b of the Criminal Code unjustifiably infringed on Section 7 Charter rights when the patient clearly consents to terminating their own life and has a "grievous and irremediable condition." MAiD legislation was introduced the next year.

Which brings us back to religious hospitals, the specific situation at St. Martha's, and "The Agreement" it had in place with the province and the regional health authority. In 2017, the government of Nova Scotia tried to excuse St. Martha's exceptionalism by insisting that not every health service is available at every publicly funded health facility. However, health law expert Dr. Jocelyn Downie[41] pointed out "there is no issue of "quality, safety, efficiency and efficacy" justifying non-provision of MAiD in any institution in Nova Scotia; "providers are willing to go to the institutions and they can bring the equipment and supplies that they need with them." Arguing "The Agreement" would never survive a challenge under principles of contract law, Downie suggested three possible solutions to St. Martha's predicament: (1) a refusal of MAiD would only be permissible if a patient could be transferred to another location without "undue harm or delay"; (2) the province could legislate a requirement that MAiD be available in all publicly funded sites (including St. Martha's); or (3) The Agreement could go unrenewed.

In 2019, St. Martha's agreed to a policy change along the line of Downie's first suggestion: MAiD is allowed in a building directly adjacent to the hospital, called the Antigonish Health and Wellness Centre.[42] A similar compromise was reached between the province of British Columbia and St. Paul's hospital in Vancouver: prospective MAiD patients are taken from the hospital itself to a "nearby" hospice. But that hospice is eleven kilometres down the road. In 2023, Sam O'Neill, a British Columbia woman diagnosed with stage 4 cervical cancer, had to make that "unnecessary and undignified" journey to receive end-of-life care. Her family is suing Providence Health Care, which operates St. Paul's, arguing that "[t]he transfer was not medically required or indicated, and was undertaken for the sole purpose of accommodating PHC's faith-based prohibition on providing MAiD where PHC provides medical services."[43]

Whether or not procedural sexual health services such as abortion, sterilization, and even long-acting reversible contraception insertion (intrauterine devices or contraceptive implants) should or could also be diverted to the Antigonish Health and Wellness Centre has yet to be disputed in court. There are St. Martha's physicians who quietly prescribe medication abortion and contraception, but this area of care remains shrouded in secrecy.

In recent years, abortion availability in faith-affiliated hospitals has come under increasing scrutiny. In May 2015, patient "C.V." was referred to a Mt. Sinai Hospital (MSH) obstetrician in downtown Toronto for fetal reduction, the practice of terminating one (or more) fetus(es) in a multiple pregnancy, such as from twins to a singleton. A fetal reduction is a different procedure than an abortion. Fetal reduction may be clinically indicated or a choice of the pregnant person. C.V. had used in vitro fertilization (IVF) and, like many IVF patients, chose to have more than one fertilized egg implanted to improve the likelihood of pregnancy success. Multiple pregnancies are, however, much more clinically complicated and carry higher risks of harm to both pregnant person and fetus. C.V.'s request for fetal reduction was refused, and she was told the policy at MSH is not to offer a reduction of twins to a singleton, except in the case of fetal anomaly, and that there were facilities in the US where this service was available. The "policy" was unwritten, although after C.V.'s case, a written policy was developed.

C.V. was not offered an alternative direct referral or even clear guiding information. C.V. then initiated an Ontario Human Rights Tribunal proceeding based on discrimination on the Section 15 grounds of family status/pregnancy. The Tribunal ruled against her, finding that Mt. Sinai's policy did not discriminate based on family status or pregnancy, but rather based on clinical criteria (number of fetuses): "A doctor is not required to perform a procedure that the doctor believes is not medically appropriate."[44] C.V. sought the procedure at Toronto's Sunnybrook Health Sciences Centre, effectively down the road from Mt. Sinai.[45]

What is now known as Mt. Sinai, a key teaching hospital in the biggest city in Canada, began in 1923 as the Hebrew Maternity and Convalescent Hospital, a thirty-bed facility created to meet the needs of Hebrew-speaking immigrants and to employ Jewish physicians other institutions refused to hire.[46] Similarly, the Sir Mortimer B. Davis Jewish General Hospital in Montreal opened in 1934 in response to an antisemitic protest across several of the city's hospitals over the Notre Dame Hospital hiring of Jewish physician Sam Rabinovitch.[47] Both Mt. Sinai (in collaboration with Toronto's Women's College Hospital) and the Jewish General Hospital now offer abortion into the second and third trimesters, however information about these services is hard to find and the most likely items to come up on a web search are published by anti-choice organizations.

As of 2022, there were 129 Catholic hospitals across Canada,[48] making up approximately 1 percent of the 1,280 hospitals in the country.[49] Notable examples include Covenant Health across Alberta, St. Paul's Hospital in Vancouver, and St. Michael's in Toronto. Several of these, however, are the only hospitals in town — as is the case for St. Martha's in Antigonish or St. Joseph's Hospital/Foyer d'Youville in Gravelbourg, Saskatchewan. In 2013, an Estevan, SK, woman's case made headlines when she was reportedly forced to travel to Regina, a two-hour drive, for termination of a non-viable pregnancy because St. Joseph's, the closest and only facility near to her home, refused.[50]

Faith-based institutions rely on the notion of religious freedom enshrined in the Charter of Rights and Freedoms, but those rights do not belong to buildings or institutions: they are *human* rights. Facilities cannot take a moral position. It is because of this that the Quebec government determined several hospitals across Montreal had to *share* responsibility for providing later gestational care; case by case, these services are distributed, with different hospitals responsible on a rotating basis. Furthermore, the religious orders that once funded many of these facilities are no longer the primary funder in any instance — the provinces/territories are. Policies or "agreements" to restrict care on religious grounds in public institutions would be difficult to defend on Charter grounds. In a small town, and taking account of the stigma that surrounds abortion, mounting a challenge is a tall order. In Antigonish, for example, the Sisters of St. Martha are a powerful philanthropic force. They donate to non-profit organizations in the area and provide significant gifts to St. Francis Xavier University (StFX).[51] Abortion seekers and health providers alike may be reluctant to challenge "The Agreement." That said, in 2018 during the early days of medication abortion implementation, StFX was the only university in Nova Scotia where the student health centre offered mifepristone prescriptions.[52] It is possible StFX was trying to fill the St. Martha's gap.

Prince Edward Island

Taking things to a macro level, for decades, the province of Prince Edward Island insisted it had a province-wide religious right to deny provision of abortion care. When the Catholic Charlottetown Hospital merged with the Prince Edward Island Hospital in 1982, renamed the Queen Elizabeth Hospital, the merger relied on an agreement that no abortions would take place inside. Then in 1988, when abortion was decriminalized federally, PEI premier Joe Ghiz put forward a resolution in rebellion, insisting that "[w]hereas the great majority of the people of PEI believe that life begins at conception … be it resolved that the Legislative Assembly of PEI oppose the performing of abortions."[53] Abortions would not be performed on the Island for thirty-five years, until a courageous and clever group of activists, under the banner of Abortion Access Now PEI (AANPEI) filed a lawsuit against the province with the help of Nijhawan McMillan Barristers in Halifax.[54] They argued the province-wide religious objection to abortion was a violation of

Charter Sections 7 (life, liberty, and security of the person), 12 (freedom from cruel and unusual punishment) and 15 (the equality provision). Under then-premier Wade MacLauchlan, PEI did not dispute their claim and promised to launch services. The Women's Wellness Program opened in January 2017 and continues to operate at the leading edge of family planning care, offering procedural and medication abortion, and is now called Sexual Health, Options and Reproductive Services (SHORS).[55]

Care Denial versus Concern about Competence

Many potential prescribers of mifepristone are not refusing to participate in prescribing out of moral objection, but rather out of concerns about competence. It is important to differentiate this from conscientious objection. A health professional who does something very infrequently, such as an IUD insertion, is necessarily less competent at the task compared to one who does it often. Most primary care providers in Canada likely did not learn about medication abortion in their preparatory training, and they do not know what is involved. Or they have never been asked by a patient for it, so they have never thought about what it would involve. Perhaps they worry if they only prescribe it a small number of times they will not know how to respond when, infrequently, things go wrong. Although medication abortion rarely results in adverse events, when it does, emergency room clinicians are most likely to encounter it. As a result, they may think the process is more complicated and riskier than the evidence suggests. Because they are not familiar with clinical developments and deregulation, they may be confused if prior ultrasound and serial blood work results were not ordered by the initial prescriber, even though these are not necessarily required under current guidelines.[56] There is considerable work to do to educate health professionals of all types about medication abortion.

With better teamwork and networking, abortion prescribing could be the domain of the people most interested in doing it. In Ontario, there are three pilot sites (Thunder Bay, Hamilton, and Toronto) where registered midwives lead provision of medication abortion, although the prescriptions they distribute are signed by family physicians. It is not that the family physicians are necessarily unwilling or unsupportive of medication abortion, it is that they recognize that normal pregnancy is the domain of their midwifery colleagues and termination is a routine outcome for normal pregnancies — it should be left to those who have expertise. In 2018, abortion prescribers across Nova Scotia united under a single toll-free number, 1-833-352-0719, so that patients anywhere in the province could self-refer and be connected to the closest health professional with the swiftest availability. These kinds of efforts to coordinate and expedite care, if promoted widely, can overcome the dangers posed by care denial, whether related to competence or moral belief, particularly in places with ambiguous regulations about requirements to refer. There are similar clearinghouse approaches in Ontario (the SHORE Centre/ChoiceConnect.ca) and BC (Options for Sexual Health). The issue, of course, is ensuring patients know about them. Legitimate health service providers face an uphill battle competing with well-funded and deftly marketed crisis pregnancy centres, whose main aim is to obscure care pathways.

* * *

Although provision of medication abortion in primary care has vastly expanded potential access, it may also expand the pool of providers who choose to deny care based on their religious beliefs. There is significant and confusing variation in regulation across Canada to limit the impact of belief-based denial of care. Not only individuals, who may argue they have Charter rights to religious freedom, but institutions, which have no such constitutional rights, impede access to services. Effective referral is ethically and clinically essential to ensure abortion seekers receive required care.

CHAPTER 6

CRISIS PREGNANCY CENTRES

> This chapter introduces crisis pregnancy centres, which are non-clinical, anti-abortion operations run by religious organizations, and describes efforts to minimize the potential harm they pose to abortion seekers.

A perennial problem in the abortion movement, particularly when headway is being made, is public relations (PR) — or rather, the lack of it. Advocacy against something bad is generally more publicly compelling and newsworthy than advocacy to promote something good; protests may make headlines, but straightforward communication about improvements in receiving care likely will not. These deficits in positive PR mean the narrative of abortion care is vulnerable to persistent and well-funded rhetoric from anti-abortionists, particularly promotion of crisis pregnancy centre (CPC) services. There are over 150 CPCs in Canada,[1] far outweighing the number of actual abortion clinics across the country.[2] CPCs are not really clinics at all, but rather serve as storefronts for religious campaigns against abortion.

Often referred to as "fake clinics," CPCs are Christian ministries devoted to steering might-be patients who are "pregnant and concerned" away from abortion. They respond to the "crisis" of unintended pregnancy by offering free pregnancy tests, "counselling," and sometimes even ultrasound. "Counselling" is in quotations, as the counsellors are not required to be credentialed as social workers or psychologists. The ultrasound, too, while presented as a medical treatment, may not be conducted by a licensed technician. The goal of offering ultrasound is simply "to get the individual to hear the 'fetal heartbeat,' which early in the pregnancy is the result of pulsating cells firing electrical signals within an embryo and not an actual heartbeat."[3] The sound of those signals can then be manipulated in discussions with the abortion seeker.

Advertising

CPCs advertise heavily, targeting youth and lower-income members of the public, focusing marketing efforts on public transit, in bus shelters, and more recently, online. Although they do not offer abortion services, they are often the first hit when a person seeking care Googles "abortion + name of province." In a vacuum of information about actual abortion services, these ads confuse and misdirect patients and providers alike.

Because of their deployment of skilful marketing techniques and abundant ads, a CPC may be more publicly known than a real abortion health service. Prominent abortion activists in Canada have most often been clinicians, lawyers, frontline workers, and academics — professionals who rarely bring PR expertise to the table. Furthermore, the costs of providing care trump costs of advertising. Family practice clinics, community organizations, and hospitals rarely need to promote services because, overwhelmingly, demand for medically necessary care is generated by patients themselves. Most health care does not require messaging to convince prospective patients that it exists and is allowed. Improvements in reproductive health care may go underappreciated, in large part because of failure to spread the word.

One of the greatest gains in abortion care over the past decade was implementation of the drug mifepristone. In Canada, promotion of drugs is prudently restricted. As a public safety measure, the 1985 Canadian Food and Drugs Act[4] prohibited direct-to-consumer advertising (DTCA) of prescription drugs. Enforcement of the Act falls to Health Canada. As Gardner, Mintzes, and Ostry[5] explain, in 1996, Health Canada relaxed interpretation of the Act, recognizing "the importance to the pharmaceutical industry and to the general public of being able to disseminate and access nonpromotional information regarding drugs for human use." This resulted in tacit approval of so-called "help-seeking" and "reminder" ads that do not explicitly explain what a drug is for but suggest you ask a health care provider about it. Indirect, subtle ads are crafted to squeak through the help-seeking/reminder loophole, like the beaming, suddenly zippy actors appearing on screen in full sun and smiles with Pfizer's blue-pill symbol then filling the screen. Everyone knows this is promoting Viagra. Prior to releasing help-seeking/reminder non-ad types of ads, drug manufacturers are supposed to submit their suggested content to the Pharmaceutical Advertising Advisory Board (PAAB) and Ad Standards Canada (ASC) for approval. Although complaints about ad content veracity can be made to

ASC, complaints about violations of the Food and Drugs Act are handled by Health Canada. This process is not fast or cheap. A company would have to anticipate significant value to going down this road.

Pharmaceutical manufacturers would be more interested in pursuing ad approval if they anticipated it would yield high consumption of their product and a strong return on their investment. Abortion pills are simply not, relatively speaking, frequently used. So, while Viagra ads long ago entered the zeitgeist, in the nine years since its approval, no one has seen a "non-ad" for Mifegymiso (the brand name for the mifepristone and misoprostol regimen for medication abortion). Absent industry or health-system-supported information about abortion in advertising spaces, whether it be print, online, or TV/radio, CPCs find space for their messages.

Charitable Status

CPCs pass themselves off as generously offering care and options, but most are staffed entirely by non-clinicians. CPCs espouse deeply anti-abortion mandates, and their materials[6] often exaggerate and falsify the risks of abortion while simultaneously failing to acknowledge the very real physical and emotional harms of continuing an unintended pregnancy, such as entrapment in violent relationships, poverty, and exposure to pregnancy complications.

Usually associated with churches and religious groups, CPCs seek and receive charitable status to boost their fundraising success. Charities can offer donors tax receipts, powerfully incentivizing donations. In Canada, registered charities must use their resources for activities and purposes that can be characterized as the relief of poverty, the advancement of education, the advancement of religion, or other purposes that benefit the community.[7] Advancing religion is a legitimate purpose for charitable status; however, most CPCs receive charitable status for "relief of poverty" work, such as distributing free diapers.[8] Largely run by volunteers and not providing actual health care, CPCs can use the ample funds generated through charitable fundraising to advertise heavily.

The question of whether a legitimate abortion clinic could qualify as a charity came under dispute on the heels of the *R. v. Morgentaler* decision in 1988, when the newly incorporated Everywoman's Health Centre[9] in Vancouver applied for charitable status. They described their services as falling under the fourth principle of the Charities Registration Act,[10] providing "other purposes that benefit the community." At the time, with abortion newly decriminalized, the Vancouver General Hospital was providing one hundred abortions a week and it was not meeting demand. Further, the hospital placed all patients under general anesthetic, did not provide counselling, and did not accept self-referrals. Everywoman's was filling an important gap in care. Although physician services at Everywoman's were funded publicly, according to the Canada Health Act and through BC provincial health insurance, other costs associated with delivery of care were approximately $150 to $250 at the time. Patients came from across BC, Alberta, and the Yukon, and a reported 15 percent were completely unable to pay these additional expenses. Private donations were essential support for the clinic's work. Everywoman's first application was denied, with the minister of national revenue explaining, "absent clear statements of public policy and absent public consensus on the abortion issue, it cannot be said that the (appellant)'s activities are beneficial to the community in a way the law regards as charitable."[11] Canada's lawlessness around abortion care was being used as a lever to refuse them charitable status.

The clinic appealed. The court determined that while a charity cannot act *against* public policy, it should not be thought to be opposing a policy when there is no policy to oppose. Further, hospitals providing "care for the sick" were providing "other benefit to the community." In the appeal, the minister's lawyers tried to argue that the abortion clinic was not equivalent in intention to a hospital, because pregnancy is not a "sickness." The court did not accept that argument. Everywoman's was registered as a charity. There are still some elements of care that may require out-of-pocket payment[12] by patients who do not have BC Medical Services Plan and private drug coverage, such as additional medications (not the mifepristone/misoprostol itself) and blood draws.

Reproductive Justice

Although they now exist all over the world, it was a Canadian who created the first CPC: "Birthright" was forged in 1968 by Louise Summerhill, in Toronto.[13] The organization continues to thrive today,[14] with over 500 branches across Canada, the US, and Africa. Summerhill, a Catholic, had seven children and sought to support women who, she believed, would feel better able to accept an unplanned pregnancy if provided with encouragement and companionship. The mission statement of

Birthright is "To offer friendship, love, and support during a time they may feel overwhelming and stressful. We offer hope and reassurance that an unexpected pregnancy does not have to be faced alone."[15] Birthright operates through volunteerism, providing "counselling" in various forms, and often providing free basic resources such as diapers, baby clothes, and furniture.[16] Summerhill believed "it is the right of every pregnant woman to give birth and the right of every child to be born."[17]

In contrast, reproductive justice theory captures not only the right to *not* have children, but the right to have children and parent them in safety.[18] It recognizes the social, political, and economic forces that keep people from being able to have kids they want to have and to raise them free from oppression and environmental degradation. It could be argued that Summerhill, an experienced mother of seven, was responding to the social discrimination, poverty, and violence that she believed prevented people from being able to have and raise their children. It's possible she saw the complexity beyond the dogma of "choice." But unlike reproductive justice action, Summerhill, and Birthright, focused on the individual's circumstances and adjusting her perceptions, not on shifting structural determinants of well-being.

The timing of Summerhill's founding of Birthright in 1968 coincided with intensifying reproductive rights discourse surrounding the federal Omnibus Bill, which would reform the Criminal Code to partially decriminalize abortion and completely decriminalize contraception in 1969. In 1968, the McGill Students Society's Birth Control Committee published the *Birth Control Handbook*, with detailed illustrations and instructions about contraception and abortion. Technically an illegal publication at the time, the handbook "exploded" in popularity, with millions of copies distributed, including in universities' official student registration packages.[19] Birthright was a strong force of resistance against this type of progress in family planning. Then the *Roe v. Wade* US Supreme Court Decision of 1973 escalated interest in anti-abortion crisis pregnancy response in that country, swiftly spreading Birthright's reach southwards. Summerhill's three daughters all went on to serve as co-presidents of the organization.[20]

Deceptive Tactics

Describing Birthright services in 1974, Catholic physician and member Dr. Eugene Diamond explained the organization's strategic approach to promotion and its position on abortion:

> The advertisement usually says merely, "Pregnant? Need Help? Call (telephone number)." Since the message is ambiguous, some persons call expecting to receive help in obtaining an abortion. To make an abortion referral would constitute formal cooperation in the clearly immoral abortion act and would, therefore, itself be immoral. The charter of the Birthright International organization specifically prohibits any and every referral for abortion no matter what the indication.[21]

Furthermore, he explains, "Birthright agencies do not become involved in birth-control counseling because they deal with women already pregnant and because birth control counseling really requires the individual attention of a competent private physician."[22]

Although Birthright describes itself as "non-political," barring support seekers from even hearing about abortion is a deeply political act that undermines reproductive autonomy. Many CPCs deliberately use language about abortion on their websites and promotional materials to strengthen the ruse. Thomsen and Morrison summarize CPC operative politics:

> They deploy a range of deceptive tactics, including opening crisis pregnancy centers near abortion clinics with the intention of confusing, and thus intercepting, those seeking abortion; obscuring their political and religious ideologies; implying that they offer abortions when they do not; and spreading false information regarding abortion, claiming incorrectly, for example, that abortion leads to breast cancer, mental health problems, and infertility.[23]

Politics is about power, and these deceptive and manipulative activities exert power over pregnant people and impact public health.

As but one example of proximal location to inspire confusion, in New Brunswick, Fredericton's Right to Life organization headquartered itself as the "Women's Care Center"[24] (note the American spelling), at 562 Brunswick St. This is next door to the Morgentaler Clinic at 554 Brunswick Street, which became known as Clinic 554 after Dr. Morgentaler's death; under both names, there has never been prominent signage indicating abortions took place therein. As a result, patients, often arriving from out of town, might be very confused by the clear

"Women's Care Center" sign on one building and the absence of a large sign on the next.

The original Women's Care Center building burnt down in July 2016. In 2017, Fredericton's City Council Planning and Development Committee authorized a rebuild, despite the architectural plans falling below the municipality's ten-metre height minimum for the commercial area.[25] The Women's Care Center reopened in 2018,[26] and while Clinic 554 permanently closed in January 2024,[27] the Women's Care Center remains open.[28]

CPCs have become increasingly stealthy. They absorb the language from the reproductive rights movement, promising "choices" and "options," and sometimes they even replicate the fonts, logos, and names of actual clinics. But once inside, abortion seekers may be questioned, shamed, and misinformed, ultimately delaying the process of obtaining care, potentially pushing the patient beyond the gestational window possible in their jurisdiction and requiring them to pursue the expense and burden of travel for care.

CPCs work *together* in a complex network. Pregnancy Care Canada,[29] the largest group of CPCs in the country, includes seventy-seven offices. Care Net,[30] an evangelical CPC conglomerate, boasts 1,100 affiliates around the world. Heartbeat International[31] has 3,000. An online scan of Care Net's Canadian affiliates include the Pregnancy Resource Center of Saint John and the Pregnancy and Wellness Center of Moncton, in New Brunswick; the Valley Care Pregnancy Centre and Tri-County Pregnancy Care Centre in Nova Scotia; dozens across Ontario; the Family Support Centre of Winnipeg and the Prairie Pregnancy Support Centre in Manitoba; the Options Pregnancy Centre in Regina, Saskatchewan; eight facilities in Alberta; and over a dozen in British Columbia. The ambiguous language they use makes it difficult for abortion seekers to differentiate actual clinics from fake.

In its FAQs, the Family Support Centre in Winnipeg responds to the question "Where can I find an abortion clinic?" with

> Just like there are hospitals throughout the city, there are places you can go to get an abortion. However, because this is one of the biggest decisions you'll ever make, we suggest that you spend some time talking to people you can trust about it … and doing lots of your own online research. Whatever you decide we'd be very happy to talk with you about it.[32]

They then suggest reading their disclaimer on a separate webpage, which explains, "It is important that you understand that we are not a professional counselling agency," and "Because the Family Support Centre is not a medical facility we do not provide for nor arrange any medical treatments."[33]

This disclaimer is notable. A 2023 study by Joyce Arthur,[34] executive director of the Abortion Rights Coalition of Canada (ARCC), and colleagues examined the content on CPC websites to identify deception and important omissions. They identified 146 CPCs across the country, 134 (94 percent) of which had charitable status. ARCC regularly updates a publicly accessible document listing CPCs and anti-choice organizations in Canada.[35] In an analysis of the content of 110 associated CPC websites, the author team found that fifty-five (39 percent) lacked any disclaimer that they do not provide or assist with arranging abortion, and sixty-one (43 percent) failed to clarify they were not actually a clinic. Furthermore, many CPCs provided misinformation about the risks of abortion, which, as earlier chapters have explored, is very safe, especially in comparison to continued unintended pregnancy.[36] Arthur et al.[37] found eight websites (6 percent) that linked abortion to elevated risk of breast cancer (unfounded); twenty-seven (19 percent) suggested additional health risks associated with abortion that are not scientifically supported; and 108 (76 percent) claimed abortion caused psychological harm, namely "postabortion distress," which is not a clinically recognized disorder. Finally, two websites (1 percent) suggested "abortion pill reversal" was possible. It absolutely is not.[38]

The Care Net and Heartbeat networks worked together to establish the Option Line, a 24/7, English-Spanish bilingual counselling "ministry" service available worldwide, constantly accessible to abortion seekers searching online about what to do. Heartbeat and Care Net help guide affiliates through the process of adding licensed medical services to their offices; indeed, anti-abortion medical doctors and nurses may volunteer or work for CPCs, lending credibility and expanding service range from a "centre" into a "clinic." Heartbeat International[39] hosts an "academy" for prospective CPC leaders to learn the ropes. It offers webpage support to teach affiliates how to accelerate traffic, and the organization will leverage big data for branches "on critical metrics to provide powerful, actionable insights at the local level." Theirs are sophisticated and expansive organizations.

Barriers to Access are Barriers to Justice

When abortion providers fail to promote their services, when public/political narratives about access are confusing, and conversations about abortion are stigmatizing[40] or secretive, the result is a serious and profound barrier to access. Abortion seekers are left very alone to navigate a health system that can be confusing at the best of times; for less socially acceptable needs, it can be dire. That is where CPCs step in, seemingly benevolent shepherds of the unknown world of pregnancy management. But rather than shepherd, they gatekeep. A 2021 survey in the US of over 850 abortion seekers found that 13 percent had visited a confirmed CPC,[41] and those who visited a CPC were twice as likely to still be pregnant and still be seeking abortion when researchers followed up four weeks later. These findings suggest CPCs can drive delays in care, which may ultimately result in denial of care as patients "age out" of the gestational capacities of clinics in their geographic area.

Thomson and Morrison[42] make note of the comparatively minor attention that reproductive justice scholars have paid CPCs, given the vast investment the anti-abortion lobby makes in their proliferation. They point out that the canonical text for reproductive justice, *Reproductive Justice: An Introduction*, by Loretta J. Ross and Rickie Solinger (2017), barely mentions CPCs. Noting the steady climb in the numbers of CPCs across Canada over the prior thirty-five-year period, Haiqi Li[43] interviewed abortion activists in Canada about their comparatively low attention to CPCs versus policies to expand abortion access. The activists shared beliefs that the liberal context in Canada weakened the threat CPCs could pose, in comparison to the US, and were therefore less of a focus for their activity.

In a unique study, sociology graduate student Sarah Rudrum[44] investigated student experiences with an on-campus CPC in Wolfville, NS — Acadia Pregnancy Support (APS). In 2014, APS gained student club status at Acadia University and secured a space to operate but lost both in 2018 after the club's practices were found to be noncompliant with the student union bylaws. Rudrum chronicled those practices, explaining that because of APS's abundant advertising across campus and the fact that the ads did not include any information about religious affiliation or positions, research participants felt comfortable contacting APS for help. Having the university name, "Acadia," in the group's name increased perceptions of legitimacy and led participants to believe APS was formally affiliated with the university.[45]

Manufactured legitimacy is CPC's main currency. They use language like "women" and "options" and "pregnancy," which sounds legitimately supportive of reproductive health; they repeat medical claims that, though completely false, are said often enough to gain validity; and they offer medicalized activities, from pregnancy testing to "counselling" or even ultrasonography that are indistinguishable to the client from clinical services from trained, regulated professionals. Despite the deception in CPC tactics, they are unregulated in Canada.

Deplatforming Strategies

One of the strategies for deplatforming CPCs is to demand the revocation of their charitable status. In 1984, an anti-choice organization named Human Life International[46] registered as a charity, with a mandate to "(i) to promote the social welfare and defend the human rights of persons born and unborn; (ii) to promote, and to assist the promotion of, natural methods of child creation; and (iii) to educate and assist the education of persons in their obligation to respect and protect human life." HLI was audited twice, in 1989 and 1993, to determine if their activities could be considered "advancement of education." The minister of national revenue determined HLI's intentions were largely to sway public opinion on a controversial issue and revoked its charitable status. Although HLI appealed, the appeal was dismissed, with the judges describing that HLI's "literature appeared to be predominantly of a tendentious or polemical character that one would not normally associate with the formal training of the mind." A year later, in 1999, another anti-choice organization, Alliance for Life,[47] also lost its charitable status after an audit of activities.

Advocates leaned in to the 2016 branding of the Canadian federal Liberals as a "feminist party" to advance a host of sexual and reproductive health goals, including political pressure against CPCs.[48] In 2018, as a result of substantial media attention to government funding of CPCs, the Justin Trudeau federal government started requiring applicant organizations to the Canada Summer Jobs program to sign an attestation of support for Canadian constitutional rights and the right to reproductive choice.[49] This tactic aimed to weed out anti-abortion organizations as well as those with homophobic and transphobic philosophies. The Canada Summer Jobs program funds minimum-wage summer positions for students and youth under thirty.

The 2021 Liberal election platform[50] claimed that, if elected, the federal government would no longer provide charitable status to CPCs, acknowledging that CPCs conduct dishonest counselling. The Canada Revenue Agency Act requires charities operating to advance a health purpose must "generally show that each health care service or product it provides effectively prevents or relieves a physical or mental health condition and meets applicable quality and safety requirements."[51] The misleading practices of CPCs would not. In October 2024, Prime Minister Trudeau announced legislation that would require CPCs to disclose on all their public facing materials whether they provide abortion support, or they would risk losing charitable status.[52]

Another approach is to simply seek to ban CPC ads, to prevent the "noise" of this marketing from confusing abortion seekers. In 2012, a University of California–San Francisco student group named End Fake Clinics ran a successful campaign to have the university ban fake advertising by CPCs on campus property.[53] The group's Facebook page was last active in 2014,[54] and the group reportedly disbanded that year as most members graduated.[55] The ban continues. Canadian efforts to remove public anti-abortion advertising will be discussed in Chapter 7, "Freedom of Expression and Assembly."

Cognizant of the consequences of little positive and genuine promotion of abortion services, a new Canadian campaign, missINFORMED,[56] deploys youthful social media skills to tackle information vacuums about abortion access. Action Canada for Sexual Health and Rights,[57] Canada's foremost nongovernmental leader in sexual and reproductive health information and advocacy, is another skilful agent of abortion promotion, creating Instagram memes. But these efforts are piecemeal, dependent on the graphic design and tech skills of a few employees or volunteers and subject to the whims of grant funding.

Continuous Support Services

CPCs might become less relevant if only their advertising were less voluminous in comparison to public information about abortion and if the "softer" services they claim to offer were available legitimately. When the formal health system fails to meet patients' needs, they are more likely to seek and encounter CPCs and fall victim to their practices. For example, if a prescriber fails to comprehensively explain the experience of medication abortion, and a patient gets home that evening with their pills, feels unsure, and the only person to answer their calls is a volunteer at a CPC, they may end up coerced out of their decision or filled with shame. This could be prevented through continuous access to support from the health system. For example, the staff nurses at SHORS PEI (Sexual Health, Options and Reproductive Services,[58] the full-service abortion clinic on the island), rotate through a 24/7 call schedule, ensuring one is always available to respond to patient questions and concerns. Although 95 percent of patients report relief[59] as their dominant feeling after their abortion experiences, that does not mean they would not appreciate post-abortion support. Although abortion is a *right*, it does not mean that it should not be provided without tenderness.

CPCs also often target "fathers" of pregnancies. For example, Ohio's "Pathway to Hope"[60] pregnancy centre website has a tab labelled "For the Guys," a fathers' one-on-one coaching service.[61] By contrast, when a support person calls an abortion clinic, be they an intimate partner, friend, or parent, they are usually told that the patient themselves must call to seek information and book services. This approach aims to ensure patient autonomy and non-coercion, critical principles of abortion care. But as a result, people trying to support abortion seekers find minimal support for themselves and their questions within the formal health system.

Abortion doulas have emerged as an alternative source of support to compensate for limited support resources available from abortion clinics and providers/prescribers.[62] The doula role is non-clinical; there is no specific, singular training program or certification process, and licences or registration with a regulatory body are not required to practice. In that way, the doula is similar to the CPC volunteer. A 2023 qualitative study among abortion doulas across Canada[63] identified about seventy doulas with public profiles online indicating their participation in abortion doula work.[64] Of those seventy, fifteen agreed to interviews. They indicated that in addition to driving patients to and from services, a dominant part of their work is offering support for abortion seekers who feel abandoned emotionally by clinicians once the physical concern of becoming unpregnant is accomplished. Culturally appropriate abortion doulas may be particularly helpful for abortion seekers from underserved groups, including those who are Black, Indigenous, and people of colour, and those from 2SLGBTQIA+ communities, to navigate systemically exclusionary health care spaces. For security reasons, most clinics do not allow companions inside; therefore, abortion clinic connections with community doulas may be minimal. Familiar with the fraudulent tactics of CPCs, clinic staff may be reluctant to engage non-registered, non-clinical support people. Further, the ethics of downloading valuable support functions on to abortion doulas, who are largely unpaid, is fraught. To resist the influence of CPCs, as well as improving PR, abortion professionals in the formal health system may need to enhance gentle aspects of care.

The enduring popularity of CPCs speaks to the sheer heft of unintended pregnancy in Canada, along with the persistent need among patients for support in navigating their management. A 2020 survey of 3,300 women in Canada found that of those who had ever been pregnant, over 60 percent of the pregnancies were unintended. Of these, 43 percent went on to complete the pregnancy, 15 percent miscarried, 33 percent had an abortion, and 2 percent opted for adoption services.[65] In Canada, over 180,000 unintended pregnancies occur every year, resulting in direct costs of $320 million.[66] A large Calgary study compared women with unintended pregnancies to those intending to become pregnant and found women with unintended pregnancies were significantly younger, less educated, had a lower household income, were less likely to be in a stable relationship, and less likely to speak English in the home. Further, a fifth did not use contraception, despite not intending to become pregnant.[67] National headway towards enhancing access will be discussed in Chapter 10, "Contraception." Improving prevention of unintended pregnancies is an important strategy to reduce the power and influence of CPCs.

* * *

Despite substantial improvements in access since decriminalization, the abortion movement continues to struggle to get the word out about what abortion is and how to get one. Well-funded and adept at public relations, crisis pregnancy centres (CPCs) can mislead and misdirect abortion seekers, delaying care. Without ample and effective public promotion of legitimate abortion care, CPCs flourish. Mechanisms such as legal restrictions on CPC registration as charities could limit the harm.

CHAPTER 7

FREEDOM OF EXPRESSION AND ASSEMBLY

> This chapter discusses the Charter rights to freedom of expression and assembly and to what extent these rights protect anti-abortion protestors.

The subterfuge of fake care presented by crisis pregnancy centres is but one robust manifestation of anti-abortion activity in Canada; other highly visible forms are the direct action of protest and the publication and promotion of anti-abortion materials. Section 2 of the Canadian Charter of Rights and Freedoms[1] protects the right to freedom of expression, to freedom of conscience and religion, and to peaceful assembly; Section 1 allows rights protected under the rest of the Charter to be reasonably limited if the limits are justified in a free and democratic society. Many of the disputes regarding Charter rights of members of the anti-abortion movement are situated on university campuses and pertain to anti-abortion student group conduct. Others relate to "protests" at the sites of abortion care and the homes of abortion providers that serve to threaten, harass, and intimidate patients and health professionals. The legal disputes over these actions demonstrate other forms of law relevant to abortion regulation and operation in Canada.

University Disputes

The extent to which universities in Canada are "under government control" is relevant to regulation of freedom of expression and assembly on campus, as the Charter applies only to government actions and policies, not those made by private institutions or individuals. How this has been interpreted has differed from province to province.

For example, in one prominent anti-abortion student group case, *Lobo v. Carleton University*,[2] the Ontario court determined that the Charter did not apply on the university campus. It started in 2010, when the now-defunct student group Carleton Lifeline, despite being denied permission to do so by university administrators, set up what they called a "Genocide Awareness Project" (GAP) exhibit in a busy outdoor area on the Carleton University campus in Ottawa.[3] Making deeply offensive connections between abortion and the Holocaust is a recurrent tactic of anti-abortion extremists.[4]

In response to the anti-abortion exhibit, administrators called police to campus, who then arrested four student members of Carleton Lifeline, charging them with trespassing. Although the charges were later dropped, two students subsequently sued the university for breaches of their Charter rights as defined in Sections 2, 9, and 15. Section 2, "fundamental freedoms," stipulates the right to freedom of conscience and religion; of thought, belief, opinion, and expression; of peaceful assembly; and of association. Section 9 stipulates that everyone has a right not to be arbitrarily detained or imprisoned; and Section 15, the equality provision, affirms the right to freedom from discrimination based on race, national or ethnic origin, colour, religion, sex, age, or mental or physical disability. In *Lobo*, the Ontario court determined that the Charter did not apply on the university campus because Carleton University was not applying a specific governmental program or policy when it sought to prevent the demonstration. The students' suit was dismissed. The Carleton University Students' Association decertified Carleton Lifeline,[5] and it lost its student group status in 2010.

In a subsequent case in Alberta, the courts determined the Charter did apply and students had the right to free assembly. The case, *Wilson v. the University of Calgary*,[6] also pertained to a GAP demonstration. For several years beforehand, the Campus Pro-Life (CPL) group had erected their display in MacEwan Hall, a high-traffic building on campus. The university put up their own signs leading to the display, stating, "The exhibit's images are extremely graphic and may be offensive to some" and that "the exhibit is protected under the relevant section of the Charter of Rights and Freedoms related to Freedom of Expression." Then in 2007, a pro-choice group of students started their own counter-protest, setting up barriers to block visibility of the GAP content. CPL objected, arguing this counter-protest could lead to physical confrontation, and asked for the university to determine a better way forward. The university suggested that in the future, CPL set up their images facing inward.

When CPL launched their 2010 campaign, they disobeyed this directive, and the signs continued to be positioned to maximize visibility. Campus security was called and asked CPL to leave the premises. The students refused. These CPL members were found by UC's academic vice-provost to have violated UC's Non-Academic Misconduct Policy by failing to comply with the direction of campus security, and they received a written warning. The students sought an appeal of the decision through the university's own process, which was denied. They then took their complaint to the Alberta court, arguing they were discriminated against. The court determined the university *should* have considered the Charter implications and allowed the students to appeal. However, by the time this decision was determined, in 2014, the affected students had all graduated. Furthermore, CPL had continued to regularly mount the GAP display on campus during the legal proceedings.

The University of Alberta and UAlberta Pro-Life (UAPL)[7] experienced a similar pattern and resulted in an affirmation of Charter rights on campus. In 2015, when UAPL mounted an exhibit of graphic anti-abortion images in the quad, a counter-protest was organized. UAPL complained that the counter-protestors were violating the university's student code. U of Alberta did not pursue the complaint. But the subsequent year, when UAPL sought to hold their demonstration again, the university charged the group $17,500 for part of the campus security costs, an unusual demand of a student group and one that would be prohibitively costly. UAPL appealed the fee and the dismissal of their code of conduct complaint, taking their case all the way to the Alberta Court of Appeal. Although the Court of Appeal dismissed the complaint, it ruled that university's regulation of anti-abortion student expression constituted a responsibility given to the university by the government, and it was therefore a government action subject to the Charter. The court reached that conclusion because it considered key purposes of university education to be teaching through free expression and fostering student debate, and not only does the university receive significant public funding but it is physically designed as "community space."

Whether universities can restrict freedom of expression remains murky. In spring 2024, during graduation preparations and celebrations, encampments sprung up on campus lawns across Canada to protest the genocide in Palestine and university complicity through financial and academic ties to Israel.[8] Both the University of Alberta and the University of Calgary brought in police forces to violently dismantle the camps that had formed in each location. Videos show police swinging batons and using tear gas, flash-bangs, and rubber bullets. Legal scholars have been quick to cite the UAlberta Pro-Life decision as evidence that the removal of the encampments constitutes serious and mass violations of Charter rights.[9] In Quebec, the court refused to grant McGill University an injunction to allow them to remove the anti-genocide encampment on its campus.[10] McGill hired a private security firm to demolish the site instead.[11] The court in Ontario did grant such an injunction to University of Toronto.[12] By summer 2024, most encampments had been disassembled and cleared away. In the last week of July, Dalhousie University in Halifax shut down entirely, even closing children's camps, while it removed the Students for the Liberation of Palestine's camp on campus, named Al Zeitoun University.[13] One potential lesson from these restrictions on anti-genocide activism is that efforts to ban anti-abortion material/action on campus may harm the reproductive justice movement more than it helps, when such actions can be leveraged against progressive protest.

Freedom of Expression and Offensive Images

While the promotional efforts of anti-choice organizations may cost them charitable status, as discussed in Chapter 6, "Crisis Pregnancy Centres," they may also prompt disputes about freedom of expression. In 2015, the Canadian Centre for Bioethical Reform (CCBR)[14] — not a registered charity — sought to mount an advertising campaign on buses in several Canadian cities. The ad depicted fetuses at seven weeks and sixteen weeks, along with the words "Abortion Kills Children" in all caps. The city transit authority in Grande Prairie, Alberta, refused to run the ad, arguing that buses are taxpayer funded and the general public would be disturbed by the ads. Further, the city had a policy in place that all ads abide by the Advertising Standards Canada's Canadian Code of Advertising Standards (the Code).[15] As described in the Chapter 2, "With Laws Come Limits," discussion of the "We Need a Law" billboard campaign, the Code requires ads be accurate and Section 14 of the Code outlines "unacceptable depictions or portrayals." Ads that "demean, denigrate or disparage any identifiable person, group of persons, firm, organization, industrial or commercial activity, profession, product or service or attempt to bring it or them into public contempt or ridicule" are unacceptable. CCBR's ads appeared to be in violation. CCBR took the city to court, insisting Grande Prairie had violated Section 2 Charter rights to freedom of expression by refusing the ad campaign. The city countered that its refusal was reasonable, that the ad constituted hate speech against women who had had an abortion and was psychologically damaging. Justice Anderson noted that the Charter right to freedom of expression is not absolute, and "as a society, we routinely restrict the audience for certain types of expression"[16] such as movies that are rated for ages eighteen and above. Further, she found the CCBR's intention was to vilify women who have had an abortion. The suit was dismissed. CCBR appealed, only to lose the appeal as well.

Peterborough, Ontario, also refused to run the same ad, although it did not have a policy in place backing its decision. When CCBR threatened to take the city to court, it gave up and allowed the campaign to run. Wanting to further strengthen its position, CCBR took the city to court anyway, seeking a court order affirming the decision to run the ad. The city did not even appear at the hearing. Judge Kent referred to the images as depicting "pre-born babies" and described CCBR as "a non-profit corporation which functions as a pro-life educational organization. It attempts to inform the public about its views of fetal development and abortion by providing literature, visual displays and oral presentations."[17] He concluded "with little difficulty" that the city's initial refusal of the ads "was not reasonable" and "interfered with the Applicant's freedom of expression" but stopped short of issuing a declaration that constitutional rights had been violated. He did issue a court order to double down on the requirement that CCBR's ad be published. The Abortion Rights Coalition of Canada (ARCC) critiqued Peterborough's capitulation as prioritizing money over ethics and putting other cities as risk by creating a dangerous precedent. ARCC concluded that "the City bears responsibility for this situation, so it must also bear the consequences of any negative effects of the ad, including reduced transit ridership and public trust."[18] Whether Peterborough showing up at the hearing would have changed the outcome is suspect, but it is clear that CCBR is willing to escalate natters to seek court orders solidifying their Charter rights. Even proactive municipal policies against these types of ads could meet a Charter challenge.

The transit authority in Greater Vancouver, TransLink, also refused the CCBR campaign, again determining that it violated the Code. In CCBR's suit against TransLink, the court determined inadequate consideration had been taken with respect to CCBR's rights to freedom of expression. The court effectively sent the decision back to the table; if TransLink was to refuse the ads, a stronger case had to be made that considered potential Charter violations, not only an advertising code.

In 2017, the Lethbridge and District Pro-Life Association (DPLA) in Alberta[19] presented a new anti-abortion ad campaign to be placed on city buses and bus shelters. Lethbridge had a pre-existing agreement with Pattison Outdoor Advertising[20] to maintain ad space for the city, requiring the company to first determine that ads be of "moral and reputable character" and in compliance with the Code. The campaign in question depicted a fetus and the words "Unborn Babies Feel Pain/ Say NO to Abortion" as well as a web address, "DoctorsonFetalPain. com." Although Pattison initially accepted the ad on the condition that DPLA's own organizational website was included, it later informed the association that the city's lawyers found the ad in violation of advertising standards. Various changes were proposed and eventually, in early 2018, the city accepted the ads, which began running in February. The city received over one hundred complaints, and Ads Standards Canada received an official complaint that the ad was both inaccurate and unacceptable. The city also received petitions with hundreds of signatures supporting DPLA's freedom of expression.

In April 2018, the city removed the ads, prompting DPLA to inquire about an appeal process — there was none. Over subsequent months, DPLA proposed new ads to Pattison and the city, none of which the city accepted, arguing the new ads did not "promote a safe, efficient, inclusive and customer-focused transit system."[21] The city maintained that the new ads continued to violate the Canadian Code of Advertising Standards for accuracy and acceptability because, in showing a fetus at a later gestational duration, the images were not representative of the fact that most abortions occur in the first trimester. Further, the city perceived scientific claims in the ads to be misleading and the content generally demeaning and disparaging towards women who have had or might have an abortion. DPLA took Lethbridge to court.

While many parallels were drawn to the arguments in *CCBR v. Grande Prairie*, Justice Gates found the Lethbridge case to be different, with the images and phrases in Grande Prairie to be hateful and extreme. He concluded that in its decision to refuse DPLA's ads, Lethbridge failed to balance its statutory objective to develop and maintain a safe and viable community with its obligations to protect Charter rights to freedom of expression. Relying on the Code is simply not enough. He sent the decision back to the table, urging the city to appoint a new third party in the decision-making role. The burden on city or even transit employees to conduct constitutional analyses with respect to ad decisions was mounting.

A very similar result stemmed from a 2022 case, when Guelph, Ontario, refused ads proposed by Guelph and Area Right to Life:[22] the city was found to have inadequately considered Section 2 in its analysis of the ads acceptability, relying too heavily on the Advertising Code. Again in 2023, when Hamilton, Ontario, turned down ads proposed by an anti-abortion organization called Association for Reformed Political Action (ARPA)[23] based on Code violations, the court sent the ads back to the city's decision-making table for deeper constitutional analysis.

A city has different Charter obligations than a private business like a local newspaper. In October 2018, the *Nelson Star* in Nelson, BC, published by Black Press Media, ran a Halloween-themed ad on behalf of the local anti-abortion Nelson Right to Life Society (NRLS). The ad's tagline stated "Is it really just your body? Choose life Mummy! An abortion will haunt you forever. A baby is the sweetest treat ever!" with an image of a pregnant woman in a T-shirt with an infant skeleton on it.[24] Complaints to the paper were swift and strong, and the editor and publisher decided to issue a moratorium on any ads addressing the issue of abortion. The next year, when NRLS submitted their ad for publication, the paper refused. NRLS applied to the BC Human Rights Tribunal, arguing they were being discriminated against based on Catholic faith, and as a remedy, they should be allowed to advertise pro-life messages and images. The complaint was dismissed by the Tribunal, which doubted discrimination could be proven and determined that Black Press Media was simply acting in its own business interests. The City of Nelson was, in the meantime, facing demands from anti-abortion organizations to have their banners hung in the city's streets. To resolve that conflict, the city opted to ban all banners from non-profits, regardless of message.[25]

Saskatchewan is "known for its classic views of canola fields and grain elevators, but another common sight is the many anti-abortion billboards along highways."[26] In the wake of the June 2022 *Dobbs v. Jackson* decision in the US, volunteers with a pro-choice non-profit group in Saskatchewan identified sixty-four anti-abortion billboards across the province.[27] They endeavoured to have the signs removed but met resistance from city mayors and councils, who determined that the statements on the signs, such as "life is sacred from conception to natural death"[28] were not discriminatory. Abortion is Healthcare Signs Inc. fundraised and mounted a counter-campaign. In November, the first sign went up — a bright orange, pink, blue, and green billboard in rural Aylesbury, outside of Regina, with a simple message: "Abortion is Healthcare." The group's leader, Rachel Regio, explained the intention of the billboard campaign was to decrease abortion stigma while increasing access.[29] Saskatchewan was the last province to provide public funding for medication abortion (mifepristone) and only has two sites for procedural abortion: in Saskatoon at the hospital, where referrals are required and care caps at twelve weeks, and in Regina, where patients can self-refer to eighteen weeks. The province is over 650,000 square kilometres and home to 1.2 million people[30] — it is far larger in geographic and population size than provinces like New Brunswick or Nova Scotia, where there are more facilities offering procedural abortion. Unfortunately, Abortion is Healthcare Signs Inc's billboard in Regina was vandalized with anti-abortion graffiti,[31] and the group's website is no longer operational.

Beyond bus ads, billboards, and banners, another tactic among anti-abortion organizations is to leaflet private residences, dropping graphic images into mailboxes. To reduce the potential harm of these flyers, particularly children's exposure to their content, the cities of London (Ontario),[32] Calgary (Alberta),[33] and New Westminster (British Columbia)[34] recently adopted bylaws requiring any distributed graphic images of fetuses first be enclosed in envelopes with a warning and identifying information about the sender. Toronto[35] city councillors Dianne Saxe and Paula Fletcher have also put forward a motion for such a bylaw. Saxe explained, "People don't get a choice, whether or not to be exposed to these disturbing images in their homes, and they feel quite strongly that it interferes with their rights of privacy and self-determination."[36]

Injunctions and Bubble Zones around Clinics

In 1989, just after the *R. v. Morgentaler* decision, the canonical Canadian TV series *Degrassi High*[37] premiered with a two-part episode, "A New Start," featuring sixteen-year-old character Erica Farrell discovering she is pregnant and seeking an abortion in Toronto. Outside of the clinic, she faces a humiliating and physically challenging clash with a throng of aggressive protestors. A staff person opens the door, welcomes her in, and once inside, assures her she is safe now.

In the context of seeking abortion services, protestors' freedom of assembly butts up against patients' and providers' rights to privacy and security of the person. The 1990s were a period of anti-abortion extremism in Canada, including assassination attempts on abortion providers and aggressive "sidewalk counselling" in front of clinics. The regularity and hostility of these types of anti-abortion violence prompted injunctions and eventually laws to protect the clinic spaces and clinicians' homes.

In 1992, the Morgentaler clinic in downtown Toronto was destroyed by a firebomb overnight. Although no one was hurt, in an affidavit,[38] Dr. Morgentaler described the impact of the explosion:

> On May 18, 1992, at approximately 3 a.m. an unidentified man drilled a hole in one of the rear doors of the clinic and poured several gallons of gasoline into the building. After waiting some minutes for the fumes to disseminate he ignited the gasoline. The subsequent explosion and fire destroyed both 85 and 87 Harbord Street. Contents in both buildings were severely damaged. The building became a hazard to public safety and was demolished under public order. The explosion and subsequent fire caused $550,000.00 damage to the building and contents at 85 Harbord Street. I do not know the total monetary damage to 87 Harbord Street. There was a suspension of patient services for 2 days after the firebombing.

The firebombing of Morgentaler's Toronto clinic and its subsequent demolition contributed to making the persistence of standalone abortion clinics into a radical political symbol of defiance. For decades afterward, abortion clinics across the country continued to deploy significant security measures to prevent terrorist infiltration, while also, as Joanna

Erdman has theorized, developing identities as "a community resource, an economic and social resource" and personification as "the someone who would/could help you in this place."[39]

In November 1994, a sniper used an AK-47 to shoot through a window into Dr. Gary Romalis's Vancouver home, hitting his femoral artery and almost causing his death.[40] Dr. Romalis had been providing abortion care since 1972, and he and his family had been subjected to prior protest around his clinic and their home. He survived the shooting, as well as a stabbing attack inside his clinic in 2000.[41] He continued his practice until his death from illness in 2014.[42] In 1995, Dr. Hugh Short was shot at home in Ancaster, Ontario. Then in 1997, Dr. Jack Fainman was shot in Winnipeg, Manitoba. The attacks had a chilling impact on care providers at the time,[43] and deep fear and secrecy among the abortion provider community persisted long after.

While these extreme acts of violence were highly anomalous and all directed at male physician providers, there were quotidian protests outside clinics that generated constant intimidation of patients and staff, mostly women. Lowe and Hayes[44] describe anti-abortion activism outside clinics as violating "social rules governing encounters with strangers in specific places and reinforc[ing] gendered hierarchies. As such, they are often experienced as acts of gendered harassment." In the late 1980s, the tactics of Operation Rescue, a militant, US-based anti-abortion organization, began to overwhelm clinics in Toronto and Vancouver. Emerging in the 1970s, Operation Rescue involved creation of what were effectively human blockades in front of clinics, physically barring people from entry. In 1989, at his own private expense, Dr. Morgentaler filed for and received an injunction to protect his Toronto clinic.

In 1994, the Attorney General of Ontario sought and received an injunction against anti-abortion protest within the vicinity of Morgentaler's clinic and all Ontario abortion clinics, hospitals providing abortion services, and the offices and homes of abortion providers (physicians) more broadly. The case *Ontario v. Dieleman*[45] is so named because one of the sixteen anti-abortion protestors expressly named in the case was named Joanne Dieleman. The judge summarized,

> The decision to abort is a profoundly personal one and its complexities pervade the entirety of that individual's life. To be trapped by the circumstances prevailing at the free-

standing clinics, in a face-to-face public encounter with a hostile stranger, justifies government concerns over the unnecessary humiliation and embarrassment inflicted on these women.

Building on the injunctions, demand for safe access zone laws emerged. Also known as bubble-zone legislation, these laws aim to protect the dignity, privacy, and security of patients and providers, reduce physical barriers to accessing care, reduce the emotional distress associated with care seeking, foster peace in the community, reduce traffic disturbances, and reduce the impact of anti-abortion activism generally, all while "minimally impacting the protestors' freedom of speech, as they are free to protest elsewhere, outside of the bubble zone or away from the clinic."[46] Unlike on a university campus, proximity to patients and care providers, and even direct interference with care delivery, generates a different level of conflict between the risk to security of (another) person posed by someone's freedom of expression or assembly. On balance, the patient must come first.

The earliest such piece of legislation in Canada, British Columbia's Access to Abortion Services Act,[47] was passed in 1995, creating a safe access zone within fifty metres of an abortion clinic or 160 metres from a doctor's residence. In September 1995, almost immediately after BC's bubble-zone law was implemented, anti-abortionist Maurice Lewis was charged for "sidewalk interference" within the bubble zone of Everywoman's Health Centre, on Commercial Drive in Vancouver. The charges against Lewis were dismissed by the provincial court, which ruled that the bubble zone ban on protest violated his Section 2 Charter rights to freedom of religion and of expression and assembly. The Crown appealed the court's decision, arguing that infringement on Section 2 rights can be permitted under Section 1, which allows limitations that can be justified in a free and democratic society.[48] Madame Justice Saunders of the BC Court of Appeal agreed, convicting Lewis. Lewis then appealed, but before his case could be heard, he died.[49]

This was not the end of his case, however. In December 1998, Gordon Watson and Donald Spratt[50] were arrested outside Everywoman's. Watson held a sign on which was written "Abortion is Murder" and Spratt carried a nine-foot cross. The pair were convicted in 2000 and then appealed, which they again lost in 2008. A coalition had formed to intervene in the case, including Everywoman's as well as the Elizabeth Bagshaw Clinic (another free-standing Vancouver-based clinic), the CARE Program (abortion clinic within BC Women's Hospital, also in Vancouver), the BC Pro-Choice Action Network Society non-profit, and the Women's Legal Education Action Fund (LEAF). While no one disputed that the Act impinged on Section 2 rights, they argued the impingement was justified under Section 1.

Then in 2009, Donald Spratt, along with Cecilia "Sissy" Von Dehn, tried to test the limits of the bubble zone law by protesting outside of Everywoman's with signs not denigrating abortion but rather rebutting restrictions on freedom of expression itself.[51] They wore sandwich boards reading, "CAUTION! YOU CAN BE ARRESTED HERE UNDER BILL 48" and "BE INFORMED! THIS AREA IS A BC LEGISLATED ACCESS ("BUBBLE") ZONE! Read "BILL 48."[52] Spratt had taped his mouth shut. They were both arrested under the provisions of Bill 48, and the court refused to indulge their attempt to find a loophole, with Mr. Justice Hall stating, "I consider that women seeking services at an abortion facility and care providers are vulnerable to harassment.... This legislation has a prophylactic function designed to de-escalate the controversy around the subject of abortion services and serves to protect the vulnerable."[53]

It was only twenty years later that a second province implemented a bubble zone, on the other coast. The Athena Health Centre in St. John's, Newfoundland, started out in 1990 as a Morgentaler Clinic, facing aggressive protests on its doorstep from the outset. Entrepreneur and nurse Rolanda Ryan took ownership of the clinic in 2010 and in 2015 moved it to its current location at 215 LeMerchant Street, inside a large house that also serves as a family practice, known as Clinic 215. The move exacerbated the protests, as did the increasingly commonplace use of smartphone cameras: patients were in danger of being videotaped.[54] Free-standing clinics like Athena may attract more anti-abortion protest than a hospital because of the specificity of abortion clinic services in comparison to the hospital behemoth. When abortion care is provided in a hospital, no one could know who enters the building as an abortion patient or an abortion provider in a facility with hundreds of patients and staff of all types going in and out every day. The hospital provides anonymity and a type of safety.

In June of 2016, Ryan sought and won a court injunction, at her own significant expense, to prevent protestors from assembling within forty metres of Athena.⁵⁵ In December of that year, the Newfoundland provincial government gave royal assent to bubble-zone legislation, the second province at the time to do so. After the legislation passed, Athena's protestors quickly moved along, setting up regularly at busy nearby intersections, maximizing their audience without directly interfering with patients or staff.

Quebec also passed legislation in 2016, by rolling protections into a broader law called An Act Respecting Health Services and Social Services,⁵⁶ which stipulates that anyone who threatens or intimidates someone when they are entering or exiting a site of abortion can be fined $500 to $5,000 (Section 531.0.1). Within fifty metres of a facility, demonstrators may not dissuade patients from obtaining services or providers from providing services (Section 16). The same Quebec law also covers things like the need to have a licence to operate a seniors' residence. Placing these bubble-zone rules within a broader law about proper operation of health facilities deradicalizes the ban on sidewalk picketers.

The BC Access to Abortion Services Act defined the access zone as within fifty metres of an abortion clinic or 160 metres from a doctor or "service provider's" residence. Nurses or other staff involved in abortion care were not specifically acknowledged or protected. The Newfoundland legislation enacted subsequently borrowed from the language of the original BC Act.⁵⁷ In 2018, nearly thirty years after Dr. Morgentaler sought the injunction to protect his Toronto clinic, the Liberal government under Premier Kathleen Wynne passed Ontario's bubble-zone legislation,⁵⁸ the Safe Access to Abortion Services Act. The Ontario Act added the definition of "a person who provides, or assists in the provision of, abortion services" to include not only physicians but also nurses, pharmacists, and regulated health professionals. It also banned photography of patients or providers. In Alberta that same year, NDP health minister Sarah Hoffman introduced the Protecting Choice for Women Accessing Health Care Act, which also banned video recording.

Five days after Ontario's Act came into effect in February of 2018, longtime anti-abortion picketer Cyril Winter was charged under the Act for protesting in front of Ottawa's Morgentaler Clinic on Bank Street. Like Spratt and Von Dehn in Vancouver, Winter sought to find a loophole to the law's applicability. He was wearing a sandwich board that read "Freedom of Expression and Religion, No Censorship," and news items about the charges characterized the Ottawa police as "facing a new quandary: When and how does the new law apply in cases that aren't clear-cut?"[59] Like Lewis, Winter died suddenly and before his first court appearance to contest the charges.[60]

Almost a year later, eighty-three-year-old priest Anthony Van Hee, another well-known anti-abortion demonstrator, was charged with "intimidating or attempting to intimidate" a person accessing abortion services outside the Ottawa Morgentaler Clinic.[61] Strategically, neither of his signs — both removed by Ottawa police — mentioned abortion. Rather, they read: "The Primacy Of Free Speech/Cornerstone of Western Civilization," while the other said, "Without Free Speech/The State Is A Corpse."[62] It was not until four years later that charges against Van Hee were dropped.[63] Van Hee's lawyers had planned to argue that the Safe Access to Abortion Services Act was overbroad.

It is not just the prickly definition of what counts as abortion protest that challenges enforcement of bubble-zone laws. The presence of enforcers — e.g. police — is also intimidating to patients and staff, particularly those belonging to groups disproportionately subject to state violence.[64] Furthermore, in the current era, when approximately half of abortion is provided through medication and prescriptions can be procured through primary care and filled at retail pharmacies, abortion provision is widely diffused. It is much less obvious where to target an anti-abortion protest.

Purpose-specific, free-standing clinics are disproportionately targeted for anti-abortion protest. Currently, Saskatchewan, the three Maritime provinces, and both Nunavut and the Northwest Territories do not have any free-standing abortion clinics. The private-pay clinic in Fredericton closed in January 2024. The Morgentaler free-standing clinic in Halifax was closed in 2003 when it became apparent the hospital-based clinic was meeting patient service needs. But anti-abortion efforts such as the annual fall "40 Days for Life" campaign featuring a "Life Chain" lineup of protestors do persist and are organized in proximity to hospitals known to provide abortions. In 2017, the New Brunswick court issued a permanent injunction against protest anywhere on the grounds of the Chaleur Hospital, located in the northern town of Bathurst, after "40 Days" protestors obstructed an ambulance. The driver had to brake suddenly to avoid a picketer who stepped off the sidewalk.⁶⁵ Although the Vitalité regional health authority that governs Chaleur applied for the injunction, hospital officials "took no position on the abortion debate but instead were concerned the safety of patients and employees was at risk."⁶⁶ In Moncton, the site of New Brunswick's two other procedural abortion facilities, Pro-Choice Moncton holds an annual counter-protest "Choice Chain" during the forty days.⁶⁷

Meghan Boudreau,⁶⁸ then a university student at Saint Mary's University, led a 2019 campaign to protect patients from anti-abortion protests like the 40 Days demonstrations frequently held outside the Victoria General Hospital in Halifax. On March 11, 2020, Nova Scotia passed Bill 242, An Act to Protect Access to Reproductive Health Care,⁶⁹ introduced by Claudia Chender, currently the leader of the provincial New Democratic Party. Eleven days later, Nova Scotia⁷⁰ declared a provincial state of emergency due to the COVID-19 pandemic. While many worried about how the pandemic would affect access to abortion,⁷¹ governments were vocal and swift to assure "operation as usual" for providers, and COVID-19 allowed for practice innovations like adoption of telemedicine, sparked comradery and appreciation, and dissuaded congregation of anti-abortion picketers.⁷²

Bubble-zone legislation to protect abortion access, like Bill 242, has been leveraged to limit other types of protest in the vicinity of health services. In May 2021, just over one year into COVID-19 pandemic protections, the Nova Scotia court issued an injunction to stop anti-vaccine and anti-lockdown protests outside of hospitals.⁷³ Then in October 2021, the government passed the Protecting Access to Health Services Act, to "establish a 50-metre safe-access bubble zone around facilities such as hospitals, mental-health services, home-care services, long-term care services, clinics, doctors' offices and pharmacies. Peaceful protests can occur outside that perimeter."⁷⁴ Penalties mirrored those for the Act to Protect Access to Reproductive Care.

On the heels of the Nova Scotia legislation, and still in the thick of anti-COVID-19 vaccine protests, in January 2022 the federal Bill C-3 came into effect, which amended the Criminal Code to criminalize the intimidation of health care workers and patients and obstruction of access to health care facilities. The new Section 423.2⁷⁵ makes it "an offence for a person to engage in any conduct with the intent to provoke a state of fear in: A person in order to impede them from obtaining health services from a health professional; A health professional in order to impede them in the performance of their duties."

At the tail end of January 2022, hundreds of vehicles and thousands of protestors converged on downtown Ottawa to protest vaccine requirements and other restrictions that had come into effect during the pandemic. The convoy occupation persisted for weeks, with protestors ceaselessly honking horns and blocking roadways. Protestors reportedly pelted ambulances with rocks and blocked their movement, requiring paramedics to request law enforcement escort.[76] By mid-February, Prime Minister Justin Trudeau invoked the Emergencies Act[77] for the first time, and police forces were deployed to clear the protestors.

Bill C-3 refers specifically to invoking fear or impeding access; peaceful protest that does neither, even if located outside an abortion facility, might not apply. As such, despite the federal law coming into play, when the NDP was elected with a majority government in Manitoba under Premier Wab Kinew in fall 2023, families minister Nahanni Fontaine re-proposed bubble-zone legislation for the province. She had tried many times before, while the NDP were in opposition.[78] As this proposal was making its way through various legislative steps, in March 2024, the Manitoba Conservative health critic, Kathleen Cook, suggested that the government plan to ban anti-abortion protestors should be expanded to incorporate all protests, including picket lines of striking workers.[79] The bill passed in June 2024.

Bubble-zone protections were never intended to restrict workers' rights, and the Canadian Civil Liberties Association has raised alarm about the potential impact of stretching these restrictions on freedom of assembly.[80] The continued democratization of access to abortion through medication abortion complicates the organization and deployment of anti-abortion protestors. Right alongside medication abortion is its ensuing expansion of professional scope, as a physician is no longer the sole health professional authorized to provide abortion. Both are useful tools to augment patient and provider safety.

*　*　*

Anti-abortion protest is a point of tension between the Charter right to freedom of expression and the need for to protect patient and health professional safety. University campuses — supposed bastions of academic freedom — have been the sites of considerable conflict and clench down over offensive anti-abortion displays. Much more terrifying, anti-abortion extremism, including the bombing of Morgentaler's Toronto clinic and sniper attacks on abortion physicians, led to the eventual establishment of bubble-zone laws to shield abortion seekers and providers from intimidation and violence. The implementation and deregulation of medication abortion has decoupled abortion from physical clinic spaces and placed it within the home, improving safety and deplatforming anti-abortion protest.

CHAPTER 8

EXPANSION OF CARE

> This chapter describes recent actions to expand access to abortion through changes to professional scope of practice, clinical activity, and attention to diversity, equity, and inclusion in services.

The past ten years has seen an explosion of activity to expand access to abortion care across Canada. The radical impact of mifepristone approval and deregulation by Health Canada was described in Chapter 4, "The Mifepristone Revolution." The persistent efforts of researchers, lawmakers, health care providers, educators, activists, and community groups have driven important, complementary changes. This chapter focuses on work to reduce logistical barriers, broaden health professionals' scope, enhance training, build capacity for later gestational duration, address the serious threats to access that emerged in the US, and improve service for patients with diverse backgrounds.

Reducing Logistical Barriers

Ten years ago, it was still necessary to seek approval from two separate physicians prior to receiving publicly funded procedural abortion care in New Brunswick. This regulation made the province effectively one of the most challenging sites to access care in the country. In 2014, Brian Gallant, a young Liberal candidate for premier, made removing this regulation an election promise, and when he won, he made good. In early 2015, not only was physician "permission" no longer necessary to receive abortion, but the province also asserted self-referral to publicly funded care would be available every weekday, launching a full-time, comprehensive abortion clinic on the fifth floor of the Moncton Hospital. Two other hospital family planning clinics, at Georges Dumont Hospital in

Moncton and Chaleur Hospital in Bathurst, operated two days and one day a week, respectively. While Gallant did not go as far as rescinding New Brunswick's refusal to publicly fund abortions in the free-standing private clinic in Fredericton, the shift to self-referral and the investment in the Moncton Hospital clinic were critical and precedent-setting shifts. As her first act as New Brunswick's first woman premier, in November 2024, Susan Holt revoked the regulation that had barred public funding for procedural abortions in free-standing clinics.

In 2016, facing the threat of a constitutional challenge from activist group Abortion Access Now Prince Edward Island (AANPEI), the PEI government agreed that their thirty-five-year ban on abortion was no longer acceptable. When the doors opened at the Women's Wellness Program in January 2017, the clinic operated by self-referral, using text and email with patients, offering 24/7 support for medication abortion, and providing free post-abortion contraception options. The program was one of the first to use gender-inclusive language and now is called Sexual Health, Options and Reproductive Services, SHORS, evoking the red sand beaches and the Atlantic coastline.

A year after that, in 2018, the Nova Scotia government agreed to support a toll-free, self-referral telephone line for abortion appointment booking from anywhere in the province. Prior to 2018, NS patients first had to seek a referral from a supportive primary care provider to be seen at any of the four procedural facilities, located in hospitals in Halifax, Truro, Kentville, and Bridgewater. The patient might strategically book in all four sites, hoping one would have an earlier appointment opening than another, resulting in duplication, no-shows, and significant system waste. From 2018 onwards, all patients could simply call 1-833-352-0719 to speak directly with a nurse at the Nova Scotia Women's Choice Clinic, who would arrange all aspects of care (blood work, ultrasound, and either a prescription for mifepristone or an appointment for a procedure), all of which was publicly funded if the patient carried a provincial health card. In 2022, after unanimous and persistent advocacy from staff, the clinic adopted the gender-inclusive name of Reproductive Options and Services (ROSE),[1] an homage to longtime physician Dr. Jacques Desrosiers.

In every province and territory, it is now possible for patients to self-refer to at least one procedural abortion provider. For example, in Saskatchewan, the clinic in Regina offers self-referral to eighteen weeks, while the site in Saskatoon requires a referral and caps services at twelve weeks. In some hospitals, abortion is provided only after a referral is made from a primary care provider to the abortion provider. Other hospitals are home to dedicated abortion clinics that can be called directly, as is the case with ROSE, SHORS, and the Moncton Hospital, Georges Dumont, and Chaleur Hospital family planning clinics. The 2017 implementation of mifepristone for medication abortion through primary care providers, which by definition does not require prior referral, has significantly altered the logistics of receiving abortion care.

Scope

In 2017, Health Canada[2] deregulated mifepristone, allowing for nurse practitioners (NP) to be authorized to prescribe it for medication abortion.[3] New Brunswick was the earliest adopter of NP prescribing, with all provinces and territories except Quebec quickly following suit (Quebec did not change until 2022). NP prescribing was supported by volumes of international evidence of the safety and efficacy of non-physician health workers, such as nurses and midwives, prescribing medication abortion, as well as performing procedural abortion.[4] Prior to these changes, abortion care had largely been conceptualized as the domain of physicians, despite the considerable roles of other professionals, including registered nurses and social workers, providing patient education and counselling, administering medications, accompanying patients through procedures, and following up. A 2019 national survey of the abortion workforce,[5] with 465 respondents, included thirty NPs. Of the 48,509 abortions respondents reported providing, 327 were provided by NPs. This was the first accounting of non-physicians as members of the abortion workforce. In the years since, it is suspected uptake among NPs has been steadily increasing.

The quick succession of provinces and territories to authorize NPs as prescribers in Canada was not complemented by similar support for registered midwives. The reason is not related to appropriateness or competence, however, as midwives are *the* provider best suited to care for normal pregnancy, and abortion is very normal. Rather, barriers include provincial legislation and regulations limiting scope of practice; midwifery compensation models; and regulation of prescribing power.[6] Midwifery legislation has often been very hard won, with PEI[7] only beginning to offer services in January 2024. The resulting patchwork legislation and regulation are often tight and inflexible, with no nimble mechanism for adjustments in scope. For example, Ontario's midwifery legislation does not give midwives authority to prescribe and/or administer medications they feel confident and competent about; rather, they must work from a limited, predefined list. The list was expanded in May 2024 to include, for the first time, vaccinations, antibiotics, antifungals, antiemetics, and contraceptives.[8] There are currently pilot programs in Toronto, Hamilton, and Thunder Bay that allow midwives in these sites to provide medication abortion through medical directives; basically, a physician or NP within the shared practice assumes liability and the midwives oversee the direct patient care. In summer 2022, the Quebec government announced it would authorize midwives to prescribe medication abortion; implementation is moving ahead slowly.[9] In spring 2024, the Canadian Association of Midwifery[10] published a national strategy for midwifery-led abortion care. Progress is being made, but nowhere in Canada are midwives routinely and independently prescribing mifepristone yet.

Registered nurses' scope could be further expanded to include prescribing of contraception and insertion of long-acting reversible contraception options such as the intrauterine device and the contraceptive implant (Nexplanon). Improving access to contraception reduces the risk of unintended pregnancy. In 2022, the BC nursing regulator made changes[11] to allow certified RNs to prescribe contraception; however, the necessary companion education process has yet to be developed and approved.[12] In Ontario, authorized RNs may prescribe "systemic" (oral or injectable) contraceptives, as well as intravaginal options like the ring (not IUDs).[13] In Quebec, nurses can issue six-month prescriptions for contraception.[14] Pharmacists are authorized to prescribe contraception in eight of Canada's ten provinces, with the exceptions of Manitoba and Ontario.[15] While the ability to prescribe contraception is a necessary first step, the most effective forms of birth control are long-acting forms — the IUD and implant — both of which must be inserted. For any successful increase in scope to have an impact, there must be accompanying changes and expansions to training.

Training

Effective integration of prescribing abortion or contraception care into other health professions is not just a matter of changing legislation; there is the entirely non-legal aspect of networking, garnering experience, and feeling supported. In 2018, the Contraception and Abortion Research

Team, under the leadership of Dr. Wendy Norman and Dr. Ruth Martin-Misener, conducted a mixed-methods (survey and interview) study across Canada to understand the experiences of NPs in the thick of implementing NP prescribing. The study found training and mentorship to be the most important enablers of NP involvement in abortion care.[16]

Abortion care is not routinely taught in the approximately one hundred undergraduate and graduate nursing and six midwifery schools across the country.[17] In 2014, Sheinfeld et al.[18] surveyed thirty-two NP programs in Canada about abortion curricula. Of the sixteen responding programs, 50 percent did not include training on pregnancy options counselling, first trimester abortion procedures, and/or post-abortion care in the clinical curriculum (applied practice), and 56 percent responded that they did not offer these topics in the didactic curriculum (classroom lectures). Of those that did offer teaching on the topics, most devoted less than one hour. A re-administration of this survey is overdue, especially since NP prescribing launched the year after Sheinfeld et al.'s survey was published.

Abortion is not necessarily taught to medical students and residents. A 2016 study among OB/GYN residency programs participants and leaders found half of the programs included abortion only if the resident were to "opt-in."[19] More than two-thirds of residents wished they had more training. In a 2018 survey of family medicine residents, 79 percent reported never having assisted in or observed abortion in their training.[20] Although surveys have found the majority of medical students hold positive views towards abortion, a very small number plan to include it in their practice[21] and abortion knowledge among medical students has been found to be quite poor.[22]

In 2020, an interdisciplinary team of instructors designed and launched an abortion education course across the faculties of Health, Medicine, and Dentistry at Dalhousie University.[23] Dalhousie requires students in its thirteen health professional programs to participate in several Interprofessional Health Education (IPHE) courses of varying length; the abortion course involves four modules of 1.5 hours each. When it launched, the course was over-subscribed, and in the ensuing five years, it has been renewed ten times and is always full. Midwives, nurses, nurse practitioners, family medicine physicians, obstetricians and gynecologists, social workers, and birth doulas are represented on the teaching team and the course is open and free for members of the public to register. The appetite for this content is highly indicative of unmet learning needs in core health professional curricula, but also of public interest. The course evaluations consistently demonstrate students lack basic knowledge about abortion and contraception and about the different interdependent roles various professionals play in the process, highlighting the need for comprehensive abortion and contraception education in basic health professional preparatory training.

Despite the important role an array of professionals could play in providing abortion and contraception care, lack of access to education limits their ability to include this care in practice. And those care roles can be diverse and comprehensive:

> Nursing responsibilities in abortion care include patient education, communication, physical, social and psychological assessment, counselling, education, treatment, support, comfort, monitoring, discharge and follow up. Nurses may act as navigators between services such as diagnostic imaging, serology, post-abortion contraception provision and social work services. They may conduct administrative tasks, develop policy or lead practice innovation, research, and advocacy.[24]

Although nurses arguably perform *most* of the work of abortion care, they rarely receive education about it, and as such they might be hard pressed to even imagine their potential contributions.

In May 2023, Health Canada's Sexual and Reproductive Health Unit awarded $3.8 million[25] to a group of projects coordinated by CART to expand access to care by generating informational resources for patients from underserved populations and by creating a new national training platform for interdisciplinary health care professionals.[26] As a partner in the project, the Canadian Association of Schools of Nursing (CASN) formed a national advisory group to create competencies[27] in abortion care for students graduating from both baccalaureate nursing and NP programs. The competencies were published in spring 2024 and address six areas: clinical assessment of a patient/client for pregnancy; trauma and violence-informed therapeutic communication; collaboration with interprofessional team members to ensure delivery of abortion care; adherence to the nursing standards of practice, scope of practice, and code of ethics; direct provision of sexual and reproductive health care; and knowledge of the history of abortion in Canada and awareness of barriers and enablers to access. A next step will be to integrate the competencies into curricula in each school.

Extending Gestational Capacity

As more people become confident and competent prescribers of medication abortion, it is likely the timeliness of abortion access will improve, reducing the demand for second and third trimester care. But for the small percentage of patients seeking care at later gestational durations, in the second trimester or beyond, access may be considerably more difficult. As discussed throughout this book, abortion access in Canada heavily intersects with geography and travel. The further along the pregnancy is, the fewer providers there are with experience to provide that care, the longer the distance a patient may need to travel, and the greater the associated costs to the patient.

Public reporting of abortion volumes and types in Canada is not comprehensive or straightforward. For example, while hospitals are required to report procedural abortion volumes, free-standing clinics are not (although many do). Given the greater complexity of care, hospitals are more likely to provide second and third trimester abortion than free-standing clinics. As such, if free-standing clinics are not reporting their service volumes, it would appear as if care at later gestations made up a greater proportion of all care than it really does. So, in 2021, the Canadian Institute for Health Information stopped collecting and reporting on gestational duration of abortion. Before then, it was estimated that at least 86 percent of abortions occurred prior to twelve weeks.[28]

The 2019 survey of the Canadian abortion workforce found 94.4 percent of the abortions provided by respondents were in the first trimester.[29] Of the 465 provider respondents, a minority, 222, all physicians, provided procedural abortion care (most of these physicians were obstetrician-gynecologists).[30] Exactly half as many of these respondents provided abortion in the second trimester (109) as in the first (219). Eighty percent of the second trimester abortion providers (STAP) were in urban centres, compared to 66 percent of first trimester abortion providers (FTAP). Among both FTAP and STAP across the country, 39 percent were situated in one province, Quebec. In sum, second trimester care was sequestered in urban centres, among about one hundred providers, a disproportionate number of whom practice in Quebec. A similar study[31] in 2012 also found geographic hurdles to care.

Care beyond eighteen to twenty weeks, midway through the second trimester, requires different techniques, training, equipment, personnel, and time. After twenty weeks, fetal demise is characterized as a stillbirth rather than a miscarriage. As discussed in Chapter 3, "Defining Miscarriage, Stillbirth and Infant Death," the administrative burden increases significantly for patients as the stillbirth must be registered with Vital Statistics. For care later in the second trimester, from twenty-four to twenty-eight weeks, providers are even fewer in number.

Since *Roe v. Wade*, Canadians have travelled to the US for abortion care, particularly later in pregnancy. Sethna and Doull[32] have critiqued the term "medical tourism" in the context of abortion, explaining, "Even when individuals travel to access medical services for reasons that have little to do with choice, tourism signifies individual agency, freedom, and mobility. These characteristics are often linked to medical tourism despite the fact that legal and extra-legal impediments blocking access to medical services compel individuals to travel." The Badgley committee (1977) reported that over 50,000 Canadian patients travelled to the US for abortions between 1970 and 1975.[33] Chantal Daigle, the young Québécoise woman who fought her abusive ex-boyfriend's court injunction preventing her from seeking abortion in 1989, won her case in the Supreme Court of Canada on principle, with the court ruling that the fetus was not a person and people whose sperm causes pregnancies had no rights to determine pregnancy outcomes. Despite the win, Daigle, by then in the second trimester, had sought a procedure in the US.

US travel, especially for second and third trimester care, continued regularly for Canadian abortion seekers. For example, patients would be commonly directed to the Boulder Clinic[34] in Colorado, opened by Dr. Warren Hern in 1973. One of very few providers openly caring for abortion patients later in pregnancy, Hern is now eighty-seven years old. He and his staff have faced decades of violence and intimidation. Boulder Clinic abortion procedures in the second and third trimester take three to four days, and the cost can be more than C$15,000. Usually, this cost would be paid by Canadian patients' home provinces, as the care is medically necessary but not available locally. On the east coast, Canadians might be sent to the Dupont Clinic[35] and Partners in Abortion Care Clinic[36] in Maryland.

When COVID-19 struck, international travel became highly restricted, if not outright prohibited. In March 2020, the US-Canadian border closed[37] to non-essential travel. What constituted "essential" certainly could have included abortion care at later gestations, but the extraordinary stigma, loss of privacy, and layers of bureaucracy to which patients would be subjected made this next to impossible. Once a vaccine became available, the border opened up to vaccinated travellers, but patients seeking later care are often extremely marginalized and may have faced barriers to vaccination.

Facing this suddenly deeply restrictive context, abortion providers in Canada got to work expanding their skills to be able to offer later care. In Prince Edward Island, which launched its first abortion clinic in January 2017, that meant progressing from a twelve-week maximum capacity for procedural abortion to fourteen weeks, then sixteen, and now, on a case-by-case basis, care is provided up to eighteen. Nova Scotia and New Brunswick both pushed their limits from sixteen to eighteen, again on a case-by-case basis. A new weekly service for care in the second trimester and beyond opened at Women's College Hospital[38] in partnership with Mt. Sinai Hospital in Toronto. The CARE program at BC Women's Hospital in Vancouver,[39] which had previously maintained a cap of twenty-four or so weeks, made changes to extend their abilities as well. While much of this advancement is not captured publicly on websites, internal networks among abortion providers allow collaboration with each other to optimize access. Each little bit makes a difference: if a patient at seventeen weeks living in Moncton does not need to leave her city anymore for Toronto, and a Torontonian patient at twenty-five weeks does not need to leave the country anymore, there are major positive impacts for these individuals and the increased capacity is passed down. At the same time as these advances reduced Canada's dependence on US services, the fall of *Roe v. Wade* and new restrictions and bans on abortions have reduced capacity among US clinics to serve out-of-country patients. As of this writing, forty-one states have abortion bans: twelve states have a total ban, and nineteen have partial bans, depending on gestational duration.[40]

The Fallout of the US *Dobbs v. Jackson* Decision

Since the June 2022 *Dobbs v. Jackson* US Supreme Court ruling, which concluded that the US Constitution did not protect the right to abortion and individual states could create their own laws about abortion, there have been queries about potentially swelling demand from US patients travelling northwards. Canadian politicians, service providers, and advocates alike expressed clear willingness to serve US patients.[41] Former minister of public safety Marco Mendocino, responsible for the Canada Border Services Agency, announced he had consulted "to ensure entry guidelines are clear, 'so that women who may not be able to access health care including access to abortion are able to come to Canada.'" Meghan Doherty, director of global policy and advocacy for Action Canada for Sexual Health and Rights, acknowledged it will be challenging for already-in-demand abortion providers in Canada and assured, "there will be a lot of people who will be working day and night to provide care that is needed." Individual everyday Canadians even took to TikTok to offer accommodations and support to any American needing to come north for abortion care.[42]

Since *Dobbs*, the number of abortions happening in the US every month has increased, not decreased.[43] How is this is possible, when bans have caused clinic closures? Simply put, the demand and supply of services increases among clinics that stay open in permissive states, even if clinics are shuttered in states with restrictions and bans. Despite the stress of these shifts, there does not appear to be much northward travel. There are several potential reasons for this. Medication abortion pills can be mailed, reducing the need to travel at all. Travel to Canada requires a passport, whereas travel interstate, or even to Mexico, does not. In 1990, as few as 5 percent of Americans had a passport; that figure is now 48 percent, still not quite a majority.[44] Getting a passport is costly and time consuming. Getting to Canada is costly and time consuming. Even if Canadian providers are welcoming, the rules of Canada's Medicare system are clear: only people with a health card are insured, others have to pay out of pocket. An abortion procedure is usually several thousand Canadian dollars.

The wave of effort to express openness to US patients may have had another impact by simply spreading the word about access to abortion for potential patients in Canada. The rhetoric shifted from emphasis on access barriers to recognition of what providers in Canada had to offer. And there was a swell of pride about services in Canada among providers and the public.

Expanding Access

In 2013, Jean-Frederic Levesque[45] published an article that defined access to health care as comprising five elements from the health system: (1) approachability, (2) acceptability, (3) availability and accommodation,

(4) affordability, (5) appropriateness. Reciprocally, patients had to have the: (1) ability to perceive, (2) ability to seek, (3) ability to reach, (4) ability to pay, and (5) ability to engage with health services. Indisputably, gains have been made in recent years to increase abortion availability, to reduce extra billing or private fees, and to enhance appropriateness by implementing medication abortion as an option. More attention is needed, however, to improve the approachability and acceptability of care, particularly for people in equity-deserving groups and with intersecting experiences of discrimination and oppression, including Indigenous people, Black people, people of colour, newcomers to Canada, people who do not speak English, people with disabilities, fat people, people in 2SLGBTQIA+ communities, people in prison, and youth. The unique situation for young people seeking abortion, particularly as it pertains to regulations governing consent to sex and consent to health care, will be discussed in Chapter 9, "Children and Youth."

A 2019 survey of almost 500 abortion providers across Canada asked whether and how they cared for diverse populations. While 91 percent indicated they had not received specific training to support diverse patients, 92 percent reported they did care for people in diverse groups. Of these, 47 percent indicated they made efforts to accommodate these patients by adjusting their care practices. These techniques included:[46] adjusting care to patient's religion and/or culture — for example, involving culturally appropriate support people such as an Indigenous midwife; adjusting language and communication such as using a telephone translation service; shifting where and when services are provided such as by using telehealth for remote First Nations communities; and providing gender-affirmative, trauma-informed care such as by using gender-neutral language. Respondents were also asked about their own gender identity: 85 percent of the abortion providers in the survey identified as women.[47]

Gender Inclusivity

Some of the strongest enduring barriers to abortion in Canada have nothing to do with legal systems and are rather a product of ingrained bias and discrimination in health care systems and among health professionals. In sexual and reproductive health services, cisnormativity and heteronormativity are particularly dominant. The perceived long fight for recognition of "women's" health needs creates resistance to recognizing how this area of care causes harm through exclusionary norms. Trans and nonbinary people can and do get pregnant, and fear of discriminatory spaces and professionals can delay decisions to seek care, even if such discrimination is prohibited by law.

The Northwest Territories was the first jurisdiction to add gender identity to its human rights code, in 2002.[48] Under the Act,[49] it is prohibited to deny a person services or employment, or to discriminate against an individual with respect to services or employment, on the basis of protected grounds. Gender identity was only added to the Canadian Human Rights Act[50] as a protected ground in 2017. Section 3 now reads,

> For all purposes of this Act, the prohibited grounds of discrimination are race, national or ethnic origin, colour, religion, age, sex, sexual orientation, gender identity or expression, marital status, family status, genetic characteristics, disability and conviction for an offence for which a pardon has been granted or in respect of which a record suspension has been ordered. Where the ground of discrimination is pregnancy or child-birth, the discrimination shall be deemed to be on the ground of sex.

In 2021, for the first time and as the first country in the world to do so, the Canadian Census asked individuals about gender identity, and over 100,000 reported being transgender or nonbinary, equivalent to roughly 0.3 percent of the 36.9 million people in the country.[51] The Statistics Canada norm to ask about gender identity is to first ask about sex assigned at birth (male or female) and then ask about current gender identity (male, female, and "please specify"). A higher proportion of young people report trans or nonbinary identity, and 50 percent of all respondents reported living in one of Canada's six largest urban centres: Toronto, Montreal, Vancouver, Ottawa-Gatineau, Edmonton, and Calgary. The cities with the highest proportion of trans and nonbinary people were Victoria, Halifax, and Fredericton.[52] On average, transgender men were younger (median age of thirty-five) than transgender women (median age forty-three). Almost two-thirds of respondents identifying as nonbinary people were under the age of thirty-five.

Trans men and nonbinary people "of reproductive age" may be at risk of unintended pregnancy and seek abortion care. The experience of pregnancy, including "regrowth of chest tissue, widening of hips, and reduced facial hair," may trigger or exacerbate gender dysphoria.[53] Trans people are, moreover, at increased risk of sexual assault, which may result in pregnancy.[54] US evidence[55] shows transgender people experience four times the risk of sexual assault in their lifetimes compared to cisgender people. A 2019 US survey[56] of 1,700 "transgender, nonbinary, and gender-expansive people who were assigned female or intersex at birth" found 12 percent had experienced pregnancy, of which 21 percent resulted in abortion. Most respondents preferred medication abortion over a procedure, finding it less invasive and more private. Another US study[57] estimated that in 2017, 500 transgender patients received abortions in hospitals across the US, of which only 23 percent provided transgender-specific care.

Appropriately, there have been recent efforts in Canada to improve service inclusivity for people of all genders who may seek abortion care. The most immediate and obvious effort involves changing gendered clinic names, like the shifts to SHORS and ROSE described previously. Some clinics, like those in the hospitals in Moncton and Dieppe, were always called something ungendered, like "Family Planning Clinic" and have not needed to make a shift. Others, like the CARE program at BC Women's Hospital in Vancouver, may have inclusive names for their clinics but not for the larger hospital or health authority.

A.J. Lowik, an assistant professor at the University of Lethbridge in Alberta, has led efforts nationally and internationally to foster trans-inclusive abortion care. Their 2021 guide to trans abortion care,[58] now available in English, French, and Spanish, emphasizes the importance of language up front. They write that trans people "use language to help make themselves understood, to make their identities intelligible to others, and to help alleviate distress and dysphoria over body parts" and that language is a source of empowerment. Language can also cause great distress. Changing a clinic name and the language used on intake forms and other written materials are basic, minimal efforts to improve approachability of abortion provision. Lowik warns that the main barrier to abortion access faced by trans and nonbinary people "continues to be the reluctance of providers to frame their services in trans-inclusive ways. This is most obviously the case for clinics with women-only policies, where providers are asked to reconcile their 'women-only' frameworks with the possibility of serving clients who do not identify as women." For instance, several Toronto clinics promote themselves as "all-female"[59] and/or as having "all-female staff."[60] Lowik concludes, "If trans men and non-binary folks can be clients, abortion services should consider them as potential employees, as well. Having staff members that reflect the diversity of your clients is important as it clearly communicates your commitment to trans-inclusive services to potential clients and to the community at large."[61]

Whether an organization or business can restrict staff or even volunteers by sex or gender was the subject of a protracted legal dispute between Kimberly Nixon, a trans woman, and Vancouver Rape Relief Society (VRRS), a non-profit transition house and crisis line serving survivors of male violence (also known as Vancouver Rape Relief and Women's Shelter.) In 1995, Nixon was accepted into VRRS's volunteer peer support training program but was asked to leave when the organization learned of her sex assigned at birth, stating, "men were not allowed in the training group."[62] Nixon filed a complaint with the BC Human Rights Tribunal, which found she had been discriminated against by being denied employment based on sex and awarded $7,500 in damages. VRRS sought judicial review of the complaint, which found no discrimination and set aside the order for damages. Nixon contested that decision, bringing it to the BC Supreme Court,[63] which overturned the Human Rights Tribunal ruling. Section 41 of the BC Human Rights Act[64] allows "charitable, philanthropic, educational, fraternal, religious or social organization or corporation that is not operated for profit" that "has as a primary purpose the promotion of the interests and welfare of an identifiable group or class of persons ... must not be considered to be contravening this Code because it is granting a preference to members of the identifiable group or class of persons." In other words, if your organization's mandate is to support women, you are not discriminating when you support only women. Other jurisdictions, including the Northwest Territories mentioned earlier, have similar clauses in their human rights codes. The BC Supreme Court determined that Section 41 "preserves the right to associate" and for "non-profit organizations who fall within the scope of [section] 41 to exercise a preference for a subgroup within their identifiable group" — that is, to treat trans women differently than cis women.

Although Nixon brought her case to the BC Court of Appeal,[65] in 2005, the appeal was dismissed. BC added gender identity to its human rights code in 2016.[66] In 2019, the City of Vancouver cut $34,000 in funding to VRRS because of its refusal to include transgender women in all services, with Councillor Christine Boyle remarking, "It is, in my opinion, unnecessary to exclude trans women from vital rape relief and anti-violence services ... trans women as women are incredibly vulnerable to violence and deserving of equal protection."[67] VRRS[68] continues its emphatic exclusion of trans women from core services.

The legacy of the VRRS case is that traditional "women's" spaces can be unsafe to gender-diverse people. Abortion services need to be intentional and dedicated to inclusion of trans and nonbinary people to combat the dominance of cisnormativity and heteronormativity in reproductive care and ensure access for all.

Indigenous Peoples

Canada has a tarnished legacy with legislation on the books in two provinces — Alberta and BC[69] — to promote sterilization of people deemed unfit; this legislation was disproportionately used against Indigenous peoples. There are current class-action lawsuits alleging forced sterilization of Indigenous women by family planning professionals as recently as 2018.[70] Sexual and reproductive health care was and remains a site of racism, colonialism, coercion, and abuse.[71] The church-run residential school regime and colonial imposition of Catholicism on Indigenous communities has had implications on values and approaches towards family planning services.[72]

In a context of recognized cultural genocide against Indigenous women,[73] public health information that celebrates legal abortion and contraception may be perceived by Indigenous people as creating "a very clear message that mainstream society does not want us to grow our nations and is actively interfering with our reproduction."[74] For Indigenous people, access to perinatal care is more urgently wanted, and yet is not "top of the agenda" for mainstream feminism in Canada. Rather than a focus on pregnancy prevention and termination, Indigenous communities seek reproductive justice in a very broad sense as a means to "renormalize reproductive influence in our own lives by repairing the relationship between knowledge of our bodies and territories." Rather than focus predominantly on abortion as a hallmark of just reproductive health systems, it is critical that such frameworks also encompass ample, culturally safe prenatal, birth, and postpartum care.

The longstanding centralization of abortion care in urban areas likewise has a disproportionate impact on Indigenous people. Compared to the general population in Canada, of whom 18 percent live in rural settings, Indigenous people are more likely to live in rural and remote settings. The 2016 Census[75] found 40 percent live "on reserve," 14 percent in rural areas that are off reserve, and 45 percent in urban areas. Among First Nation communities, 70 percent have less than 500 inhabitants, and only 4 percent have more than 2,000.

While physical access to care is an issue, so are softer skills and aspects of care provision. A leader in this area of emerging scholarship,[76] Dr. Renee Monchalin,[77] and her colleagues conducted interviews with fifteen Indigenous people of Anishinaabe, Cree, Dene, Haudenosaunee, Inuit, Métis, and/ or Mi'kmaq Nations in 2021 to discuss their experiences of abortion. Most valued having options of where to have the abortion, to have a support person present, and wished they had had access to more post-abortion support, specifically from Indigenous support people. To improve access for Indigenous people, these elements of acceptability must be integrated into care delivery.

People in Prison

People experiencing incarceration in Canada — including pretrial custody, provincial and federal sentences, and immigration detention — face multiple threats to sexual and reproductive health. Women are the fastest growing population in prisons in Canada, and Indigenous women make up 50 percent of federally sentenced women.[78] Most incarcerated women are of reproductive age. Although the federal system, which incarcerates approximately 700 women on any given day, does have a Mother Child Program allowing children to live with their mothers to age four, only a handful of people qualify for it each year.[79] Survey research found 57 percent of women in a provincial prison had experienced an abortion,[80] much higher than the Canadian average of one in three. Most have experienced unintended pregnancy, and most have unmet needs for contraception.

Prisons are disproportionately located out of urban centres, resulting in geographic barriers to health care. While travel is a burden for anyone who requires it to access abortion, it is that much more onerous for a person facing escort by multiple officers, in shackles and/ or handcuffs, with violations to confidentiality and privacy inherent in the bureaucracy and logistics of the travel process. A study of distances[81] between prisons and procedural abortion centres in Canada found 13 percent of the prisons were located between 300 and 738 kilometres away from abortion facilities. Medication abortion is arguably highly inappropriate in a context of constant surveillance, limited access to menstrual products, social isolation, and unreliable access to emergency services.

Bans on use of the internet, costly telephone services, and limited visitation result in barriers to health information and dire loneliness among prisoners. Correctional procedures and security standards may result in patients being denied a supportive companion in labour and birth, let alone to an abortion clinic. When seeking services, people who have experienced incarceration report experiencing stigma, judgment, and coercion from family planning care providers.[82]

At 104 per 100,000 people, the rate of incarceration in Canada is higher than what is average among Western countries.[83] Yet health professionals rarely receive dedicated training in care for incarcerated people, and few sexual and reproductive health service centres have policies governing care for this population. The United Nations Minimum Standards for the Treatment of Prisoners,[84] known as the Mandela Rules, require prisoners to receive care equal to that available in communities. Dedicated content in health professional curricula and policy affirmations of provider responsibilities to treat incarcerated patients with dignity, confidentiality, and compassion would support providers as well as correctional officers and patients with respect to expectations surrounding appropriate care.

Newcomers

Research about the abortion experiences of newcomers, refugees, and immigrants to Canada is sparse, and furthermore, race-disaggregated data is not generally collected in health services, impeding understanding of experiences among people of colour. A 2014 Alberta study found newcomer women are not presenting for abortion care in disproportionate numbers,[85] while an Ontario study found highly varying rates of abortion among immigrants depending on country of origin.[86] A BC study found newcomers were less likely to use hormonal contraception before their abortion than non-newcomers.[87] This is an area in dire need of greater scholarship, attention, and action. The 2019 abortion workforce study did not ask about provider racial identity.

People with Disabilities

Patients with disabilities seeking abortion care are also understudied. Canadian researchers have found that contrary to myth, people with disabilities do not have lower rates of pregnancy than people without disability; in fact, adolescents with disabilities are more likely to experience pregnancy than those without,[88] and people with disabilities are more likely to experience rapid, repeat pregnancy than those without.[89] Patients with disabilities report barriers to sexual and reproductive care, including encountering health professionals reluctant to discuss sexual and reproductive health with them, physically inaccessible treatment settings, and lack of information adapted to their specific circumstances and needs.

People without Health Insurance

One of the greatest challenges with the current legislative framework governing abortion is that, although it is completely decriminalized and 100 percent publicly funded if you have a health card, people without a health card are excluded from that blanket coverage. International students and temporary foreign workers are large groups of people very likely to be living without the security of Medicare: in 2023, Canada welcomed 800,000 international students[90] and issued 700,000 temporary foreign worker permits, up from 300,000 the year before.[91] International students live in Canada for years, pursuing postsecondary education and spending tens of thousands of dollars in elevated tuition fees. Temporary foreign workers are essential contributors to countless sectors, especially the agriculture and food industries.

The portability principle in the Canada Health Act means that Canadians travelling between provinces will have their services covered even if they present a health card from another province. If a person moves to a province or territory as a newcomer to Canada or as a Canadian returning from a period abroad, that province or territory can institute a wait time of no more than three months to receiving a health card. As scholar Y.Y. Chen explains, how the provinces and territories have rolled this out varies greatly. In Newfoundland, PEI, Ontario, Manitoba, Saskatchewan, Alberta and Nunavut, there is no waiting period for newcomers and returning Canadians, but there are for other types of people. In Nova Scotia, international students must wait thirteen months before they can apply for a health card, whereas next door in New Brunswick, eligible students receive coverage on their first day of classes. In Quebec, there is no waiting period for children or if the service needed is related to pregnancy; otherwise it is three months. In the Northwest Territories, there is no waiting period for returning Canadians, but international students wait three months. In the Yukon, children do not wait at all, but returning Canadians and new residents sit out for three months. In BC, it is a three-month wait, regardless of a person's status.[92] Waiting periods are often justified as a way to mitigate so-called "health tourism," where people travel to Canada solely to access health services. However, Medicare is only available to people with proof of Canadian residency. Experts in this area, like Y.Y. Chen, argue there is no evidence of significant health tourism in Canada.[93]

Some suggest that in the interim, a person could get private health insurance to cover their needs. However, pregnancy is a pre-existing condition, which may interfere with an individual's eligibility. Furthermore, people without a health card may face multiple social, familial, employer, and knowledge barriers to accessing sexual and reproductive health services. The direct and indirect costs of unintended pregnancy are complex and substantial. Elimination of the waiting period is a minimum action that could be taken across all jurisdictions to reduce barriers to care.

* * *

The past decade has seen massive advancements in abortion access across Canada, including the implementation of mifepristone, expansion of scope among health professionals, the introduction of telemedicine, reduced logistical barriers, enhanced training and mentorship, gender inclusion efforts, and expanded access to later gestational care. More is required to address the underappreciated and underserved needs of equity-deserving groups, including Indigenous peoples, those in prison, newcomers, individuals with disabilities, and those without health insurance. These diverse identities intersect, with one population potentially crossing all: youth.

CHAPTER 9

CHILDREN AND YOUTH

> This chapter explains the unique considerations facing children and youth who seek abortion, including consent for health care and consent to sexual activity.

If the decision to have an abortion is the patient's, what happens when the patient is a child? While only a very small percentage of abortion patients are adolescents, the implications of being denied an abortion or of being forced to continue an unintended pregnancy, for any reason, are particularly severe for youth. In 2021, the Canadian Institute for Health Information[1] reported that of the 97,211 abortions for which they have records, there were 2,012 among people aged seventeen or younger, approximately 2 percent.[2] Youth seeking abortion services may have intersecting experiences of discrimination that deepen their vulnerability and the important role that controlling fertility has on their ability to thrive.

Across Canada, the fertility rate among adolescents varies significantly by jurisdiction. On average nationally, there are 4.4 children per 1,000 girls and women ages fifteen to nineteen.[3] In Ontario, there are 3.0, and in Nunavut, there are 67.2. Adolescents who experience pregnancy are at high risk of a rapid repeat pregnancy[4] and benefit greatly from unfettered access to contraception, as will be discussed in Chapter 10, "Contraception."

Youth and people who have never been pregnant before are at higher risk of not recognizing they are pregnant and being further along in pregnancy when they seek care.[5] Abortion is always on a timer: although there may not be any gestational limits in law in Canada, there are logistical limitations that can be prohibitive. Youth may already be at a disadvantage navigating the convolutions of the health care system because they start the process later in pregnancy.

Youth face barriers to privacy and confidentiality not only in their homes, but even sometimes by law, which will be discussed below. Just finding out what to do once an unwanted pregnancy is detected can be daunting; social media and web searching may lead youth to crisis pregnancy centres or other less deliberate, but nonetheless problematic, inaccurate information. It is difficult to have a medication abortion, with significant pain and bleeding, without arousing notice from parents or guardians in the home. It is challenging to travel to an appointment, let alone a series of appointments for blood work, ultrasound, and a procedure, without support. Even though abortion care is covered by a Medicare card and parents will never see the "bill," the care is likely to be on a health record, and youth may worry about who will see and share that information. Post-abortion contraception is usually not freely available, and youth may have to reveal their needs to use their parent/guardians' private medication insurance to pay for birth control. Furthermore, patient age introduces distinct regulatory and legislative considerations when health providers suspect a child seeking care is facing harm from older youth or adults. Health providers have a duty to report suspected child abuse or neglect to provincial/territorial child welfare departments.

Consent to Health Services

In the US, where 9 percent of abortion patients are adolescents,[6] most states require parental/guardian involvement in abortion care, such as requiring at least one parent be informed and/or consent to the procedure beforehand. Three states require *two* parents' consent prior to offering care.[7] This is not so in Canada, where abortion is treated as a regular health service. Consent is navigated in the same way all health decision making among minors is navigated — without the politicization of the service itself. It doesn't matter if the prescription is for penicillin or medication abortion; the process is the same. This was not always the case.

As discussed in Chapter 2, "With Laws Come Limits," after the 1969 Omnibus Bill partially decriminalized abortion, Section 251 of the Criminal Code required a hospital therapeutic abortion committee (TAC) of three physicians to determine if a patient's request for abortion care was warranted for maternal or fetal health reasons. The Badgley committee was struck by the federal government in the 1970s to analyze to what extent TACs limited equity in access to abortion across the country. Following comprehensive study of the issue, the Badgley committee found that

> uncertainties in provincial laws had been allowed to affect the hospitals' consent requirements for carrying out abortions. In provinces where the age of consent to other medical procedures was lower than the age of majority, for example, a substantial number of hospitals required a woman to have reached the age of majority in order to consent to having an abortion.[8]

The age of majority, when a child officially becomes an adult, differs among the provinces and territories. The age of majority is eighteen in six provinces: Alberta, Manitoba, Ontario, PEI, Quebec, and Saskatchewan; and nineteen in four provinces and the three territories: British Columbia, New Brunswick, Newfoundland, Northwest Territories, Nova Scotia, Nunavut, and Yukon. The age of consent for medical procedures, however, could be sixteen or fourteen, introducing a window of two to five years where consent was treated differently for abortion than it would be for other care, because of the judgment of the TAC. Effectively, it was more acceptable to force childbearing on the child than to relieve them of it, despite the safety of legal abortion compared to birth.

The 1988 *R. v. Morgentaler* decision ended the TAC era and the requirement that patients subject themselves to TAC judgment. To this day, the shame, stigma, and secrecy around abortion may confuse patients, parents, and health professionals about whether or how youth consent for abortion is any different from other forms of health care.

Informed consent for health services is characterized by three things: having the capacity to make decisions, having received adequate information to make the decision, and having made the decision voluntarily and without coercion. Unless the patient is in an emergent situation or unconscious, health professionals must ascertain every patient's informed consent before proceeding with treatment. As the Canadian Paediatric Society[9] explains, the wide variation in physical and psychological development between individual children and across the period from infancy to adolescence complicates a health professional's determination of the capacity of a pediatric patient to consent to receiving health services.

Provinces and territories still have different ways to define the age of majority as well as different legislation pertinent to age of consent to health services. The strictest is in Quebec,[10] where the age of majority is eighteen — the province's Civil Code requires children aged thirteen or younger have the consent of a parent or guardian to receive health care, regardless of the health professional's assessment of capacity. Between ages fourteen and seventeen, a minor in Quebec must have parental consent for care that is not required for health, such as cosmetic surgery.

In five provinces, there is no minimum age stipulated for autonomous consent to treatment; rather, all patients require assessment as to whether they have the capacity to understand the relevant information and appreciate the foreseeable consequences.[11] These provinces include Saskatchewan, Ontario, Nova Scotia, PEI and the Yukon. In four other jurisdictions — BC, New Brunswick, the Northwest Territories, and Nunavut — while there is no minimum age for consent to treatment, there are additional considerations when assessing the capacity of a youth. For example, in New Brunswick, where the age of majority is nineteen, youth ages sixteen to eighteen may consent to medical treatment as if they were at the age of majority. If they are younger than sixteen, however, the NB Medical Consent of Minors Act[12] stipulates that they can consent if

> in the opinion of a legally qualified medical practitioner, dentist, nurse practitioner, midwife or nurse attending the minor, (a) the minor is capable of understanding the nature and consequences of the medical treatment, and (b) the medical treatment and the procedure to be used is in the best interests of the minor and his continuing health and well-being.

Basically, it is up to the health professional to determine what is in the best interests of the child, and it is not always clear how they would do that.

The "best interests of the child" is a legal principle. If a matter pertains to a child and, for example, a law could be interpreted two ways, it must be dealt with in a way that centres the consideration of the child's well-being. The United Nations Convention on the Rights of the Child, which Canada signed in 1991,[13] requires that in "all actions concerning children, whether undertaken by public or private social welfare institutions, courts of law, administrative authorities or legislative bodies, the best interests of the child shall be a primary consideration." If requiring a child seek parental permission for a procedure might risk that child losing their parents' support, even experiencing violence or homelessness as a result, such a requirement is not in the child's best interest.

In Alberta,[14] where the age of majority is eighteen, patients under the age of eighteen are presumed to *not* have capacity to consent and parents or guardians usually determine what is in their best interests. In Manitoba and Newfoundland and Labrador, where the age of majority is eighteen and nineteen, respectively, patients under the age of sixteen are presumed to *not* have capacity to consent. Patients aged sixteen and seventeen are considered "mature minors." So, for example, to receive an immunization, the fifteen-year-old patient requires parental consent.[15] This requirement may be contested; a child has the right to present evidence that they are able to make the decision on their own accord. How serious the consequences would be to the child is considered when determining whether they can consent to or refuse treatment. The "mature minor doctrine," which "allows children who are sufficiently mature to make their own treatment decisions"[16] was recognized in Canada in 2009 by the Supreme Court's decision in a Manitoba case known as *A.C. v. Manitoba*.

A.C. was fourteen years old when she was admitted to hospital for internal bleeding stemming from Crohn's disease, a gastrointestinal disorder. Her physicians determined she required a blood transfusion to survive; however, the girl and her parents refused to consent to the procedure. She had previously signed an advance directive indicating she would never, as a Jehovah's Witness, consent to blood transfusion. Because the refusal of treatment was interpreted as placing the child in danger, the province "apprehended" the girl, meaning she was removed from the care of her parents and placed in state care. Provincial and territorial child protection law[17] governs why and how children are taken into state or foster care and, for children under sixteen, under what circumstances the state can act as a child's guardian and provide or not provide consent on their behalf to health services. The best interests of the child must be considered, including the child's religious convictions and the value of a child's development of autonomy. In A.C.'s case, Manitoba's Department of Child and Family Services sought and received court authorization under Section 25 (8) of the Manitoba Child and Family Services Act, requiring her to receive the blood transfusion.

She received three units of blood and made a full recovery.[18]

A.C.'s parents appealed the ruling, arguing it violated the child's Section 7 Charter rights to life, liberty, and security of the person, as well as Section 15 rights to freedom from discrimination. The Supreme Court of Canada upheld the court ruling, finding that Manitoba's Child Protection law balanced

> society's interest in ensuring that children receive necessary medical care on the one hand, with the protection of their autonomy interest, to the extent this can be done, on the other ... [it] is a legitimate response to heightened concerns about younger adolescents' maturity and vulnerability to subtle and overt coercion and influence.[19]

Further, the Supreme Court found the distinction Manitoba makes between children under and over sixteen is not "discriminatory" based on age but aimed at protecting the vulnerable. The Act allows children to "lead evidence" to prove they have capacity to make health decisions, while also allowing the state to intervene when the situation is very serious and the child's decision could have life-altering, or life-ending, consequences. Justice Abella proposed a "sliding scale of scrutiny, with the child's views becoming increasingly persuasive as the child achieves the intelligence and awareness required to understand fully the interests engaged."[20] The consequences of the A.C. v. Manitoba decision is that a youth's capacity to consent to health services must be assessed individually; there is no blanket law. As such, a youth's capacity to consent to abortion is assessed individually, with the care provider making a judgment based on the child's development, maturity, understanding, communication skills, and other markers of capacity.

Gender Diversity and Consent to Treatment

The rights of 2SLGBTQIA+ people have long been enmeshed in the rights to reproductive autonomy and abortion. The Omnibus Bill of 1969 not only partially decriminalized abortion, but decriminalized homosexual relationships for the first time. In spring and summer 2023, an anti-trans "parental rights" in education movement emerged in several Conservative-led provinces that could impact youth consent to treatment. In New Brunswick and Saskatchewan, the governments introduced policy and passed legislation, respectively, forcing schoolteachers to get parental consent to use gender diverse youths' preferred names and pronouns. Gender-conforming children who opt to use nicknames were not to be subjected to the same process. Alberta's Conservative provincial government went further, passing three discriminatory laws in fall 2024: the Education Amendment Act, the Health Statutes Amendment Act, and the Fairness and Safety in Sport Act. The first bill requires children under sixteen to have parental consent if they want to change their names or pronouns at school, and no student will learn about sex education, gender identity, and sexual orientation in school unless their parents opt *in*. The second prohibits "top" and "bottom" surgery for minors. The last restricts participation in female-designated competitive sports teams to people assigned female at birth.[21] As one of her first acts when elected New Brunswick's first female premier in fall 2024, Susan Holt announced an end to the discriminatory policy in that province.[22]

Access to gender-affirming treatment is deeply tied to trans youth survival. A 2017 survey of trans youth found 65 percent of those aged fourteen to eighteen had seriously considered suicide, with rates higher among trans boys than trans girls.[23] Only a quarter of respondents reported generally good mental health status. The authors conclude, "National mental health policies should include a focus on transgender youth as a population at extreme risk and develop strategies to promote positive mental health and reduce the mental health disparities for transgender youth." While Smith would ban hormone therapy for gender affirmation among trans youth, most forms of contraception to prevent pregnancy are also hormone therapies, are widely recommended and prescribed among adolescents, and would remain accessible according to the usual consent-to-treatment regime. The Canadian Paediatric Society recognizes that by age seventeen, half of children are sexually active and contraception should be a key part of the care from all health care providers supporting this age group.[24] Trans and gender-diverse youth are a growing population, increasing needs for gender-affirming expertise among health professionals.

The most recent census found one in every 300 people in Canada identified as trans or non-binary,[25] and a recent US study among school-age children found 9 percent identified differently than their sex assigned at birth.[26] Rates of access to a primary health care provider, comfort discussing trans health issues, and receipt of gender-affirming care among trans people in Canada varies widely by province:[27] the Trans PULSE Canada survey of almost 3,000 people from 2016 to 2019 found 44 percent of respondents had unmet health needs. Smith's proposal will exacerbate access issues and has arguably already contributed to worsening stigma about trans care.

There is worry that if gender-affirming care can be treated differently, abortion would be next. Alberta's legislation met a swift promise of legal action from Egale Canada and a provincial organization, the Skipping Stone Foundation. The Canadian Civil Liberties Association[28] fought New Brunswick's education policy in that province until it was reversed by Premier Holt, while UR Pride, a Regina-based 2SLGBTQIA+ rights organization, is taking Saskatchewan to court over its pronoun law.[29] Gender identity is one of the core protected grounds under the Alberta Human Rights Code.[30] Since 2017, the Canadian Human Rights Act[31] has included gender identity as prohibited grounds for discrimination.

While treating abortion differently than other types of health care is suspect, a youth's decision to seek abortion may have unique stakes that make it especially problematic to require parent involvement. The child could be a victim of sexual violence perpetrated by the parent or guardian. The parent or guardian could reject the child or turn them out of the house for participating in sexual activity. Allowing the child to make these decisions for themselves, without informing or engaging parents or guardians, may protect them from significant harm.

Duty to Report Harm to a Child

When a youth seeks care, while the care provider may feel confident the patient is able to consent to the procedure, they may be concerned about the child's legal ability to consent to the sexual activity that resulted in pregnancy. Or, they may observe signs that the child is subject to other forms of harm or neglect. In all provinces and territories, child protection legislation stipulates every person has the obligation to report harm or suspected harm against children to child protection authorities.[32] Failing to report is a crime and can result in being fined or sent to jail.[33] Health care providers have a strong professional duty to report and are enmeshed in identifying child maltreatment because it is so frequently associated with a need for health services. Protecting youth from harm by making reports is complicated: children may avoid care seeking if they worry their family will be investigated and they will be removed from the family home. The longer seeking abortion care is delayed, the more complicated things become from a logistical perspective, and abortion is always safest the earlier it is experienced.

The legal age of consent to sexual activity is proscribed according to the ages of people participating and is restricted by federal law; sexual activity with people under age sixteen can be considered "statutory rape" depending on the age of the individuals involved. Under the Canadian Youth Criminal Justice Act,[34] youth under the age of twelve cannot be charged with a crime. If a child is under age twelve and the person they had sex with is any age over twelve, the child cannot have consented to the sexual activity, the sex was nonconsensual, and the older person could be found to have committed sexual assault.[35] If the youth is twelve or thirteen, consent is possible if the partner is no older than two more years, less a day. If the youth is fourteen or fifteen, consent is possible if the partner is no older than five more years, less a day. At sixteen or seventeen, the youth can consent to sex with any person older than them unless that person is in a position of authority (for example, a teacher, or coach). At age eighteen, the person's ability to consent to sex is no longer restricted by their age under federal law. Consent is defined in the Criminal Code (Section 273.1)[36] as "the voluntary agreement of the complainant to engage in the sexual activity in question." It is not valid if the person is unconscious, or if someone is using their power to induce a person to have sex, or if they cannot consent because they are incapacitated (e.g., due to drug or alcohol consumption).

Family planning providers may ask very young patients about their partners and their sexual activity to understand patient needs and in an attempt to protect patients from sexual violence perpetrated by older youth or adults. This is not because, as in many US states, abortion is more "permitted" if the pregnancy occurred because of rape or incest, but because of the laws in place in Canada that criminalize sexual violence and obligate reporting suspicion of violence against children. Youth are particularly vulnerable to sexual violence, incest, human trafficking, and intimate partner violence. Although health care providers may feel profound concern for adult patients that they suspect are experiencing gendered violence, and they may counsel and support them, the obligation to report such concerns extends only to children. While the duty to report is meant to prevent harm, systemic racism permeates the child welfare system, and racialized and Indigenous children and families are reported at disproportionate rates and make up a disproportionate number of children in state care.[37]

Incest

Section 155.1 of the Criminal Code[38] stipulates that "[e]very one commits incest who, knowing that another person is by blood relationship his or her parent, child, brother, sister, grandparent or grandchild, as the case may be, has sexual intercourse with that person." In Canada, police-reported data show that parents commit approximately half of all sexual offences against children and youth, and girls are victimized more often than boys.[39] The rates of sexual offenses against girls peak at age fourteen. Furthermore, only a tiny percentage of sexual offences are reported to police and counted in national statistics; intra-family sexual violence is likely to be especially hidden and underreported.[40] That secrecy is particularly profound for children and youth in small towns and rural communities, where there is little anonymity.

Human Trafficking

Women and girls make up 96 percent of victims of human trafficking in Canada. There are various types of human trafficking — sex trafficking and forced labour,[41] forced marriage, and organ trafficking[42] — with sex trafficking as the most common.[43] Child protection is a precursor to most trafficking: over half of all victims were or had been involved in child protection care. A quarter of police-reported human trafficking cases involve children aged seventeen and under.[44] According to government data, 91 percent of trafficking is initiated by a person known to the victim; over a third are trafficked by an intimate partner.[45] Sex trafficking is inherently gendered violence and can result in unintended pregnancy and the need for abortion. Family planning professionals need to be attuned to what trafficking is, what it is not, and youths' particular vulnerability to it. They must offer not only contraception and abortion services but also resources for safety planning and support.

Intimate Partner Violence

Intimate partner violence (IPV), including sexual violence as well as physical and emotional harm, occurs fairly frequently among youth and is a common reason for seeking abortion. In Canada, reasons for abortion are not required and are not usually reported. The Turnaway Study, a landmark study of abortion experience in the US, found that one-third of patients seeking abortion did so for "Partner As Reason." Of these, 80 percent reported their partners to be violent, and the abortion was a way to protect themselves from further entrenchment in the relationship.[46] In Canada, 44 percent of women aged fifteen or over have experienced IPV; 80 percent of IPV victims are women and girls. Almost one third of people experiencing IPV are between the ages of fifteen and twenty-four. Further, women under twenty-five years of age are more likely than those twenty-five and older to have been sexually assaulted, physically assaulted, and emotionally, financially or psychologically abused by an intimate partner.[47]

Female Genital Mutilation/Cutting

Finally, family planning providers may encounter evidence of female genital mutilation or cutting (FGM/C). This is considered a form of aggravated assault under the Criminal Code. A recent study of health professionals in Canada found 90 percent wanted more information[48] or training to be able to respond to FGM/C. Statistics Canada has estimated that between 95,000 to 161,000 girls and women currently residing in Canada are at risk of experiencing or have experienced FGM/C. FGM/C is abuse and, if observed in a child, would be grounds for a health provider to contact child welfare authorities; the young person's fear of this could be a barrier to seeking abortion care.

* * *

Anyone denied an abortion faces serious and long-term risks of physical, social, and economic harm; for youth, the impact may be even worse. Youth with intersecting identities, such as youth with disabilities, youth in 2SLGBTQIA+ communities, newcomers to Canada, Indigenous youth, and youth in visible minority groups all experience intersecting types of oppression and may need abortion. Youth may face barriers to care because of exposure to social media misinformation, not having the sexual health education to prevent pregnancy and identify they are pregnant early, and because they lack resources and independence to seek care confidentially. Although consent for abortion is treated no differently in Canada than age and capacity to consent to health care generally, youth may not know they do not need their parents' permission for care. Depending on their age and the position of power potentially occupied by a sexual partner, the law may determine their sexual activity to be nonconsensual, and family planning professionals have a duty to report suspected violence against a child. Youth are disproportionately vulnerable to gendered violence, including sexual assault, incest, human trafficking, intimate partner violence, and female genital mutilation and cutting. Fear of child welfare involvement may result in youth avoiding care seeking. Youth require comprehensive sexual health education, respect for their capacity, and care from professionals who understand the risks of sexual violence and offer patient-centred support.

CHAPTER 10

CONTRACEPTION

> This chapter explains the important role of contraception in discussions about abortion and describes efforts to enhance access through universal funding.

Counselling and patient decision making about post-abortion contraception are underappreciated and inherent aspects of abortion care. Before every abortion procedure or prescription for mifepristone, ideally a patient is asked about what birth control options they have used in the past, what they have considered using after the abortion, whether they would like additional information to help them decide, and if they want a prescription or same-day, post-procedure, long-acting, reversible contraception (LARC) insertion. People with a uterus are at risk of unintended pregnancy for approximately thirty-seven years of their lives,[1] and people seeking abortion are, by definition, people who can get pregnant: they are a priority population for support with pregnancy prevention.

Access to contraception is recognized by the United Nations as a human right.[2] In 2016, the United Nations Committee on the Elimination of Discrimination against Women (CEDAW) severely criticized Canada for inequalities in access to abortion and contraception.[3] Contraception was only legalized in Canada in 1969, as part of the Pierre Trudeau government's Omnibus Bill that also partially decriminalized abortion. As previously discussed, decriminalization was but one step towards affirming access; the Canadian Levesque model of access includes the concepts of approachability, acceptability, availability and accommodation, affordability, and appropriateness.[4] Approachability and acceptability depend on health system connections with communities and nonjudgmental, supportive professional norms and behaviours. Efforts have been made in recent years to improve availability of contraception by expanding the scope of pharmacists, nurses, and midwives to include contraception-prescribing authority. Appropriateness is enhanced when more options are available, such as the recent implementation of the contraception implant.[5] The greatest barrier to contraception in Canada arguably remains cost, particularly the unequal burden of that cost. At $30 a month for thirty-seven years, a person can spend over $13,000 on birth control pills in their lifetime.

An Issue of Gender Equality

Economic barriers to prescription contraception are plainly an issue of gender equity because only people with a uterus seek pregnancy prevention. When upwards of 40 percent of all pregnancy is unplanned, and most unplanned pregnancies result in birth, the life consequences land disproportionately on people with a uterus. Negative effects of unintended parenthood include entrenchment in violent relationships, inability to pursue education and employment goals, increased risk of poverty, and physical harms that include complications from pregnancy and birth.[6] Furthermore, unfulfilled educational and employment goals impact civic and economic participation in society.

In recent years, the sexed and gendered nature of "period poverty" has gained widespread recognition. Not only do hygiene products cost thousands of dollars over the thirty-seven years over which a person menstruates,[7] people who menstruate are also responsible for the costs of over-the-counter pain medication, laundry, replacing permanently soiled clothing and linens, and days lost from work due to intolerable symptoms of dysmenorrhea. Recognizing the productivity and economic losses of period inequality, in December 2023 the Canadian federal government rolled out requirements that pads and tampons be freely available to employees in all federally regulated environments, including government offices, postal services, and even banks.[8] Countless municipal and provincial governments have followed suit, and many employers, schools and universities, and other large organizations ensure at the very least that their bathrooms, for all genders, are stocked.

Contraception is used to support menstrual regulation and minimize menstrual pain — in that sense, it should be part of the period poverty discourse. Approximately 20 percent of users of the hormonal (levonorgestrel) IUD (known in Canada under the brand name Mirena) will experience amenorrhea (the cessation of menstruation) in the first year,[9] with rates increasing after that. Short-acting, combined hormonal contraception formulations such as the pill, patch, or ring can be taken continuously, without the "sugar pill" week or "off week." This practice has been found to reduce "headaches, genital irritation, tiredness, bloating, and menstrual pain."[10] Contraception is another expenditure contributing to period poverty: it has yet to become freely available to all.

Contraception Economics

Canada is the only country in the world with a "universal" health care system that is without a pharmacare program.[11] "Universal" is a peculiar descriptor for a system with such a gap, but it is one of the five principles of the Canada Health Act:[12] public administration, portability, accessibility, comprehensiveness, and universality. What "universal" refers to is not that all common health services be covered, but that everyone registered in the health system through a provincial or territorial health card is entitled to care under uniform conditions. So, you do not get preferential access just because you are wealthy. The principle of "comprehensiveness" also fails to pull common pharmaceutical prescriptions into the Medicare basket — only medically necessary physician-provided or hospital-based services are currently included under Medicare. A tubal ligation surgical procedure, provided by a surgeon in a hospital setting, is covered. A packet of birth control pills dispensed by a community pharmacist is not.

The exclusion of prescription drugs from public coverage has severe consequences for economic equality: only adults with strong employment and robust health insurance benefit packages, and their spouses and children, experience reliable coverage and can confidently seek pharmaceutical treatment for health needs. Beyond that slim slice of the working population, coverage is complex and patchy. People on social assistance usually have coverage from their provincial/territorial government, and lower-income individuals may apply for means-tested provincial/territorial programs, but each program may have variable co-pay requirements and each is attached to a formulary — a list of covered products — which may or may not include the drug the patient needs.

Contraception options are often discussed in "tiers" of effectiveness. The top tier includes sterilization (permanent), such as tubal ligation, hysterectomy, or, for people with a penis, vasectomy. The top tier also includes long-acting reversible contraception (LARC) options, the contraceptive implant (Nexplanon) and the hormonal or copper intrauterine device (IUD). Second tier options include short-acting hormonal methods like the Depo-Provera injection (which works for three months at a time), the cervical ring (for three weeks), the patch (for one week), and the pill (for one day). Third tier options are non-hormonal, including physical barrier methods (male condom, female condom, diaphragm, or cervical cap), fertility awareness tracking and phone apps, and withdrawal. These are the least effective.

The more effective a type of contraception is, the more it costs. Fertility awareness methods, which can be free, result in approximately twenty-four pregnancies per hundred people per year.[13] Compare that with condoms, which cost less than $1 each, and the result is eighteen. The pill/patch/ring, which each cost about $30/month, result in six. Finally, the hormonal IUD and contraceptive implant (Nexplanon), at $350–$450 each, result in fewer than one. Yet the IUD is actually the most cost-effective options because, although the up-front cost is steep, since it only needs replacing every five to seven years, and the cost is spread out over time, it works out to less than $5 a month.[14] Even this method, at $5/month for thirty-seven years of fertility, would cost over $2,000. For oral contraceptive pills, the cost goes up to over $13,000.

In April 2023, British Columbia became the first province in Canada to incorporate universal contraception into its budget.[15] The decision came after years of vigorous evidence collection and strong advocacy. In 2015, the Contraception and Abortion Team (CART-GRAC) at UBC, led by Dr. Wendy Norman, set out to survey reproductive-age people (aged fourteen to forty-nine) across BC.[16] Researchers went door-to-door, in all corners of the province, and spoke with 1,671 people. No survey of this type had ever been conducted before. They found that 81 percent of respondents reported vaginal intercourse in the past year and had had an average of ten sexual partners during their lives. At least 89 percent were actively trying to avoid pregnancy, and that number rose to 98 percent among the teenagers in the sample. For those who had been pregnant in the past five years, 40 percent of their pregnancies were unintended. The need for effective contraception was apparent. Yet 27 percent of respondents were not using any method of contraception at all, and among the teenagers, that number rose to 60 percent. The researchers estimated that at these low rates of use of effective contraception methods, approximately 24,000 unintended pregnancies would occur every year in the province, resulting in 14,000 births. This is in keeping with a 2015 model of unintended pregnancy Canada-wide, which estimated that 180,000 unintended births happen annually, at a direct cost of $320 million.[17]

In 2019, CART went on to analyze elements of the Canadian Community Health Survey to demonstrate a clear association between lower household income (under $80,000) and reduced (and even no) uptake of contraception options among sexually active youth (aged fifteen to twenty-four).[18] Money clearly matters in terms of ability to prevent pregnancy. It is very difficult to counsel a patient about contraceptive "choices" when the choices are completely constrained by affordability. CART estimated that a universal subsidy for contraception would reduce the rate of unintended pregnancy by 13 percent within four years.[19] Among youth, it could reduce it by 20 percent.

The BC program for free contraception launched in 2023 with a three-year budget of $119 million,[20] or $39.7 million per year, which is the equivalent of $7.50 per person in the province of 5.3 million people. As of December 2023, at least 188,000 people had made use of the program, including 37,000 who used it to cover the cost of emergency contraception.[21] It is estimated it will take about four years to achieve a "steady state," where the public savings from avoiding system costs of unintended pregnancies equal the cost of public investment in contraception. After that, economic modelling[22] suggests the province can anticipate starting to, on balance, *save* money overall — approximately $5 per person per year, or over $25 million annually.

The BC program covers sixty different products and is straightforward to use. The patient seeks a prescription, takes the prescription and their health card number to a pharmacy, and pays nothing.[23] If the prescription is for LARC, an appointment must then be made with a health professional for the insertion. Generally, across Canada, LARC is only inserted by physicians or nurse practitioners, although numerous studies have demonstrated the efficacy of nurses and midwives in LARC insertion.[24]

BC's program is *not* what is called a "fill-the-gap" approach: every single person is eligible, not just those without other recourse (such as an employer-provided insurance plan or existing provincial coverage for people on social assistance). Fill-the-gap fails people who have coverage but for whom the coverage is inappropriate: they are required to pay up front, for example, and seek reimbursement. Or the insurance is in their parent or spouse's name, and their discovery of records of contraception could have potentially serious negative consequences, including violence. Or the coverage plan involves an arduous amount of paperwork and is so poorly promoted as to be effectively unknown, as is the case with many provincial plans. In Canada, there are over one hundred public drug insurance plans and over 100,000 private ones.[25] The complexity is bewildering.

In November 2023, shortly after the election of an NDP provincial government, Manitoba's new premier, Wab Kinew, announced plans for a BC-like universal program in that province, with a budget of $11 million.[26] The population of Manitoba is approximately 1.5 million people, with the annual cost again hovering around $7.50 per person. The program launched in October 2024.

Universal Coverage

Pharmacare, the inclusion of prescription medicine in the Medicare basket, has been a federal political promise for decades. In February 2024, the Liberal federal government under Prime Minster Justin Trudeau, in partnership with the New Democratic Party, announced Bill C-64, "An Act Respecting Pharmacare," to create a pharmacare program specifically for contraception and medications for the treatment of diabetes.[27] Although initially positioned as a fill-the-gaps model to supplement private insurance, it evolved to include language for universal, single-payer, first-dollar coverage. It was proposed to start with diabetes medication and contraception, presented as prudent, with more types of medication to be included over time. After all, over 50 percent of people in Canada have a uterus, and those people may seek pregnancy prevention for up to thirty-seven years. Almost one in two people in Canada has a diagnosis of diabetes.[28] All-cause mortality for people living with diabetes is twice as high as it is for those living without.[29] The impact of coverage for contraception and diabetes medication could be huge. Bill C-64 received royal assent by the Senate of Canada in October 2024.[30] Diabetes Canada[31] has suggested the bill could have been improved by emphasizing comprehensiveness and choice among therapies, ensuring it has the flexibility to adapt as improvements and innovations are made to treatment options, and securing robust consultation among key stakeholders, including patients and Indigenous peoples.

There is a nationwide model already in place for presenting a health card at the community pharmacy and receiving a prescription without personal charge: the model created to publicly fund mifepristone. As discussed in Chapter 4, "The Mifepristone Revolution," beginning with New Brunswick in 2017 and culminating in Saskatchewan in 2019, every province and territory made the decision to publicly fund medication abortion through their jurisdictional health card systems. And as discussed in Chapter 8, "Expansion of Care," any person without a health card, such as migrant workers and international students, could fall through the cracks.

Another consideration with Bill C-64 was that, as with implementation of free mifepristone, improving affordability of contraception is likely to increase demand for prescriptions. In recent years, efforts have been made to expand prescribing authority for birth control. Pharmacists can prescribe in eight provinces; Ontario, Manitoba, and the territories all have yet to adopt pharmacist prescribing of birth control. Midwives gained the authorization to prescribe contraception in Ontario in 2024.[32] Soon, registered nurses with specific training will be authorized.[33] In BC, nurses may be certified to prescribe if they first complete a six-week course in contraception management offered by the BC Institute of Technology.[34] There is also a BC framework for certification of midwifery prescriptions.[35] In Quebec, nurses can prescribe a six-month course of birth control pills.[36] Again, as the most effective contraceptive methods are the IUD and implant, beyond expanding prescribing authority, availability would improve by regulating nurses and midwives to insert LARC.[37] Regulated midwifery practice in Canada is usually tightly defined as encompassing care of "normal pregnancy." Ironically, prevention of pregnancy, like its termination, is not necessarily conceptualized as a part of normal pregnancy care.

Disinformation

Beyond cost, the other serious challenge with contraceptive counselling is the extent to which mis/dis/information is shared on social media, particularly among youth. A 2020 study of tweets about contraception found more than half of all mentions were negative.[38] As Schneider-Camp and Takhar explain, social media "consolidates the social constructions of hazards" associated with contraception and delegitimizes health professionals in comparison to peer influencers.[39] Anecdotes shared online are treated as scientific facts.[40] A large study of contraception content on TikTok found half of relevant videos addressed the creator's personal experience, in most cases the sharing of anecdotes about side effects.[41] Only 19 percent of creators "appeared" to be health care professionals, and only through their handles or even just their attire.

The availability of factual information is a critical component to accessible health care; it falls under Levesque's first principle of approachability. If a person does not know about something, they certainly do not know how to start seeking it out. In 2023, Action Canada for Sexual Health and Rights conducted a cross-Canada analysis of access to birth control by province and territory, called the Contraception Policy Atlas.[42] Newfoundland and Labrador scored the poorest overall, with New Brunswick and the Yukon next in line. In all three jurisdictions, governments do not share any public information about birth control on their websites. This information vacuum contributed significantly to the overall poor scores.

While multimillion-dollar budgets for free contraception are one thing, and adjusting scope-of-practice regulations in health professions is arduous, it is not complicated or expensive to add content on public departmental websites to direct and support contraception-seekers. This should be the bare minimum expected from health authorities, and factual information is essential to ensuring access to health services.

* * *

Access to contraception is recognized as a human right by the United Nations. Post-abortion contraception is an integral component of abortion care, and optimal contraception services include early and thorough information about options, informed consent, and equity in affordability. The financial, social, and physiological burdens of contraception are disproportionately borne by people with uteruses, just as the burdens of unintended pregnancy are faced unequally. British Columbia and Manitoba lead the country with the recent implementation of universal contraception coverage. Extending pharmacare to all is a necessity that must be paired with improved public education about contraception and expansion of health professional scope to widen the pool of prescribers.

CHAPTER 11

INTERNATIONAL LAW

> This chapter argues that as a signatory to international laws, Canada has indicated its support for the right to abortion.

While the specific rights to abortion or even to health may not be enshrined in Canadian law, Canada has signed multiple international treaties affirming the right to health. International law legally defines how a state is obliged to treat the people who live within its boundaries. Canada's participation in several such international obligations supports protection for access to free, safe, and legal abortion services for all.

A key function of the United Nations is to uphold international law. The 1946 World Health Organization (WHO)[1] Constitution established the WHO as a specialized agency in relation to the United Nations.[2] As the WHO Constitution stipulates, "The enjoyment of the highest attainable standard of health is one of the fundamental rights of every human being without distinction of race, religion, political belief, economic or social condition." Further, it specifies that "[g]overnments have a responsibility for the health of their peoples which can be fulfilled only by the provision of adequate health and social measures." Canada was the third member state to ratify the WHO Constitution, and in 1946, a Canadian, Dr. George Brock Chisholm, became the WHO's first director general.[3]

Two years later, on December 10, 1948, forty-eight countries, including Canada,[4] joined together at the Paris UN General Assembly to proclaim the Universal Declaration of Human Rights.[5] The Declaration set out, for the first time, fundamental human rights and their protection. Article 2 asserts, "Everyone is entitled to all the rights and freedoms set forth in this Declaration, without distinction of any kind, such as race, colour, *sex,* language, religion, political or other opinion, national or social origin, property, birth or other status" (my emphasis), while Article 25 insists, "Everyone has the right to a standard of living adequate for the health and well-being of himself and of his family, including food, clothing, housing and medical care and necessary social services."

The Declaration was followed by two treaties: the International Covenant on Civil and Political Rights (ICCPR)[6] and the International Covenant on Economic, Social and Cultural Rights (ICESCR).[7] Both treatises share identical language across several articles, affirming human rights to self-determination, to determine political affiliations, and to pursue economic, social, and cultural experiences. The ICCPR asserts the inherent human right to life. The ICESCR was adopted by the United Nations General Assembly in 1966, and it entered into force in 1976, the year Canada "acceded" (agreed) to it. In 1985, a body to monitor compliance was established — the Committee on Economic, Social and Cultural Rights (CESCR). Article 12 of the ICESCR recognizes "the right of everyone to the enjoyment of the highest attainable standard of physical and mental health." This would include the right to abortion — to enjoy a physically and mentally healthy unpregnant body — but it could also include the right to the food, housing, and other requirements for health.

The signing of an international treaty does not mean it is an enforceable law in the signing state; it would need to be translated into legislation to be binding. It was only in 1977 that Canada created its own federal human rights law, the Canadian Human Rights Act.[8] The current Act prohibits discrimination based on race, national or ethnic origin, colour, religion, age, sex, sexual orientation, gender identity or expression, marital status, family status, genetic characteristics, disability, and conviction for an offence for which a pardon has been granted. In the case of discrimination in relation to pregnancy or childbirth, "the discrimination shall be deemed to be on the ground of sex." Barriers to care required in pregnancy, including abortion, could be understood as an experience of discrimination based on sex. In 1977, the federal government also created the Canadian Human Rights Commission, which receives complaints based on the Act, and the Canadian Human Rights Tribunal, which acts like a court to hear arguments as to the merits of the complaints.

In 1979, the United Nations General Assembly in New York City adopted the Convention on the Elimination of All Forms of Discrimination against Women (CEDAW).[9] Canada signed on in 1980, and it became an international treaty in 1981. Article 10 requires that states provide "Access to specific educational information to help to ensure the health and well-being of families, including information and advice on family planning." Article 12 explains states' obligation to "take all appropriate measures to eliminate discrimination against women in the field of health care in order to ensure, on a basis of equality of men and women, access to health care services, including those related to family planning." Finally, Article 14 stipulates states ensure rural women "have access to adequate health care facilities, including information, counselling and services in family planning." CEDAW is monitored by the Committee on the Elimination of Discrimination against Women.

In 2016, in its report on Canada, the Committee on the Elimination of Discrimination against Women expressed concern about unequitable disparities in access to abortion and contraception in Canada.[10] It recommended that Canada

> (a) Ensure access to legal abortion services in all provinces and territories;
> (b) Ensure that the invocation of conscientious objection by physicians does not impede women's access to legal abortion services;
> (c) Make affordable contraceptives accessible and available to all women and girls, in particular those living in poverty and/or in remote areas.

There has yet to be a follow-up report. If there were, perhaps it would take note of British Columbia and Manitoba's remarkable programs to introduce free contraception for all, as well as the alarming consequence that affordable pregnancy prevention is now dependent on the province in which a person lives.

Every five years, Canada must answer questions posed by the CESCR.[11] In 2016, it was asked about the legal framework regulating abortion, any ethnic-based or regional discrepancies in access to legal abortion services, how expenses for abortion are covered, and any disparities among jurisdictions. Action Canada for Sexual Health and Rights made a submission[12] to the CESCR calling attention to the persistent barriers to access to abortion that existed in Canada despite decriminalization under *R. v. Morgentaler*. Action Canada's report referenced the concentration of abortion providers along the US border in urban centres, that only one in six hospitals provided abortion, that rural people faced unique barriers, and that there continued to be a complete absence of services in PEI. Canada also submitted a report, acknowledging that despite an absence of legal restrictions on abortion, regional differences persisted.[13] At the time, PEI did not have services. The only services in Newfoundland, a geographically vast province, were in the capital of St. John's. And it recognized that although New Brunswick had long maintained a requirement that two physicians approve each publicly funded procedural abortion, that requirement ceased in 2015. In response, CESCR concluded its report with a recommendation that Canada ensure access to abortion in all provinces and territories and ensure physicians' conscientious objection not be an impediment.[14] The Committee also recommended affordable contraceptives be "accessible and available to all, and in particular those living in remote areas and those living in poverty."

As this book has described, 2016 was a turning point in Canada's abortion access trajectory. Unquestionably, a reassessment today by CEDAW and CESCR would spark different conclusions. Both reports immediately preceded the 2017 implementation of mifepristone, which has undoubtedly improved access to abortion. They preceded a constitutional challenge launched against PEI that resulted in the 2017 launch of procedural and medication abortion services on PEI through the Women's Wellness Program in Summerside and Charlottetown (now SHORS). They came before the 2019 decision of the Ontario Court of Appeal in *Christian Medical and Dental Society of Canada v. College of Physicians and Surgeons of Ontario*,[15] which affirmed the legal requirement for physicians to make a timely referral for services they themselves objected to providing. And they were published long before the 2024 announcement by the federal government of Bill C-64, An Act Respecting Pharmacare, which intended to extend universal coverage for the cost of contraception across Canada.[16] The reports urged action, and action was irrefutably taken.

However, it is not certain the extent to which mifepristone, while likely revolutionary in impact, has indeed reduced disparities in access based on axes of marginalization, including income and rurality. It is entirely possible access continues to favour those with the most resources, the highest incomes, and the greatest privileges. Without question, migrants without Medicare cards still face cost barriers. We do not know how many health professionals weaponize their religious beliefs and turn away prospective patients who are themselves too ashamed or confused to complain. We do not know if and how Bill C-64 will materialize into a truly universal umbrella to cover all contraceptive needs in Canada. We do know, at least, that PEI's abortion program is stellar.[17]

The Office of the High Commissioner for Human Rights is mandated by the UN to protect human rights around the world. Its 2022–2023 management plan includes stipulations to "deepen understanding of the impact of discrimination on health rights," "to raise awareness among health workers of their role as human rights defenders and protect those who defend and promote human rights, including sexual and reproductive rights," and "promote and support protection of health-related human rights."[18] While the plan sounds idealistic and vast, some might ask what the UN can do, in practice, when it encounters health-based human rights violations.

A recent case shows how access to essential health care in Canada can be argued under international law. Nell Toussaint was born in the Caribbean country of Grenada in 1969.[19] At thirty years old, encouraged by a relative, she came to Canada as a visitor. She never left. From 1999 to 2008, she worked regularly as a housekeeper and in factories. She did not receive residency status or have a legal entitlement to work in Canada during that time. Nonetheless, several of her employers made deductions from her wages for taxes. In 2005, she hired an immigration consultant, at considerable personal expense, to assist her in gaining legal status in Canada. The consultant "turned out to be dishonest and provided no useful service."[20]

Without legal status in Canada, she never gained access to Medicare, public insurance for health service. She paid for things on her own, when she could, and sometimes received care pro bono. By 2006, she was unwell. Untreated, her diabetes progressed and her health rapidly deteriorated. In 2008, she could no longer work, and by 2009, the situation became life-threatening. Her diagnoses included uncontrolled diabetes, pulmonary embolism, renal dysfunction, proteinuria, retinopathy, peripheral neuropathy, hyperlipidaemia, and hypertension. Toussaint eventually lost her sight, had a leg amputated, and experienced brain injury and kidney failure.[21]

She received pro-bono assistance from another immigration consultant to apply to the Interim Federal Health Benefit Program (IFHP) — a special program in Canada to cover immigrants, including refugee claimants, resettled refugees, persons detained under the Immigration and Refugee Protection Act, and victims of trafficking in persons. Toussaint fit under none of these four categories of eligible applicants. She was denied.

Toussaint sought judicial review of the decision by the Federal Court, arguing that in denying her IFHP application, the federal government was violating her Section 7 Charter right to security of the person, as well as her Section 15 right to non-discrimination. The court agreed there was evidence that her security of the person was violated, but the violation of her rights was acceptable because "denying financial coverage for health care to persons who have chosen to enter or remain in Canada illegally is consistent with fundamental justice."[22] She turned to the Federal Court of Appeal, hoping they would see that this decision violated Article 6 of the ICCPR, the inherent right to life.

Again, the Federal Court of Appeal recognized that her exposure to health risk was so great as to constitute a violation of the right to life, but they placed responsibility on Toussaint's shoulders, insisting it was a result of her decision to remain in Canada without legal status.[23] She tried to appeal to the Supreme Court of Canada and was denied.[24]

In 2013, Toussaint became eligible for the IFHP based on spousal sponsorship for permanent residency status, and she began receiving health care under Ontario Health Insurance Plan (OHIP). But she would not rest. She submitted a complaint to the Human Rights Committee of the United Nations. Article 26 of the ICCPR asserts, "The law shall prohibit any discrimination and guarantee to all persons equal and effective protection against discrimination on any ground such as race, colour, sex, language, religion, political or other opinion, national or social origin, property, birth or other status." She aimed to win access to IFHP for illegal immigrants for at least the costs of health care required to live, as well as compensation for the psychological distress and inhumane treatment she endured.

It took five years, but in 2018, the UN Human Rights Committee sided with Toussaint, finding that Canada had failed in its international human rights obligations. It chastised Canada for excluding her from IFHP, reasoning the IFHP restrictions and their myopic interpretation in light of her life-threatening illnesses were "not an objective, proportionate or reasonable means of deterring illegal immigration."[25] The UNHRC instructed the Canadian government to ensure migrants' access to essential health care when their lives are at risk and to pay Toussaint for the harm done. Canada refused.

Two years later, in 2020, Toussaint filed a lawsuit against the federal government for $1.2 million in damages in the Ontario Court.[26] By 2022, ten nongovernmental organizations, including Amnesty International, the Canadian Civil Liberties Association, and the Canadian Health Coalition joined the lawsuit as intervenors. The Canadian government sought to have the case thrown out on grounds of jurisdiction, and further, they called her claim "frivolous and vexatious." Canada insisted Toussaint was characterizing herself as having a right to any health care anywhere in the world. And circularly, Canada argued that because no Canadian law incorporates international law, including the right to free health care regardless of citizenship status, and because international law cannot be directly enforced in Canada unless so incorporated into Canadian law, the Ontario Court should not allow the suit to proceed. Justice Perell disagreed, disgustedly calling Canada out for "a dog whistle argument that reeks of the prejudicial stereotype that immigrants come to Canada to milk the welfare system."[27] Perell's decision opened the door for Toussaint's suit to proceed. However, Toussaint died shortly thereafter, on January 9, 2023.

Toussaint's fierce advocacy has been characterized as not only paving the way for the health rights of migrants, but for many groups experiencing oppression to argue their Charter rights to things not explicitly mentioned in the Charter but necessary for life and security of the person, such as health, housing, and food.[28] In March 2020, as a response to the COVID-19 pandemic, Ontario implemented Physician and Hospital Services for Uninsured Persons (PHSUP) funding.[29] The fund's intention was to encourage uninsured people to seek treatment in order to reduce the potential burden of disease spread. This is, arguably, exactly what Toussaint had in mind: not necessarily all health care for everyone anywhere on earth, like the Canadian government attempted to characterize her as demanding, but at least the care needed to keep people in Canada alive. Like prevention and treatment for infectious disease, prevention of pregnancy and termination of unintended pregnancy are services that reduce future health and social harms.

The PHSUP covered medically necessary care in hospitals and physician-provided services in community clinics. Abortion fits that bill. COVID-19 vaccines, which are not necessarily administered in hospital or by physicians, were also covered for the otherwise uninsured. In March 2023, Conservative premier Doug Ford and health minister Sylvia Jones announced the program's end.[30] The Ontario Medical Association, sharply criticizing the decision, reported that under the program, 7,000 doctors billed for 400,000 patient services, and cost about $15 million over the course of three years. The Ontario government claimed there were "other ways" for the uninsured to seek coverage, but applications for a health card require submission of "three separate original identification documents: one proving they have Canadian citizenship or eligible immigration status, one proving they live in Ontario and another confirming their identity."[31] Hardly an easy task for people without these papers, living rough, facing language barriers, and with disabilities or mobility restrictions.

* * *

The *R. v. Morgentaler* Supreme Court decision in 1988 affirmed that, while not explicitly mentioned in the Charter, access to abortion is necessary to ensure protection of Section 7 rights to life, liberty, and security of the person. While the right to abortion is not explicitly enshrined in Canadian law, Canada has signed on to United Nations international treaties that effectively require its access be ensured, but Canada has faced international criticism for gaps, including lack of public funding for contraception and regional disparities in abortion access. Undocumented people, omitted from the Canada Health Act, are at greatest risk of being barred from health services. Toussaint's legacy, and her preventable, premature death, established just how obviously free services are needed for protection of the right to health, regardless of immigration status. In 2025 — a time of escalating xenophobia, white nationalism, and populist racism — securing free family planning services for undocumented people in Canada should be one of the greatest priorities of the abortion movement.

CONCLUSION

ONWARD

In many ways, abortion in Canada could not be more straightforward: it is safe, it is common, and for over thirty-seven years, it has been completely decriminalized.[1] But taking the service out of the criminal-legal system has not actually made it *lawless*. This book has traced the webs of laws and regulations in which abortion is entangled. Abortion is richly considered by lawmakers, care providers, and by advocates and abortion seekers themselves.

Despite countless attempts to reintroduce abortion law since the *R. v. Morgentaler* decision in 1988, people in Canada have become increasingly comfortable with abortion as a social norm. As of this writing, only 11 percent of people in this country oppose the right to choose.[2] Canada's abortion "lawlessness" is neither chaos, nor is it an assertion of access. It protects patients, the public, and practitioners from arbitrary criminal boundaries that could be subject to persistent lobbying and changes for the worse. It creates space and allows energy to be devoted to other struggles.

From 1988 to 2016, not much changed dramatically in Canada with respect to access, although much was happening behind the scenes. After a prolonged delay, the 2017 implementation and deregulation of mifepristone for medication abortion massively expanded the availability and acceptability of abortion for people across the country. Now patients can choose to have an abortion as well as *how* to have an abortion. Now nurse practitioners, family doctors, and even some midwives can prescribe mifepristone. Abortion seekers can pick it up at the community pharmacy, just like they do penicillin and antacids. Integration of abortion into primary care is deeply impactful: it diversifies the face of abortion provision, normalizes abortion care into the quotidian routine of family practice, and improves readiness of access like no other policy remedy has done before. The abortion workforce is ballooning, and the need for second and third trimester care is decreasing, a harbinger of enhanced patient safety and reduced cost, inconvenience, and travel. What a coup!

But the anti-abortion movement is active and enthused by the rapid deterioration of abortion care across the border in the US. While there have been some legal wins asserting the obligation to refer, disapproving health professionals wield their religious convictions as grounds to deny care. Buoyed by charitable status, crisis pregnancy centres proliferate. They leverage search engine optimization strategies to be the first hit when an abortion seeker searches online to find out what to do about unintended pregnancy. This can delay access to care, and withholding information about abortion suggests one should feel shame about seeking it. Outside of irregular bubble-zone protections, sidewalk picketers rely on Charter Section 2 protections of freedom of expression and assembly to distribute anti-abortion propaganda and interfere with people just trying to get into the doors of abortion clinics to give or get care.

Despite these threats, there are hearty efforts nationwide to advance abortion access. Logistical barriers like exceptions to reciprocal billing, two-doctor approval in New Brunswick, and the "wink-wink, nudge-nudge" tacit ban on abortion in PEI are all things of the past thanks to sustained advocacy. Scope of practice in relation to family planning keeps expanding. Not only can nurse practitioners prescribe mifepristone, but pharmacists can prescribe birth control, and some midwives and nurses can too. Providers across the country have stretched their skills to be able to extend gestational capacities, whether it be from twelve weeks to sixteen, or sixteen to eighteen, or beyond. Finally recognizing the unconscionable exclusion of abortion from core health professional training, more and more opportunities — and expectations — for education are available.

The fall of *Roe v. Wade*, while striking profound empathy in Canada for US colleagues, sparked inspiration and action. Canadian abortion care professionals rolled up their sleeves to attend to gender-exclusionary language, queer-friendly spaces, colonialism and racism, and access for people in state custody. Abortion doulas hung out shingles to provide unwavering full-spectrum support. There is a long road ahead to get this right, but the approach is changing. There is less defensiveness, more humility, and more understanding among abortion team members that feeling safe in an abortion clinic is more than bulletproof glass in the reception room. Patients need providers who look like them, are embedded in their communities, and care about what happens next in their lives. This change is not something a law can bring about; it requires commitment and self-awareness among the abortion workforce.

There are at least two groups for whom urgent legal changes are needed: youth and uninsured people. Uneven and unclear age of medical consent laws across Canada generate confusion and result in violations of confidentiality and possibly exclusion from care. Any restrictions on public funding of abortion, such as the blanket exclusion of people who do not qualify for a public insurance health card, are unethical, clinically dangerous, and, in the long run, fiscally irresponsible. Access to abortion is recognized as a requirement to enjoy the constitutional right to life, liberty, and security of the person. No one should be forced to pay out of pocket for that right to be protected.

Neither should anyone be paying privately for pregnancy prevention. An obviously sexed and gendered situation, the exclusion of birth control from Medicare results in profound inequity. Universal funding for contraception makes sense in every possible way, and it could save governments and taxpayers millions of dollars every year. Avoiding unintended pregnancy allows people to fulfill their education goals, gain and maintain meaningful employment, contribute to their communities, and, perhaps most importantly, escape gendered violence. The originators of the reproductive justice movement recognized bodily autonomy and reproductive freedom are not just about access to abortion, but rather about all the intersections between reproductive health and social, economic, and political justice. To have children when we are ready and able, we need access to pregnancy prevention tools like birth control pills. But the project of reproductive justice is more complex: we need to recognize gender inequities and the remedies that allow us to thrive. Universal coverage of contraception positions people with a uterus to govern their bodies, families, careers, and futures. It is basic and also big-picture thinking.

Canada has signed on to several international treaties that protect women from discrimination and assert the right to health. Canada's global leadership as an early and comprehensive adopter of abortion decriminalization should be mirrored in its actions to ensure the widest possible access to abortion and contraceptive care for all people who can get pregnant. At a minimum, migrants must have access to funded services, and birth control must be free for all.

So much has been accomplished in recent years that deserves to be recognized and heralded. People in Canada have moved mountains to improve abortion access in many ways. These organizers, researchers, care professionals, lawyers, and policymakers are at it still. Onward.

ACKNOWLEDGEMENTS

This book is my attempt to bring together an "Abortion 101" for Canada, an introductory survey to the service and the politics that have so gripped my attention since adolescence. Countless people have contributed to this book, through the lawsuits they launched, and I cited, the studies they led, and I read, and the care they provided, and I admired. But I will start with thanking my mother, Beth Paynter, who proofed every page before it got anywhere near my editor. Mom models curiosity, courage of conviction, and public service like no one I have ever met. She and my father, Jacques, an icon of care and skill, support my dreams and my family with zest and deep love.

Thank you to Fazeela Jiwa, the editor in question, and an extraordinary one at that, for welcoming this work and steering it forwards. I immensely appreciate the work of my research staff, Anja McLeod and Clare Heggie, to make this book a reality. There is not one single thing you cannot do. My friend and colleague Dr. Benjamin Perryman critiqued and reviewed every word, and his suggestions served to clarify my arguments and immeasurably strengthen this book. Thank you, dear friend.

I am profoundly privileged to work in near constant collaboration with some of the country's most dedicated sexual and reproductive health researchers in the Contraception and Abortion Research Team at UBC, led by Dr. Wendy Norman. I cannot imagine where I would be or what I would do without your mentorship and alliance. I estimate CART is responsible for half of the references in this book.

The other half may be attributable to the Abortion Rights Coalition of Canada, under the sharp stewardship of Joyce Arthur, and Action Canada for Sexual Health and Rights, currently headed by Frederique Chabot. These organizations, and Abortion Care Canada (formerly National Abortion Federation Canada), are the beating heart of sexual and reproductive health advocacy in this country. This book would certainly not exist without their labour.

Nearly everything I get up to is a partnership or project with Wellness Within: An Organization for Health and Justice, now led by Natasha Hines and Kristen Turtle. The board shows persistence, is genuinely open, and celebrates small wins. That is how a movement thrives.

In 2022, I left Halifax after fourteen years of immersion in a community of activists, scholars, and carers. My dearest Halifax friends have hosted me for countless visits back, made their way again and again to my new home in Fredericton to raise a glass together, and held me up when I would otherwise have been very squarely knocked down. I treasure you.

My witty, loyal, and capable siblings Emma and Willem, sister-in-law Erinn Bailey, and niece Ella are the strongest forces of support and fun. How grateful am I for your companionship.

Thank you to my partner Annie Mallory, a legend of kindness and joy, and to my kids, Freyja and Aggie, with their wildly independent minds and ways. Freyja beamed at me when she saw over my shoulder that I was writing the acknowledgements, wisely aware of what it means to get far enough into a manuscript to share thanks. I hope my brilliant daughters get to experience a richer world of reproductive justice. Better is always possible.

ENDNOTES

Introduction

1. Jacques Poitras, "Rising Use of Abortion Pill Shifting the Landscape," *CBC News*, May 21, 2023, cbc.ca/news/canada/new-brunswick/abortion-pill-expert-1.6859533.
2. Madeleine Ennis, Regina M. Renner, Bimbola Olure, Wendy V. Norman, Stephanie Begun, Lisa Martin, Lisa H. Harris, Lauren Kean, Meghan Seewald, and Sarah Munro, "Experience of Stigma and Harassment Among Respondents to the 2019 Canadian Abortion Provider Survey," *Contraception* 124 (2023).
3. Jason Herring, "'Deeply Concerning': Smith Suggests Privatizing Major Hospitals in 2021 Video," *Calgary Herald Online,* May 10, 2023, calgaryherald.com/news/politics/smith-suggests-privatizing-major-alberta-hospitals-in-2021-video.
4. Tanya E. Surette, "Privileging Heteronormativity in Alberta's Comprehensive Health and Sanctioned Religious Curriculum: A Critical Discourse Analysis," *Alberta Journal of Educational Research* 65, no. 2 (2019).
5. Quinn Keenan, "'A Little Bit Disconcerting': Alberta Scores Poorly in Poverty Report," *CTV News Calgary Online,* September 26, 2023, guelph.ctvnews.ca/calgary/article/a-little-bit-disconcerting-alberta-scores-poorly-in-poverty-report/.
6. UN OHCHR (United Nations Human Rights, Office of the High Commissioner), "International Covenant on Civil and Political Rights," December 16, 1966, ohchr.org/en/instruments-mechanisms/instruments/international-covenant-civil-and-political-rights.

Chapter 1

1. Wendy V. Norman, "Induced Abortion in Canada 1974–2005: Trends Over the First Generation with Legal Access," *Contraception* 85, no. 2 (2012).
2. CIHI (Canadian Institute for Health Information), "Induced Abortions in Canada," March 2025, cihi.ca/en/induced-abortions-in-canada.
3. Gretchen Sisson and Katrina Kimport, "Fact and Fictions: Characters Seeking Abortion on American Television, 2005–2014," *Contraception* 93, no. 5 (2016).
4. Ushma D. Upadhyay, Leah Coplon, and Jessica M. Atrio, "Society of Family Planning Committee Statement: Abortion Nomenclature," *Contraception* 126 (2023).
5. Lara Bullens, "The Long and Winding History of the War on Abortion Drugs," *France 24,* April 26, 2023, france24.com/en/health/20230426-the-long-and-winding-history-of-the-war-on-abortion-drugs.
6. Nicole Fallert, "What Does the Mifepristone Case Mean for Plan B? The Difference Between the Two Explained," *USA Today,* March 26, 2024, yahoo.com/news/does-mifepristone-case-mean-plan-170622727.html.

7   Amanda Black and Edith Guilbert, "Canadian Contraception Consensus," *SOGC Clinical Practice Guideline* 37, no. 10 (2015).
8   Laura Eggertson, "Plan B Comes Out from Behind the Counter," *Canadian Medical Association Journal* 178, no. 13 (2008).
9   Michelle C. Chan, Sarah Munro, Laura Schummers, Arianne Albert, Frannie Mackenzie, Judith A. Soon, Parkash Ragsdale, Brian Fitzsimmons, and Regina Renner, "Dispensing and Practice Use Patterns, Facilitators and Barriers for Uptake of Ulipristal Acetate Emergency Contraception in British Columbia: a Mixed-Methods Study," *CMAJ Open* 178, no. 13 (2008).
10 Chan et al., "Dispensing and Practice Use Patterns."
11 Honor MacNaughton, Melissa Nothnagle, and Jessica Early, "Mifepristone and Misoprostol for Early Pregnancy Loss and Medication Abortion," *American Family Physician Journal* 103, no. 8 (2021).
12 K. Louie, E. Chong, S. Ginde, L. Kuehl, S. Washington, M. Gatter, B. Winikoff, "A Survey Study of Marijuana Use for Pain Management During First-Trimester Medical Abortion," *Contraception* 94, no. 4 (2016).
13 Norman, "Induced Abortion in Canada."
14 CIHI, "Induced Abortions."
15 CIHI, "Induced Abortions."
16 Margot Sanger-Katz, Claire Cain Miller, and Quoctrung Bui, "Who Gets Abortions in America?" *New York Times*, December 14, 2021, nytimes.com/interactive/2021/12/14/upshot/who-gets-abortions-in-america.html.
17 Rachel K. Jones, "People of All Religions Use Birth Control and Have Abortions," *Guttmacher Institute Online*, October 2020, guttmacher.org/article/2020/10/people-all-religions-use-birth-control-and-have-abortions.
18 Sanger-Katz et al., "Who Gets Abortions in America?"
19 CIHI, "Induced Abortions."
20 Statistics Canada, "Births, 2022," 2023, 150.statcan.gc.ca/n1/daily-quotidien/230926/dq230926a-eng.htm.
21 CIHI (Canadian Institute for Health Information), "Hospital Stays in Canada, 2022–2023," February 2024, cihi.ca/en/hospital-stays-in-canada-2022-2023.
22 Regina M. Renner, Madeleine Ennis, Damien Contandriopoulos, Edith Guilbert, Sheila Dunn, Janusz Kaczorowski, Elizabeth K. Darling, Arianne Albert, Claire Styffe, Wendy V. Norman, "Abortion Services and Providers in Canada in 2019: Results of a National Survey," *CMAJ Open* 10, no. 3 (2022).
23 Ushma D. Upadhay, Sheila Desai, Vera Zlidar, Tracy A. Weitz, Daniel Grossman, Patricia Anderson, and Diana Taylor, "Incidence of Emergency Department Visits and Complications after Abortion," *Journal of Clinical Obstetrics and Gynecology* 125, no. 1 (2015).
24 Laura Schummers, Elizabeth Darling, Sheila Dunn, Kimberlyn McGrail, Anastasia Gayowsky, Michael R. Law, Tracey-Lea Laba, Janusz Kaczorowski, and Wendy V. Norman, "Abortion Safety and Use with Normally Prescribed Mifepristone in Canada," *New England Journal of Medicine* 386, no. 1 (2021).
25 American College of Obstetricians and Gynecologists, "Abortion Access Fact Sheet," n.d., acog.org/advocacy/abortion-is-essential/come-prepared/abortion-access-fact-sheet.
26 Peter Frank, Roseanne Mcnamee, Philip C. Hannaford, Clifford R. Kay, and Sybil Hirsch. "The Effect of Induced Abortion on Subsequent Fertility," *BJOG: An International Journal of Obstetrics and Gynaecology* 100, no. 6 (1993).
27 Janice Hopkins Tanne, "Abortion Does Not Raise Risk of Breast Cancer, US Study Finds," *British Medical Journal* 334 (2007).

28 University of California San Francisco, "The Turnaway Study," Advancing New Standards in Reproductive Health, n.d., ansirh.org/research/ongoing/turnaway-study.
29 University of California San Francisco, "The Mental Health Impact of Receiving vs. Being Denied a Wanted Abortion," *Advancing New Standards in Reproductive Health*, July 22, 2018, ansirh.org/research/brief/mental-health-impact-receiving-vs-being-denied-wanted-abortion.
30 University of California San Francisco, "Turnaway."
31 Julianne Toohey, "Depression During Pregnancy and Postpartum," *Journal of Clinical Obstetrics and Gynecology* 55, no. 3 (2012).
32 Renner et al., "Abortion Services and Providers."
33 Kevin W. Coughlin, "Medical Decision-Making in Paediatrics: Infancy to Adolescence," *Paediatrics & Child Health* 23, no. 2 (2018).
34 Medical Consent of Minors Act, SNB 1976, c M-6.1, laws.gnb.ca/en/document/cs/M-6.1.
35 Clare Heggie, Lin Tong, Aishwarya Heran, Ishika Bhambhani, Shelley McKibbon, and Martha Paynter, "The Role of Doulas and Community Birth Workers in Abortion and Contraception Care: An International Scoping Review," *Contraception* 136 (2024).
36 Christabelle Sethna and Marion Doull, "Far from Home? A Pilot Study Tracking Women's Journeys to a Canadian Abortion Clinic," *Journal of Obstetrics and Gynaecology Canada* 29, no. 8 (2007).
37 Christabelle Sethna and Marion Doull, "Accidental Tourists: Canadian Women, Abortion Tourism, and Travel," *Women's Studies* 41, no. 4 (2012).
38 Christabelle Sethna and Marion Doull, "Spatial Disparities and Travel to Freestanding Abortion Clinics in Canada," *Women's Studies* 38 (2013).
39 Wendy V. Norman, "Abortion Health Services in Canada," *Canadian Family Physician* 62, no. 4 (2016).
40 Diana Greene Foster, M. Antonia Biggs, Lauren Ralph, Caitlin Gerdts, Sarah Roberts, and M. Maria Glymour, "Socioeconomic Outcomes of Women Who Receive and Women Who Are Denied Wanted Abortions in the United States," *American Journal of Public Health* 108, no. 3 (2022).
41 Bethany G. Everett, Kyl Myers, Jessica N. Sanders, and David K. Turok. "Male Abortion Beneficiaries: Exploring the Long-Term Educational and Economic Associations of Abortion Among Men Who Report Teen Pregnancy," *Journal of Adolescent Health* 65, no. 4 (2019).

Chapter 2

1 Marie-Danielle Smith, "Canada Has No Abortion Right Law. Does It Need One?" *CBC News*, June 28, 2022, cbc.ca/news/canada-abortion-law-1.6503899.
2 Smith, "Canada Has No Abortion Right Law."
3 Barbara Surk and Nicholas Garriga, "France Becomes the Only Country to Explicitly Guarantee Abortion as a Constitutional Right," *AP News Online*, March 4, 2024.
4 Tanja Ignjatovic, "Yugoslavia Pioneered Abortion Rights in Constitution Long Before France," *Balkan Insight Online*, March 8, 2024, balkaninsight.com/2024/03/08/yugoslavia-pioneered-abortion-rights-in-constitution-long-before-france/.
5 South African Government, "Constitution of the Republic of South Africa, 1996 — Chapter 2: Bill of Rights," 1996, gov.za/documents/constitution/chapter-2-bill-rights.

6   Smith, "Canada Has No Abortion Right Law."
7   Center for Reproductive Rights, "The World's Abortion Laws," n.d., reproductiverights.org/maps/worlds-abortion-laws/.
8   South African Legal Information Institute, "Choice on Termination of Pregnancy Act 1996," November 22, 1996, parliament.gov.za/storage/app/media/ProjectsAndEvents/womens_month_2015/docs/Act92of1996.pdf.
9   *Le Monde*, "Enshrining Abortion Access in the French Constitution is a Win for Feminism and Democracy," March 4, 2024, lemonde.fr/en/opinion/article/2024/03/04/enshrining-abortion-in-the-french-constitution-is-a-win-for-feminism-and-democracy_6583154_23.html.
10 Republique Française, "Voluntary Termination of Pregnancy (IVG)," April 25, 2024, service-public.fr/particuliers/vosdroits/F1551?lang=en.
11 Pamela Druckerman, "Where France Differs on Abortion," *The Atlantic*, June 30, 2022, theatlantic.com/ideas/archive/2022/06/france-abortion-rights-roe-united-states/661447/.
12 République Française, "Law No. 2001-588 of July 4, 2001 Relating to Voluntary Termination of Pregnancy and Contraception (1)," *Légifrance*, July 7, 2001.
13 Marge Berer, "Abortion Law and Policy Around the World," *Health and Human Rights Journal* 19, no. 1 (2017).
14 Irish Statute Book, "Health (Regulation of Termination of Pregnancy) Act 2018," Government of Ireland, December 20, 2018, irishstatutebook.ie/eli/2018/act/31.
15 Health Service Executive, "When You Can Have an Abortion," *Republic of Ireland*, 2022, www2.hse.ie/conditions/abortion/how-to-get/when/.
16 An Roinn Slàinte Department of Health, "Notifications in Accordance with Section 20 of the Health (Regulation of Termination of Pregnancy) Act 2018," *Annual Report 2019*, Government of Ireland, June 30, 2020, gov.ie/en/publication/2e8ff-notifications-in-accordance-with-section-20-of-the-health-regulation-of-termination-of-pregnancy-act-2018-annual-report-2023/.
17 Megan Specia, "How Savita Halappanavar's Death Spurred Ireland's Abortion Rights Campaign," *New York Times*, May 27, 2018, nytimes.com/2018/05/27/world/europe/savita-halappanavar-ireland-abortion.html.
18 Joanna Mishtal, "Abortion Policy Implementation in Ireland: Lessons from the Community Model of Care," *PLoS One* 17, no. 5 (2022).
19 Alexa MacLean, "Anti-abortion Billboard Raising Concerns in Dartmouth," *Global News Online*, August 9, 2018, globalnews.ca/video/4379560/anti-abortion-billboard-raising-concerns-in-dartmouth/.
20 Ad Standards, "The Canadian Code of Advertising Standards," n.d. adstandards.ca/code/.
21 Ad Standards, "The Canadian Code."
22 ARCC (Abortion Rights Coalition of Canada), "Submitting Complaints Against Anti-Choice Ads," February 11, 2024, arcc-cdac.ca/submitting-ad-complaints/.
23 ARCC, "Submitting Complaints."
24 *R. v. Morgentaler* 1988 1 SCR 30, decisions.scc-csc.ca/scc-csc/scc-csc/en/item/288/index.do.
25 *Canada (Attorney General) v. Bedford*, 2013 3 SCR 1101, decisions.scc-csc.ca/scc-csc/scc-csc/en/item/13389/index.do.
26 Criminal Code R.S.C., 1985, c. C-46, laws-lois.justice.gc.ca/eng/acts/c-46/.
27 Heather Rivers, "London Transit Reinstates Anti-Abortion Law Bus Ads," *London Free Press*, November 9, 2020, lfpress.com/news/local-news/london-transit-reinstates-abortion-law-bus-ad-following-legal-settlement.

28   Hilary Beaumont, "Duelling Abortion-Themed Bus Ads Come to Halifax," *The Coast,* January 23, 2014, thecoast.ca/news-opinion/duelling-abortion-themed-bus-ads-come-to-halifax-4217256.
29   Julia Wong, "Crowdsourcing Campaign Launched to Counter Pro-Life Bus Ads," *Global News,* January 17, 2014, globalnews.ca/news/1091247/crowdsourcing-campaign-launched-to-counter-pro-life-bus-ads/.
30   We Need A Law, "International Standards Abortion Law," n.d., weneedalaw.ca/initiatives/international-standards-abortion-law/.
31   SRHR (Sexual and Reproductive Health and Rights), "Abortion Care Guideline," World Health Organization (WHO), 2022, srhr.org/abortioncare.
32   Action Canada for Sexual Health & Rights, "Why We Don't Need a New Abortion Law in Canada," 2022, actioncanadashr.org/news/2022-06-24-why-we-dont-need-new-abortion-law-canada.
33   Offences Against the Person Act 1861 C. 100 24 and 25 Vict. UK Public General Acts, September 22, 2019, legislation.gov.uk/ukpga/Vict/24-25/100/contents.
34   Caroline M. de Costa, "The King Versus Aleck Bourne," *Medical Journal of Australia* 191, no. 4 (2009), 230.
35   D. Seaborne Davies, "The Law of Abortion and Necessity," *Modern Law Review* 2, no. 2 (1938).
36   Davies, "The Law of Abortion and Necessity," 126.
37   de Costa, "The King Versus Aleck Bourne," 230.
38   J. Macnaghten, *Rex v. Bourne*, Central Criminal Court, July 18–19, 1938, 1, law.utoronto.ca/sites/default/files/documents/reprohealth/united_kingdom_1938_bourne.pdf.
39   Howard A. Palley, "Canadian Abortion Policy: National Policy and the Impact of Federalism and Political Implementation on Access to Services," *Journal of Federalism* 36, no. 4 (2006).
40   David Fraser, "Indecency, Abortion Offences Added to list of 'Unjust' Canadian Historic Convictions," *National Observer,* March 8, 2023, nationalobserver.com/2023/03/08/news/indecency-abortion-offences-added-list-unjust-canadian-historic-convictions.
41   York YWCA: Women's Collection, "Abortion Caravan Demands," May 1970, riseuparchive.wpenginepowered.com/wp-content/uploads/AbortionCaravan-May1.970-DemandsAndBrief.pdf.
42   Beth Palmer, "'Lonely, Tragic, but Legally Necessary Pilgrimages': Transnational Abortion Travel in the 1970s," *University of Toronto Press Journals* 92, no. 4 (2011).
43   *Roe v. Wade,* 410 US 113 (1973).
44   W.D. Thomas, "The Badgley Report on the Abortion Law," *Canadian Medical Association Journal* 116, no. 9 (1977).
45   Thomas, "The Badgley Report."
46   Thomas, "The Badgley Report."
47   Robin Badgley, "Report of the Committee on the Operation of the Abortion Law," Ottawa: Ministry of Supplies and Services (1997), 3, law.utoronto.ca/sites/default/files/documents/reprohealth/badgley-report-480-pages-first-half.pdf.
48   Badgley, "Report of the Committee," 31.
49   Badgley, "Report of the Committee," 19.
50   Badgley, "Report of the Committee," 24.
51   Badgley, "Report of the Committee," 30.
52   Badgley, "Report of the Committee," 32.
53   Minister of Health, "Canada Health Act Annual Report," Government of Canada, 2015.

54　Canada Health Coalition, "Canada Health Act at 40 — A Research Roundtable," *University of Ottawa Centre for Health Law, Policy and Ethics*, June 20, 2024.
55　Health Canada, "About Canada's Health Care System," Government of Canada, October 10, 2023, canada.ca/en/health-canada/services/canada-health-care-system.html.
56　CIHI (Canadian Institute for Health Information), "National Health Expenditure Trends, 2022 — Snapshot," November 3, 2022, cihi.ca/en/national-health-expenditure-trends-2022-snapshot.
57　Beth Ryan, "Abortions Now Funded in Newfoundland," *Canadian Medical Association Journal* 158, no. 7 (1998).
58　Health Minister Diane Marlean to all Ministers of Health, "RE: Canada Health Act," January 6, 1995, arcc-cdac.ca/media/2020/07/HC-letter-Jan1995.pdf.
59　Health Canada, "Canada Health Act Annual Report 2022–2023," Government of Canada, February 26, 2024, canada.ca/en/health-canada/services/publications/health-system-services/canada-health-act-annual-report-2022-2023.html.
60　Patrick Butler, "NL's only Abortion Clinic Almost Closed Earlier this Year," *CBC News*, July 20, 2022, cbc.ca/news/canada/newfoundland-labrador/abortion-clinic-nl-near-closure-1.6525340.
61　Government of New Brunswick, "Chapter M-7: Medical Services Payment Act," December 13, 2023, laws.gnb.ca/en/document/cs/M-7.
62　Martha Paynter, "Finally, New Brunswick is Being Sued for Unlawful Restrictions on Abortion Access," *Briarpatch Magazine*, January 18, 2021, briarpatchmagazine.com/articles/view/finally-new-brunswick-is-being-sued-for-unlawful-restrictions-on-abortion-access.
63　*CBC News*, "Morgentaler Abortion Clinic in Fredericton to Close," April 10, 2024, cbc.ca/news/canada/new-brunswick/morgentaler-abortion-clinic-in-fredericton-to-close-1.2604535.
64　*CTV News*, "New Brunswick's Only Clinic that Provides Procedural Abortions Outside of Hospital Setting Closes," filmed January 31, 2024, youtube.com/watch?v=btmyy7fDpVg.
65　Government of New Brunswick, "New Brunswick Government Budget Information," 2024, gnb.ca/content/gnb/en/corporate/promo/budget.html.
66　Canadian Civil Liberties Association, "CCLA Announces Victory and Discontinues Abortion Access Challenge in New Brunswick," press release, January 13, 2025, ccla.org/press-release/ccla-announces-victory-and-discontinues-abortion-access-challenge-in-new-brunswick/.
67　Jacques Poitras, "Holt Government Repeals Ban on Funding Abortions Outside Hospitals," *CBC News*, November 7, 2024, cbc.ca/news/canada/new-brunswick/holt-government-abortions-funding-1.7376879.
68　Niagara Reproductive Justice, "Abortion Cost Breakdown By Clinic," 2023, niagarareproductivejustice.com/docs/abortion-cost-breakdown-by-clinic/.
69　Health Canada, "Annual Report 2022–2023."
70　*Doe et al. v. The Government of Manitoba*, 2004 MBQB 285, ca.vlex.com/vid/jane-doe-v-man-680912821.
71　Women's Health Clinic, "Anniversary Timeline: Jane's Clinic Advances Abortion Care," n.d., womenshealthclinic.org/anniversary-timeline.
72　Olivier Bourque, "Judge Orders Quebec to Reimburse Abortion Costs," *Globe and Mail*, August 18, 2006, theglobeandmail.com/news/national/judge-orders-quebec-to-reimburse-abortion-costs/article1101922/.
73　National Abortion Federation, "Quebec Decides not to Appeal Abortion Ruling," September 18, 2006, prochoice.org/quebec-decides-not-to-appeal-abortion-ruling/.

74 Catherine Dunphy, *Morgentaler: A Difficult Hero: A Biography* (Random House of Canada, 1996).
75 Madeline Weld, "Henry Morgentaler: March 19, 1923–May 29, 2013," *Humanists International,* June 2, 2013, humanists.international/2013/06/henry-morgentaler-march-19-1923-may-29-2013/?lang=fr.
76 Leslie MacKinnon, "A Crusader's Legacy: How Henry Morgentaler Changed Canada's Laws," *CBC News,* May 30, 2013, cbc.ca/news/politics/a-crusader-s-legacy-how-henry-morgentaler-changed-canada-s-laws-1.1369361.
77 The Fédération du Québec Pour le Planning des Naissances, "Quebec History," *The Morgentaler Decision,* January 28, 2013, morgentaler25years.ca/the-struggle-for-abortion-rights/quebec-history/.
78 Henry Morgentaler, "Report on 5641 Outpatient Abortions by Vacuum Suction Curettage," *Canadian Medical Association Journal* 109, no. 12 (1973).
79 Judy Rebick, "What It Was Like to Fight at an Illegal Abortion Clinic in Toronto During the 1980s," *This Magazine,* June 13, 2018, this.org/2018/06/13/what-it-was-like-to-fight-at-an-illegal-abortion-clinic-in-toronto-during-the-1980s/.
80 *R. v. Morgentaler* 1988 1 SCR 30.
81 The Canadian Press, "Mulroney-era Documents Reveal Struggle with Abortion Laws," *CBC News,* November 17, 2013, cbc.ca/news/politics/mulroney-era-documents-reveal-struggle-with-abortion-laws-1.2430081.
82 The Canadian Press, "Mulroney-era Documents."
83 The Canadian Press, "Mulroney-era Documents."
84 The Canadian Press, "Mulroney-era Documents."
85 Tim Bousquet, "The Houses Around Colonial Honda are Being Prepped for Demolition," *Halifax Examiner,* May 16, 2016, halifaxexaminer.ca/housing/the-houses-around-colonial-honda-are-being-prepped-for-demolition/.
86 *R. v. Morgentaler* 1988 1 SCR 30.
87 *CBC News,* "Morgentaler Closes Halifax Abortion Clinic," November 29, 2003, cbc.ca/news/canada/morgentaler-closes-halifax-abortion-clinic-1.376738.
88 Nova Scotia Health, "ROSE Clinic (Reproductive Options and Services)," n.d., nshealth.ca/clinics-programs-and-services/rose-clinic-reproductive-options-and-services.
89 Lianne McTavish, "Abortion in New Brunswick," *Journal of the History of the Atlantic Region* 44, no. 2 (2015).
90 *PEI (Minister of Health and Social Services) v. Morgentaler,* 1996 CanLII 3713 (PE SCAD), canlii.org/en/pe/pescad/doc/1996/1996canlii3713/1996canlii3713.html?resultIndex=1.
91 *Borowski v. Canada (Attorney General)* 1989 1SCR 342, decisions.scc-csc.ca/scc-csc/scc-csc/en/item/421/index.do.
92 *Tremblay v. Daigle* 1989 2 SCR 530, decisions.scc-csc.ca/scc-csc/scc-csc/en/item/515/index.do.
93 *Tremblay v. Daigle.*
94 *Dobson (Litigation Guardian of) v. Dobson* 1999 2 SCR 753, decisions.scc-csc.ca/scc-csc/scc-csc/en/item/1716/index.do.
95 Laura Payton, "MP's Motion on Sex Selection Stirs Abortion Debate," *CBC News,* December 5, 2012. cbc.ca/news/politics/mp-s-motion-on-sex-selection-stirs-abortion-debate-1.1188154.
96 ARCC (Abortion Rights Coalition of Canada), "Position Paper #24: Sex Selection Abortions," n.d., arcc-cdac.ca/media/position-papers/24-Sex-Selection-Abortions.pdf.

97 Laura Payton, "Sex-Selective Abortion Motion Blocked Again," *CBC News*, March 28, 2013, cbc.ca/news/politics/sex-selective-abortion-motion-blocked-again-1.1365452.

98 Brian Platt, "House of Commons Defeats Bill to Ban Sex-Selective Abortion, but Two Thirds of Conservatives Vote in Favour," *National Post*, June 2, 2021, nationalpost.com/news/politics/house-of-commons-defeats-bill-to-ban-sex-selective-abortion-but-two-thirds-of-conservatives-vote-in-favour.

99 *CBC News*, "Ban on 'Entertainment' Ultrasounds Urged," June 13 2012, cbc.ca/news/canada/ban-on-entertainment-ultrasounds-urged-1.1242522.

100 *CBC News*, "Health PEI Misses Ultrasound Wait-Time Targets Amid Shortage, Growing Demand," January 6, 2020, cbc.ca/news/canada/prince-edward-island/pei-long-ultrasound-wait-times-1.5416735.

101 House of Commons Canada, "Bill C-311: An Act to Amend the Criminal Code (Violence Against Pregnant Women)," January 31 2023, parl.ca/legisinfo/en/bill/44-1/c-311.

102 Criminal Code, Section 223, 1985, laws-lois.justice.gc.ca/eng/acts/C-46/section-223.html.

103 The Canadian Press, "Conservative Bill Defeated Amid Concerns It Would Promote Fetal Rights," *Global News*, June 14, 2023, globalnews.ca/news/9769739/conservatives-violence-against-pregnant-women-fetal-rights/.

104 Laura Jane McLeod, Katherine E. McLeod, Jessica Liauw, Alison Carter Ramirez, Mary Coll-Black, and Fiona G. Kouyoumdjian, "Antenatal Obstetrician Care Among People who Experience Incarceration in Ontario: A Retrospective Cohort Study," *Journal of Obstetrics and Gynaecology Canada* 45, no. 5 (2023).

105 Alison Carter Ramirez, Jessica Liauw, Alice Cavanagh, Dustin Costescu, Laura Holder, Hong Lu, and Fiona G. Kouyoumdjian, "Quality of Antenatal Care for Women who Experience Imprisonment in Ontario, Canada," *Journal of the American Medical Association (JAMA) Network Open* 3, no. 8 (2020).

106 Alison Carter Ramirez, Jessica Liauw, Dustin Costescu, Laura Holder, Hong Lu and Fiona G. Kouyoumdjian, "Infant and Maternal Outcomes for Women who Experience Imprisonment in Ontario, Canada: A Retrospective Cohort Study," *Journal of Obstetrics and Gynaecology Canada* 42, no. 4 (2020).

Chapter 3

1 Statistics Canada, "Data Quality, Concepts and Methodology: Vital Statistics — Stillbirth Database," 2004, 150.statcan.gc.ca/n1/pub/84f0211x/2004000/4068009-eng.htm.

2 K.S. Joseph, Lily Lee, Laura Arbour, Nathalie Auger, Elizabeth K. Darling, Jane Evans, Julian Little, Sarah D. McDonald, Aideen Moore, Phil A. Murphy, Joel G. Ray, Heather Scott, Prakesh Shah, Michiel VanDenHof, and Michael S. Kramer, "Stillbirth in Canada: Anachronistic Definition and Registration Processes Impede Public health Surveillance and Clinical Care," *Canada Journal of Public Health* 112, no. 4 (2021).

3 Joseph et al., "Stillbirth in Canada."

4 Statistics Canada, "Vital Statistics Death Database — Glossary."

5 Joseph et al., "Stillbirth in Canada."

6 Joseph et al., "Stillbirth in Canada."

7 Statistics Canada, "Live Births and Fetal Deaths (Stillbirths), by Type of Birth (Single or Multiple)," 2023, open.canada.ca/data/en/dataset/2715a5f7-e101-4757-a263-a59b0ef3ac03.

8   K.S. Joseph, Brooke Kinniburgh, Jennifer A. Hutcheon, Azar Mehrabadi, Melanie Basso, Cheryl Davies, and Lily Lee, "Determinants of Increases in Stillbirth Rates from 2000 to 2010," *Canadian Medical Association Journal* 185, no. 8 (2013).
9   Public Health Agency of Canada, "Chapter 7: Loss and Grief. 1.2: Loss During Pregnancy," in *Family-centred Maternity and Newborn Care: National Guidelines*, December 13, 2020, canada.ca/en/public-health/services/maternity-newborn-care-guidelines.html.
10 Joseph et al., "Stillbirth in Canada."
11 CDC (Centers for Disease Control and Prevention), "Data and Statistics on Stillbirth," n.d., cdc.gov/stillbirth/data-research/index.html.
12 Line Leduc, "Guideline No. 394 — Stillbirth Investigation," *Journal of Obstetrics and Gynaecology Canada* 42, no. 1 (2020).
13 Christy Burden, Danya Bakhbakhi, Alexander Edward Heazell, Mary Lynch, Laura Timlin, Charlotte Bevan, Claire Storey, Jennifer J. Kurinczuk, and Dimitrios Siassakos, "Parents' Active Role and Engagement in the Review of their Stillbirth/Perinatal Death 2 (PARENTS 2) Study: A Mixed-Methods Study of Implementation," *British Medical Journal* 11, no. 3 (2020).
14 BC Vital Statistics Agency, "Facts and Fiction of Online Death Registration," Ministry of Health, June 2011, slideshare.net/fsabc/bc-vital-statistics-agency#7.
15 Government of British Columbia, "Vital Statistics Act: Chapter 479," 1996, bclaws.gov.bc.ca/civix/document/id/complete/statreg/00_96479_01.
16 Statistics Canada, "Vital Statistics — Stillbirth Database (CVSS)," n.d., www23.statcan.gc.ca/imdb/p2SV.pl?Function=getSurvey&SDDS=3234.
17 Ministry of Government and Consumer Services, "Handbook on Medical Certification of Death & Stillbirth," *Office of the Registrar General*, December 2019, publications.gov.on.ca/store/20170501121/Free_Download_Files/300146.pdf.
18 Statistics Canada, "Data Quality, Concepts and Methodology: Definitions," 2012, 150.statcan.gc.ca/n1/pub/84f0210x/2008000/technote-notetech1-eng.htm.
19 E. Paul Kirk, "Psychological Effects and Management of Perinatal Loss," *American Journal of Obstetrics and Gynaecology* 149, no. 1 (1984).
20 Melanie Human, Sulina Green, Coen Groenewald, Richard D. Goldstein, Hannah C. Kinney, and Hein J. Odendaal, "Psychological Implication of Stillbirth for the Mother and her Family: A Crisis-Support Approach," *Social Work* 50, no. 4 (2014).
21 Joseph et al., "Stillbirth in Canada."
22 Wellness Within, "Accessing Abortion in Canada," n.d., static1.squarespace.com/static/5a17715d8dd04195b6708c76/t/62b9fa0be614e479268adcf4/1656355352734/Abortion+pamphlet.pdf.
23 Alberta Health Services, "Termination of Pregnancy," *Provincial Women's Health Committee*, May 2017, static1.squarespace.com/static/5a17715d8dd04195b-6708c76/t/62b9fa0be614e479268adcf4/1656355352734/Abortion+pamphlet.pdf.
24 Cabbagetown Women's Clinic, n.d., cabbagetownwomensclinic.com/.
25 Government of Canada, "EI Maternity and Parental Benefits," October 2023, canada.ca/en/services/benefits/ei/ei-maternity-parental/special-circumstances.html.
26 Government of Prince Edward Island, "Bereavement Leave (Death in the Family)," June 6, 2024, princeedwardisland.ca/en/information/workforce-advanced-learning-and-population/bereavement-leave-death-in-the-family.
27 Government of Nova Scotia, "Leaves from Work: Pregnancy Leave, Leave for End of Pregnancy and Parental Leave," *Labour, Skills and Immigration*, n.d., novascotia.ca/lae/employmentrights/leaves.asp.

28 Katie Dangerfield, "Paid Pregnancy Loss Leave Included in Budget 2023. But Who Can Get It?" *Global News,* March 30, 2023, globalnews.ca/news/9586724/pregnany-loss-paid-leave-federal-budget/.
29 Criminal Code, Section 223, 1985.
30 *CBC News,* "Andrea Giesbrecht gets 8 ½ Years for Concealing Remains of 6 Infants," July 14, 2017, cbc.ca/news/canada/manitoba/judge-rejects-andrea-giesbrecht-delay-motion-1.4204123.
31 Russell Fung, Jose Villar, Ali Dashti, ... and International Fetal and Newborn Growth Consortium for the 21st Century, "Achieving Accurate Estimates of Fetal Gestational Age and Personalized Prediction of Fetal Growth Based on Data from an International Prospective Cohort Study: A Population-Based Machine Learning Study," *Lancet Digital Health* 2, no. 7 (2020).
32 Katie Watson and Cara Angelotta, "The Frequency of Pregnancy Recognition Across the Gestational Spectrum and its Consequences in the United States," *Perspectives on Sexual and Reproductive Health* 54, no. 2 (2022).
33 *R. v. ADH* 2013 3 SCR 269, decisions.scc-csc.ca/scc-csc/scc-csc/en/item/13051/index.do.
34 *CBC News,* "Wal-Mart Baby Abandonment Case Heard at Supreme Court," October 11, 2012, cbc.ca/news/canada/saskatchewan/wal-mart-baby-abandonment-case-heard-at-supreme-court-1.1220913.
35 Louie Rosella, "Woman Acquitted of Concealing her Newborn's Death," *Mississauga News,* September 23, 2014, mississauga.com/news/woman-acquitted-of-concealing-her-newborns-death/article_21e6dd80-47ce-5a94-beb5-9e7b104c1d3a.html.
36 *R. v. Levkovic* 2014 CR 06 1253, decisions.scc-csc.ca/scc-csc/scc-csc/en/item/13031/index.do.
37 *R. v. Levkovic* 2014 CR 06 1253.
38 *Toronto Star,* "Former GTA Stripper Acquitted of Concealing Dead Baby's Body," September 24, 2014, thestar.com/news/gta/former-gta-stripper-acquitted-of-concealing-dead-baby-s-body/article_982671e2-dd8e-537d-ba2d-64b62beec83b.html.
39 Stephanie Voudouris, "If it's About Pregnancy, it's About Women: Ivana Levkovic v. Her Majesty the Queen," *The Court* (York University), October 18, 2012, yorku.ca/osgoode/thecourt/2012/10/18/if-its-about-pregnancy-its-about-women-ivana-levkovic-v-her-majesty-the-queen/.
40 *R. v. Sullivan* 1986 55 CR (3d) 48.
41 LEAF (Women's Legal Education & Action Fund), "R. v. Sullivan: Case Summary," n.d., leaf.ca/case_summary/r-v-sullivan-1991/.
42 *R. v. Sullivan* 1991 1 SCR 489, decisions.scc-csc.ca/scc-csc/scc-csc/en/item/733/index.do.
43 BCCNM (British Columbia College of Nurses & Midwives), "Practising Midwifery in BC," n.d., bccnm.ca/Public/BecomingAMidwife/Pages/practising_midwifery.aspx.
44 CAM (Canadian Association of Midwives), "Discover Midwifery Across Canada," 2021, canadianmidwives.org/about-midwifery/.
45 *CBC News,* "Midwife Jailed for Contempt of Court," July 25, 2002, cbc.ca/lite/story/1.319144.
46 Jason Proctor, "BC 'Childbirth Activist' Charged with Manslaughter in Newborn's Death," *CBC News,* January 7, 2025, cbc.ca/news/canada/british-columbia/gloria-lemay-charged-manslaughter-1.7425173.
47 Canadian Association of Midwives, "Year of Midwifery Regulation," *Canadian Association of Midwives,* October 19, 2016, canadianmidwives.org/year-of-regulation/.

48 Government of Yukon, "Midwifery Integration Amendments Act Receives Assent," October 24, 2022, yukon.ca/en/news/midwifery-integration-amendments-act-receives-assent.
49 Government of Prince Edward Island, "Midwives Regulations," *Legislative Counsel Office,* April 1, 2024, princeedwardisland.ca/sites/default/files/legislation/r10-1-5-1-regulated_health_professions_act_midwives_regulations.pdf.
50 Carol-Anne Vallée, Ana Clara Sosa Cazales, Brian Fitzsimmons, and Wendy V. Norman, "Abortion Care in BC: Evolving Practice and Next Steps," *British Medical Journal* 65, no. 4 (2023).

Chapter 4

1 Bela Ganatra, "Health Worker Roles in Safe Abortion Care and Post-Abortion Contraception," *Lancet Global Health* 3, no. 9 (2015).
2 Christina Rørbye, Mogens Nørgaard, and Lisbeth Nilas, "Medical versus Surgical Abortion: Comparing Satisfaction and Potential Confounders in a Partly Randomized Study," *Human Reproduction* 20, no. 3 (2005), 834–38.
3 Laura Eggertson, "Plan B Comes Out from behind the Counter," *Canadian Medical Association Journal* 178, no. 13 (2008).
4 FDA (US Food and Drug Administration), "Plan B One-Step (1.5 mg levonorgestrel) Information," December 23, 2022, fda.gov/drugs/postmarket-drug-safety-information-patients-and-providers/plan-b-one-step-15-mg-levonorgestrel-information.
5 Shoppers Drug Mart, "Plan B," n.d., shop.shoppersdrugmart.ca/p/BB_369536000022.
6 Lauren Vogel, "Rethink Weight Limits on Morning-after Pill," *Canadian Medical Association Journal* 187, no. 10 (2015), 719–20.
7 Ottawa Public Health, "Emergency Contraception," September 2018, ottawapublichealth.ca/en/public-health-topics/resources/Documents/Emergency-contraception_accessible_EN.pdf.
8 WHO (World Health Organization), "World Health Organization Model List of Essential Medicines — 23rd List, 2023," in *The Selection and Use of Essential Medicines 2023: Executive Summary of the Report of the 24th WHO Expert Committee on the Selection and Use of Essential Medicines* (Geneva: World Health Organization, 2023).
9 Melissa J. Chen and Mitchell D. Creinin, "Mifepristone With Buccal Misoprostol for Medical Abortion: A Systematic Review," *Obstetrics and Gynecology (New York, 1953)* 126, no. 1 (2015).
10 Andrea Carson, Emma Stirling-Cameron, Martha Paynter, Sarah Munro, Wendy V. Norman, Kelley Kilpatrick, Stephanie Begun, and Ruth Martin-Misener, "Barriers and Enablers to Nurse Practitioner Implementation of Medication Abortion in Canada: A Qualitative Study," *PloS One* 18, no. 1 (2023).
11 Jennifer L. Kerns, Katherine Brown, Siripanth Nippita, and Jody Steinauer, "Society of Family Planning Clinical Recommendation: Management of Hemorrhage at the Time of Abortion," *Contraception* 129 (2024).
12 CIHR (Canadian Institutes of Health Research), "Funding Decisions Database; Detailed Information — How Far is Too Far? Study," December 15, 2023, cihr-irsc.gc.ca/decisions/p/project_details.html?applId=488394&lang=en.
13 American College of Obstetricians and Gynecologists (ACOG), "Facts Are Important: Understanding Ectopic Pregnancy," n.d., acog.org/advocacy/facts-are-important/understanding-ectopic-pregnancy.

14 American College of Obstetricians and Gynecologists (ACOG), "FAQ: Ectopic Pregnancy," April 2020, acog.org/womens-health/faqs/ectopic-pregnancy.
15 Laura Schummers, Elizabeth K. Darling, Sheila Dunn, Kimberlyn McGrail, Anastasia Gayowsky, Michael R. Law, Tracey-Lea Laba, Janusz Kaczorowski, and Wendy V. Norman, "Abortion Safety and Use with Normally Prescribed Mifepristone in Canada," *New England Journal of Medicine* 386, no. 1 (2022).
16 Wendy V. Norman, Edith R. Guilbert, Christopher Okpaleke, Althea S. Hayden, E. Steven Lichtenberg, Maureen Paul, Katharine O'Connell White, and Heidi E. Jones, "Abortion Services in Canada: Results of the 2012 National Survey," *Contraception* 90, no. 3 (2014).
17 Willow Clinic: Willow Reproductive Health Care, "Welcome to Willow," n.d., willowclinic.ca/.
18 Pfizer Canada, "Methotrexate Injection USP" (2024), webfiles.pfizer.com/file/b0c8bdd6-1dd2-4d93-be0e-1dc79307a115?referrer=ccb731e5-4f2d-4f4a-b2dc-e5e912145fc6.
19 Kevin K. Ogilvie and Art Eggleton, *Prescription Pharmaceuticals in Canada: Off-label Use* (Ottawa: Standing Senate Committee on Social Affairs, Science and Technology Senate, January 2014), publications.gc.ca/site/eng/461021/publication.html?wbdisable=true.
20 Ellen R. Wiebe, "Abortion Induced with Methotrexate and Misoprostol," *Canadian Medical Association Journal* 154, no. 2 (1996), 165–70.
21 Esperanza Mantilla-Rivas, Ashleigh Brennan, Agnes Goldrich, Justin R. Bryant, Albert K. Oh, and Gary F. Rogers, "Extremity Findings of Methotrexate Embryopathy," *Hand* 15, no. 1 (2020).
22 Elizabeth G. Raymond et al., "Medication Abortion with Misoprostol-Only: A Sample Protocol," *Contraception* 121 (2023).
23 Vancouver Island Women's Clinic, n.d., viwc.ca.
24 Sexual Health Options Resources Education (SHORE) Centre, n.d., shorecentre.ca.
25 Ellen Wiebe and Alanna Just, "How Cannabis Alters Sexual Experience: A Survey of Men and Women," *Journal of Sexual Medicine* 16, no. 11 (2019).
26 Ellen Wiebe, Stefanie Green, and Kim Wiebe, "Medical Assistance in Dying (MAiD) in Canada: Practical Aspects for Healthcare Teams," *Annals of Palliative Medicine* 9, no. 6 (2020).
27 Jeff Lee, "Defending Patients' Right to Choose," *Vancouver Sun Online*, March 13, 2016, vancouversun.com/health/defending-patients-right-to-choose-in-bc.
28 Elizabeth Bagshaw Clinic, "Reproductive & Abortion Care Clinic," n.d., bagshawclinic.ca.
29 Dorothy Shaw, "Dr. Gary Romalis, 1937–2014," *BCMJ* 56, no. 3 (April 2014).
30 Annick Cojean, "Etienne-Emile Baulieu, inventeur de la pilule abortive: 'J'ai toujours voulu aider les femmes,'" *Le Monde*, May 7, 2023.
31 CBC Archives, "The Birth Control Pill Was Unstoppable in the 1960s: Legal or Not, There Was No Turning Back Once It Was Approved," October 11, 2018, cbc.ca/archives/the-birth-control-pill-was-unstoppable-in-the-1960s-1.4856941.
32 Pam Belluck, "The Father of the Abortion Pill," *New York Times*, January 17, 2023, nytimes.com/2023/01/17/health/abortion-pill-inventor.html.
33 Robin Herman, "In France, A New Method of Abortion," *Washington Post*, September 27, 1988.
34 Herman, "In France, A New Method."
35 Institut Professeur Baulieu, "Le Pr. Etienne-Emile Baulieu, un pionnier de la recherche hormonale," n.d., institut-baulieu.org/biographie/.

36 WHO (World Health Organization), "The Selection and Use of Essential Medicines: Report of the WHO Expert Committee, 2005 (including the 14th Model List of Essential Medicines)," *World Health Organization Technical Report Series*, 933 (2006).
37 Kelly Grant, "'Unusual' Delay on Health Canada Ruling on Abortion Pill, Professor Says," *Globe and Mail*, December 24, 2014, theglobeandmail.com/life/health-and-fitness/health/unusual-delay-on-health-canada-ruling-on-abortion-pill-professor-says/article22196745/.
38 *Globe and Mail*, "Why the Abortion-pill Delays, Health Canada?" January 15, 2015, theglobeandmail.com/opinion/editorials/why-the-abortion-pill-delays-health-canada/article22473282/.
39 University Health Network Newsroom, "Dr. Joel Lexchin, 'A Legend' in Emergency Medicine, Retires," November 10, 2022.
40 Grant, "'Unusual' Delay."
41 Sheena Goodyear, "RU-486: What You Need to Know about the Recently Approved Abortion Pill," *CBC News*, July 30, 2015, cbc.ca/news/canada/ru-486-what-you-need-to-know-about-the-recently-approved-abortion-pill-1.3173657.
42 Grant, "'Unusual' Delay."
43 NAF Canada (National Abortion Federation), "About NAF Canada," n.d., prochoice.org.
44 Christine Troskie, Judith A. Soon, Arianne Y. Albert, and Wendy V. Norman, "Regulatory Approval Time for Hormonal Contraception in Canada, the United States and the United Kingdom, 2000–2015: A Retrospective Data Analysis," *CMAJ Open* 4, no. 4 (2016).
45 Joanna N. Erdman, Amy Grenon, and Leigh Harrison-Wilson, "Medication Abortion in Canada: A Right-to-Health Perspective," *American Journal of Public Health (1971)* 98, no. 10 (2008).
46 Dustin Costescu and Édith Guilbert, "No. 360-Induced Abortion: Surgical Abortion and Second Trimester Medical Methods," *Journal of Obstetrics and Gynaecology Canada* 40, no. 6 (2018).
47 A.F. Nabhan, G. Mburu, F. Elshafeey, R. Magdi, M. Kamel, M. Elshebiny, Y.G. Abuelnaga et al. "Women's Reproductive Span: A Systematic Scoping Review," *Human Reproduction Open* 2 (2022).
48 Erdman et al. "Medication Abortion," 1768.
49 Martha Paynter, "Nexplanon, A 3-year Birth Control Implant, Is Now Approved for Use in Canada," *The Conversation*, June 1, 2020, theconversation.com/nexplanon-a-3-year-birth-control-implant-is-now-approved-for-use-in-canada-139658.
50 Morena Luigia Rocca, Anna Rita Palumbo, Federica Visconti, and Costantino Di Carlo, "Safety and Benefits of Contraceptives Implants: A Systematic Review," *Pharmaceuticals (Basel, Switzerland)* 14, no. 6 (2021), 548.
51 Sarah Munro et al. "Perspectives Among Canadian Physicians on Factors Influencing Implementation of Mifepristone Medical Abortion: A National Qualitative Study," *Annals of Family Medicine* 18, no. 5 (2020).
52 Wendy V. Norman and Judith A. Soon, "Requiring Physicians to Dispense Mifepristone: An Unnecessary Limit on Safety and Access to Medical Abortion," *Canadian Medical Association Journal* 188, no. 17–18 (2016).
53 Wendy V. Norman et al. "Could Implementation of Mifepristone Address Canada's Urban–Rural Abortion Access Disparity: A Mixed-Methods Implementation Study Protocol," *BMJ Open* 9, no. 4 (2019).
54 Munro et al., "Perspectives Among Canadian Physicians."

55 The Canadian Press, "Health Canada Eases Restrictions on Abortion Pill Mifegymiso," *CBC News,* November 7, 2017, cbc.ca/news/health/mifegymiso-abortion-pill-health-canada-1.4391267.
56 *CBC News,* "Health Canada Says Ultrasound No Longer Mandatory before Mifegymiso Prescribed for Abortion," April 16, 2019, cbc.ca/news/health/mifegymiso-ultrasound-1.5100405.
57 ACOG (American College of Obstetricians and Gynecologists), "Management of Stillbirth: Obstetric Care Consensus No, 10," *Obstetrics and Gynecology (New York, 1953)* 135, no. 3 (2020).
58 Ogilvie and Eggleton, *Prescription Pharmaceuticals in Canada: Off-label Use.*
59 Wendy V. Norman, Edith Guilbert, Christopher Okpaleke, E. Steven Lichtenberg, Maureen Paul, Katharine O'Connell White, and Heidi E. Jones, "Abortion Services in Canada: Results of the 2012 National Survey," *Contraception* 90, no. 3 (2014).
60 Regina M. Renner, Madeleine Ennis, Damien Contandriopoulos, Edith Guilbert, Sheila Dunn, Janusz Kaczorowski, Elizabeth K. Darling, Arianne Albert, Claire Styffe, and Wendy V. Norman, "Abortion Services and Providers in Canada in 2019: Results of a National Survey," *CMAJ Open* 10, no. 3 (2022).
61 Antoni Nerestant, "Access to Abortion Pills in Quebec Too Difficult, Doctors Say," *CBC News,* June 30, 2022, cbc.ca/news/canada/montreal/abortion-pill-medical-procedure-college-physicians-1.6505665.
62 *CBC News,* "It's Now Much Easier for Pregnant Quebecers to Access Abortion Pill," July 14, 2022, cbc.ca/news/canada/montreal/abortion-pill-access-quebec-1.6520492.
63 Renner et al., "Abortion Services."
64 Edith Guilbert and Geneviève Bois, "Évaluation de l'accès à l'avortement Médicamenteux Dans Les Cliniques d'avortement Du Québec En 2021 — Partie I," *Journal of Obstetrics and Gynaecology Canada* 45, no. 2 (2023).
65 Edith Guilbert and Geneviève Bois, "Évaluation de l'information Transmise Sur l'avortement Médicamenteux Dans Les Cliniques d'avortement Du Québec En 2021 — Partie 2," *Journal of Obstetrics and Gynaecology Canada* 45, no. 2 (2023).
66 "Abortion: The Unfinished Revolution" (conference proceedings, University of Prince Edward Island Charlottetown, PEI, August 7–8, 2014), projects.upei.ca/cmacquarrie/files/2014/04/FinalProgram.pdf.
67 CIHI (Canadian Institute for Health Information), "Induced Abortions in Canada," March 20, 2025, cihi.ca/en/induced-abortions-in-canada.
68 Céline Miani, "Medical Abortion Ratios and Gender Equality in Europe: An Ecological Correlation Study," *Sexual and Reproductive Health Matters* 29, no. 1 (2021), 215.
69 *CBC News,* "Morgentaler Closes Halifax Abortion Clinic."
70 Regina Renner, Madeleine Ennis, Lauren Kean, Melissa Brooks, Brigid Dineley, Helen Pymar, Wendy V. Norman, and Edith Guilbert, "First and Second-Trimester Surgical Abortion Providers and Services in 2019: Results from the Canadian Abortion Provider Survey," *Journal of Obstetrics and Gynaecology Canada* 45, no. 12 (2023).
71 WHO (World Health Organization), "Quality Abortion Care," n.d., who.int/health-topics/abortion#tab=tab_3.
72 Sharmani Barnard, Caron Kim, Min Hae Park, and Thoai D Ngo, "Doctors or Mid-Level Providers for Abortion," *Cochrane Database of Systematic Reviews* 2015, no. 7 (2015).
73 Martha Paynter, Wendy V. Norman, and Ruth Martin-Misener, "Nurses Are Key Members of the Abortion Care Team: Why Aren't Schools of Nursing Teaching

Abortion Care?" *Witness: The Canadian Journal of Critical Nursing Discourse* 1, no. 2 (2019).

74 CASN (Canadian Association of Schools of Nursing), "Entry-to-Practice Abortion Care Competencies for Undergraduate Nursing and Nurse Practitioner Education in Canada," 2024, casn.ca/2024/03/entry-to-practice-abortion-care-competencies-for-undergraduate-nursing-and-nurse-practitioner-education-in-canada/.

75 Andrea Carson, Emma Stirling Cameron, Martha Paynter, Wendy V. Norman, Sarah Munro, and Ruth Martin-Misener, "Nurse Practitioners on 'the Leading Edge' of Medication Abortion Care: A Feminist Qualitative Approach," *Journal of Advanced Nursing* 79, no. 2 (2023).

76 Madeleine Ennis, Regina M. Renner, Bimbola Olure, Wendy V. Norman, Stephanie Begun, Lisa Martin, Lisa H. Harris, Lauren Kean, Meghan Seewald, and Sarah Munro, "Experience of Stigma and Harassment among Respondents to the 2019 Canadian Abortion Provider Survey," *Contraception* 124 (2023), 110083.

77 Aaron Winter, "Antiabortion Extremism and Violence in the United States," in *Extremism in America,* ed. George Michael (University Press of Florida, 2013).

78 ARCC (Abortion Rights Coalition of Canada), "Anti-choice Violence and Harassment," Position paper 73, April 2018, 3, arcc-cdac.ca/media/position-papers/73-Anti-choice-Violence-Harassment.pdf.

79 Gordon Bagley, "Bombing of Toronto Abortion Clinic Raises Stakes in Bitter Debate," *Canadian Medical Association Journal* 147, no. 10 (1992).

80 David Rohde, "Sniper Attacks on Doctors Create Climate of Fear in Canada," *New York Times,* October 29, 1998, nytimes.com/1998/10/29/nyregion/sniper-attacks-on-doctors-create-climate-of-fear-in-canada.html.

81 Jessica Maxwell, "Hamilton Abortion Doctor Shot in 1995 Featured in New Season of True-crime Podcast," *CBC News,* May 21, 2022, cbc.ca/news/canada/hamilton/someone-knows-something-abortion-wars-hugh-short-1.6457934.

82 Jack Fainman and Roland Penner, "A Shot in the Dark: They Shoot Doctors, Don't They?" *Winnipeg Free Press,* November 12, 2011, winnipegfreepress.com/arts-and-life/entertainment/books/2011/11/12/a-shot-in-the-dark-2.

83 Rohde, "Sniper Attacks."

84 Daniel Myran, Jillian Bardsley, Tania Hindi, and Kristine Whitehead, "Abortion Education in Canadian Family Medicine Residency Programs," *BMC Medical Education* 18, no. 121 (2018).

85 US Department of Justice: Civil Rights Division, "Recent Cases on Violence Against Reproductive Health Care Providers," May 30, 2023, justice.gov/crt/recent-cases-violence-against-reproductive-health-care-providers.

86 Cojean, "Etienne-Emile Baulieu, inventeur."

87 Rajwant Minhas, Joan Chung Yan Ng, Jason Tan, Hilary Wu, Sarah Stabler, Jessica Beach, Kyle Collins, Shaylee Peterson, Kieran Shah, and Sam Louie, "Should Developed Countries, Including Canada, Provide Universal Access to Essential Medications through a National, Publicly Funded and Administered Insurance Plan?" *Canadian Journal of Hospital Pharmacy* 69, no. 2 (2016).

88 Sarah Baddeley, "LEAF Halifax Advocacy for Access to Medical Abortion," *Canadian Bar Association,* March 29, 2018, cba.org/sections/women-lawyers/member-articles/leaf-halifax-advocacy-for-access-to-medical-abortion/?lang=en-ca.

89 Julien Gignac, "New Brunswick Becomes First Canada Province to Offer Free Abortion Pill," *The Guardian,* April 5, 2017, theguardian.com/world/2017/apr/05/canada-free-abortion-pill-new-brunswick.

90 Adam Hunter, "Sask. to Provide Universal Coverage for Abortion Pill Mifegymiso," *CBC News*, June 07, 2019, cbc.ca/news/canada/saskatchewan/sask-covers-abortion-pill-mifegymiso-1.5166420.

91 Giuseppina Di Meglio and Elisabeth Yorke, "Universal Access to No-Cost Contraception for Youth in Canada," *Paediatrics & Child Health* 24, no. 3 (2019).

92 Alexandra Gero, Rebecca G. Simmons, Jessica N. Sanders, and David K. Turok, "Does Access to No-Cost Contraception Change Method Selection among Individuals Who Report Difficulty Paying for Health-Related Care?" *BMC Women's Health* 22, no. 1 (2022).

93 Brett Bundale, "Abortion Pill Still Largely Out of Reach for Women in Nova Scotia," *CityNews,* January 23, 2018, toronto.citynews.ca/2018/01/23/abortion-pill-still-largely-out-of-reach-for-most-women-in-nova-scotia/.

94 British Columbia. "Medical Services Commission Payment Schedule," Ministry of Health, May 1, 2021. 2.gov.bc.ca/assets/gov/health/practitioner-pro/medical-services-plan/msc-payment-schedule-may-2021.pdf.

95 Charlene Lyndon, "Abortion Access," October 9, 2023, static1.squarespace.com/static/568eb5bbd82d5eecf06026c4/t/655be3f305c2fd53e526272b/1700520948117/EZMSA+BN+for+HC-+Abortion+access.pdf.

96 CFS (Canadian Federation of Students), "Win for International Students' Access to Health Care in Nova Scotia, Further Action Still Needed," n.d. (blog). cfs-fcee.ca/blog/win-for-international-students-access-to-health-care-in-nova-scotia-further-action-still-needed.

97 Québec, "Connaître les conditions d'admissibilité à l'assurance maladie," *Régie de l'assurance maladie,* n.d., ramq.gouv.qc.ca/fr/citoyens/assurance-maladie/connaitre-conditions-admissibilite.

98 CBIE (Canadian Bureau for International Education), "International Students in Canada at All Levels of Study," n.d., cbie.ca/infographic/.

99 Regina M. Renner, Madeleine Ennis, Ama Kyeremeh, Wendy V. Norman, Sheila Dunn, Helen Pymar, and Edith Guilbert, "Telemedicine for First-Trimester Medical Abortion in Canada: Results of a 2019 Survey," *Telemedicine Journal and E-Health* 29, no. 5 (2023).

100 Renner et al., "Telemedicine for First-Trimester."

101 Renner et al., "Telemedicine for First-Trimester."

102 Edith Guilbert, Dustin Costescu, Marie-Soleil Wagner, Regina Renner, Wendy V. Norman, Sheila Dunn, Brian Fitzsimmons, Konia Trouton, Jeanne Bernardin, Amanda Black, Julie G. Thorne, and M.A. Gomes, "Canadian Protocol for the Provision of Medical Abortion via Telemedicine," *Society of Obstetricians and Gynaecologists of Canada (SOGC),* n.d., sogc.org/common/uploaded%20files/canadian%20protocol%20for%20the%20provision%20of%20ma%20via%20telemedicine.pdf.

103 Charlotte Ellertson, Batya Elul, Shuha Ambardekar, Lindy Wood, Julie Carroll, and Kurus Coyaji, "Accuracy of Assessment of Pregnancy Duration by Women Seeking Early Abortions," *Lancet (British Edition)* 355, no. 9207 (2000).

104 Lauren J. Ralph et al. "Accuracy of Self-Assessment of Gestational Duration among People Seeking Abortion," *American Journal of Obstetrics and Gynecology* 226, no. 5 (2022).

105 Abigail R. Aiken, Evdokia P. Romanova, Julia R. Morber, and Rebecca Gomperts, "Safety and Effectiveness of Self-Managed Medication Abortion Provided Using Online Telemedicine in the United States: A Population Based Study," *Lancet Regional Health — Americas* 10 (2022), 100200.

106 Abigail R. Aiken, Patricia A. Lohr, Jonathan Lord, N. Ghosh, and Jennifer Starling, "Effectiveness, Safety and Acceptability of No-test Medical Abortion (Termination of Pregnancy) Provided via Telemedicine: A National Cohort Study," *BJOG: An International Journal of Obstetrics and Gynaecology* 128, no. 9 (2021).
107 Aiken et al., "Effectiveness, Safety and Acceptability of No-test Medical Abortion."
108 Tim I.M. Korevaar et al. "Reference Ranges and Determinants of Total hCG Levels during Pregnancy: The Generation R Study," *European Journal of Epidemiology* 30, no. 9 (2015), 1058.
109 Maria P. Velez, Jonas Shellenberger, and Joel G. Ray, "Accuracy of Serum Human Chorionic Gonadotrophin for Estimating Gestational Age in the First Trimester of Pregnancy: Population-Based Study," *Journal of Obstetrics and Gynaecology Canada* 45, no. 5 (2023).
110 Jillian C. Burk and Wendy V. Norman, "Trends and Determinants of Postabortion Contraception Use in a Canadian Retrospective Cohort," *Contraception* 100, no. 2 (2019).
111 Corinne H. Rocca, Suzan Goodman, Daniel Grossman, Kara Cadwallader, Kirsten M.J. Thompson, Elizabeth Talmont, J. Joseph Speidel, and Cynthia C. Harper, "Contraception after Medication Abortion in the United States: Results from a Cluster Randomized Trial," *American Journal of Obstetrics and Gynecology* 218, no. 1 (2018).
112 CAPS (Canadian Abortion Providers Support), "Medication Abortion in Canada," *Society of Obstetricians and Gynaecologists of Canada*, n.d., caps.sogc.org/.
113 Enav Z. Zusman, Sarah Munro, Wendy V. Norman, and Judith A. Soon, "Pharmacist Direct Dispensing of Mifepristone for Medication Abortion in Canada: A Survey of Community Pharmacists," *BMJ Open* 12, no. 10 (2022).
114 Enav Z. Zusman, Sarah Munro, Wendy V. Norman, and Judith A. Soon, "Dispensing Mifepristone for Medical Abortion in Canada: Pharmacists' Experiences of the First Year," *Canadian Pharmacists Journal* 156, no. 4 (2023).
115 "How Long Do Abortion Pills Last?" *Women Help Women* (blog), November 23, 2022, womenhelp.org/en/page/1510/how-long-do-abortion-pills-last.
116 Zusman et al., "Dispensing Mifepristone."
117 CPhA (Canadian Pharmacists Association), "CPhA Statement on Abortion Access," May 5, 2022, pharmacists.ca/news-events/news/cpha-statement-on-abortion-access/.
118 CPhA (Canadian Pharmacists Association), "New Resources to Help Pharmacists Provide Services for Contraception and Medication Abortion," n.d., pharmacists.ca/news-events/news/new-resources-to-help-pharmacists-provide-services-for-contraception-and-medication-abortion/.
119 Nicole Ireland, "Ontario Pharmacists Association Says Ability to Prescribe Birth Control Should be Next," *The Canadian Press*, October 3, 2023, thecanadianpressnews.ca/health/ontario-pharmacists-association-says-ability-to-prescribe-birth-control-should-be-next/article_5c847261-dcce-5508-9ca2-e42f922b0d61.html.
120 Food and Drugs Act (R.S.C., 1985, c. F-27).
121 David M. Gardner, Barbara Mintzes, and Aleck Ostry, "Direct-to-Consumer Prescription Drug Advertising in Canada: Permission by Default?" *Canadian Medical Association Journal* 169, no. 5 (2003), 425–27.
122 Annette Choi and Way Mullery, "How Safe is the Abortion Pill Compared with Other Common Drugs?" *CNN Online*, June 13, 2024, cnn.com/health/abortion-pill-safety-dg/index.html.

123 Schummers et al., "Abortion Safety and Use with Normally Prescribed Mifepristone in Canada."
124 Catherine E. Kennedy, Ping Teresa Yeh, Karima Gholbzouri, and Manjulaa Narasimhan, "Self-testing for Pregnancy: A Systematic Review and Meta-analysis," *BMJ Open* 12 (2022).
125 Women on Waves, "Who are We?" n.d., womenonwaves.org/en/page/650/who-are-we.
126 Aid Access, "Get Abortion Pills Online," n.d., aidaccess.org/en/.
127 Women on Web, "Who We Are," n.d., womenonweb.org/en/page/521/who-we-are.
128 Lena Marions, Kristina Gemzell Danielsson, Marja-Liisa Swahn, and Marc Bygdeman, "Contraceptive Efficacy of Low Doses of Mifepristone," *Fertility and Sterility* 70, no. 5 (1998): 813–16.
129 Carrie N. Baker, "A Once-a-Week Contraceptive Pill, Without Side Effects? Yes, Mifepristone," *Ms Magazine,* February 8, 2024, msmagazine.com/2024/02/08/contraceptive-pill-mifepristone/.
130 Abigail Brooks and Dasha Burns, "How a Network of Abortion Pill Providers Works Together in the Wake of New Threats," *NBC News,* April 7, 2024, nbcnews.com/health/health-news/network-abortion-pill-providers-works-together-wake-new-threats-rcna146678.
131 *CBC News,* "Nurses in Ontario Will Soon Be Able to Prescribe Birth Control, Province Announces," November 6, 2023, cbc.ca/news/canada/toronto/registered-nurse-prescriptions-1.7019731.
132 Joanna Erdman, "Put Abortion Pills into People's Hands," *Policy Options,* May 11, 2022, policyoptions.irpp.org/magazines/may-2022/abortion-pills-canada/.
133 Matthew Perrone, "First Over-the-counter Birth Control Pill Gets FDA Approval in US," *CBC News,* July 13, 2023, cbc.ca/news/health/united-states-over-counter-birth-control-approval-1.6905541.

Chapter 5

1 Joyce Arthur, "Christian Doctors Angry They Can No Longer Abandon Their Patients," *Rabble,* April 3, 2015, rabble.ca/columnists/christian-doctors-angry-they-can-no-longer-abandon-their-patients/.
2 William P. Marshall, "Third-Party Burdens and Conscientious Objection to War," *Kentucky Law Journal* 106 (2019).
3 Jeremy Kessler, "The Legal Origins of Catholic Conscientious Objection," *William and Mary Bill of Rights Journal* 31, no. 2 (2022).
4 Kessler, "The Legal Origins," 362.
5 Kessler, "The Legal Origins," 362.
6 Audiey Kao, "History of Oral Contraception," *Virtual Mentor* 2, no. 6 (2000).
7 Udo Schuklenk, "Conscientious Objection in Medicine: Accommodation versus Professionalism and the Public Good," *British Medical Bulletin* 126, no. 1 (2018).
8 Christian Fiala and Joyce H. Arthur. "There Is No Defence for 'Conscientious Objection' in Reproductive Health Care," *European Journal of Obstetrics & Gynecology and Reproductive Biology* 216 (2017), 255.
9 Carolyn McLeod, "Referral in the Wake of Conscientious Objection to Abortion," *Hypatia* 23, no. 4 (2008).
10 McLeod, "Referral in the Wake," 31.
11 Paynter et al., "Nurses Are Key Members."
12 Nova Scotia Legislature, Bill No. 323, An Act to Provide a Common Legislative Foundation for Regulated Health Professions, 1st Session, 64th General Assembly Nova Scotia (2023), nslegislature.ca/legislative-business/bills-statutes/bills/assembly-64-session-1/bill-323.

13 Ontario, Nursing Act, S.O. 1991, c. 32, ontario.ca/laws/statute/91n32.
14 Ontario, Midwifery Act, S.O. 1991, c. 31, ontario.ca/laws/statute/91m31.
15 Ontario, Medicine Act, S.O. 1991, c. 30, ontario.ca/laws/statute/91m30.
16 CON (College of Nurses of Ontario), Practice Standard: Nurse Practitioner. Pub. No. 49045 ISBN 978-1-77116-173-2 (2023).
17 CIHI (Canadian Institute for Health Information), Nurse Practitioner Scopes of Practice Vary across Canada's Provinces and Territories [infographic], 2020, cihi.ca/en/nurse-practitioner-scopes-of-practice-vary-across-canadas-provinces-and-territories.
18 Canadian Medical Association (CMA), "Code of Ethics and Professionalism," 2018, cma.ca/cma-code-ethics-and-professionalism.
19 National Association of Pharmacy Regulatory Authorities (NAPRA), "Model Standards of Practice for Pharmacists and Pharmacy Technicians in Canada" (Ottawa: National Association of Pharmacy Regulatory Authorities, 2022).
20 Canadian Nursing Association (CNA), *Code of Ethics for Registered Nurses* (Ottawa: Canadian Nursing Association, 2017), cna-aiic.ca/en/nursing/regulated-nursing-in-canada/nursing-ethics.
21 CNA, *Code of Ethics*, 35.
22 CMA (Canadian Medical Association), "CMA Policy Summary: Induced Abortion," *Canadian Medical Association Journal* 139, no. 12 (1988), 1176A–1176B.
23 Sanda Rodgers and Jocelyn Downie. "Abortion: Ensuring Access," *Canadian Medical Association Journal* 175, no. 1 (2006), 9.
24 Jeff Blackmer, "Clarification of the CMA's Position Concerning Induced Abortion," *Canadian Medical Association Journal* 176, no. 9 (2007).
25 Ryan du Toit and Catriona Ida Macleod, "Demanding Doctorability for Abortion on Request: A Conversation Analysis of Pre-abortion Counselling in Public Hospitals in the Eastern Cape, South Africa," *BMJ Sexual & Reproductive Health* 50, no. 4 (2024).
26 Jocelyn Downie, Carolyn McLeod, and Jacquelyn Shaw, "Moving Forward with a Clear Conscience: A Model Conscientious Objection Policy for Canadian Colleges of Physicians and Surgeons," *Health Law Review* 21, no. 3 (2013).
27 Yukon Medical Council, "Moral or Religious Beliefs Affecting Medical Care," n.d., yukonmedicalcouncil.ca/pdfs/medical_practice/Moral_or_Religious_Beliefs_Affecting_Medical_Care.pdf.
28 College of Physicians and Surgeons of Nova Scotia, "Obligations for Services for Patients," 2024. cpsns.ns.ca/resource/obligations-for-services-for-patients.
29 ARCC (Abortion Rights Coalition of Canada), *Canadian Policies and Laws on "Conscientious Objection" in Health Care*, Position Paper #95 — Appendix (Vancouver: Abortion Rights Coalition of Canada, August 2023).
30 Elizabeth Payne, "Some Ottawa Doctors Refuse to Prescribe Birth Control Pills," *Ottawa Citizen*, January 31, 2014, ottawacitizen.com/news/local-news/some-ottawa-doctors-refuse-to-prescribe-birth-control-pills.
31 CPSO (College of Physicians and Surgeons of Ontario), *Human Rights in the Provision of Health Services*, approved by Council September 2008; reviewed and updated March 2015, September 2023.
32 Paola Loriggio, "Doctors Must Give Patients Referrals for Services They Oppose, Says Ontario Appeal Court," *CityNews*, May 15, 2019, toronto.citynews.ca/2019/05/15/court-to-rule-on-whether-doctors-have-to-give-referrals-for-services-they-oppose/.
33 Canadian Charter of Rights and Freedoms, Constitution Act, 1982, laws-lois.justice.gc.ca/eng/const/page-12.html.

34 *Christian Medical and Dental Society of Canada v. College of Physicians and Surgeons of Ontario*, 2019 ONCA 393 (CanLII), canliiconnects.org/en/commentaries/67256.
35 St. Martha's Regional Hospital Foundation, "St. Martha's Regional Hospital," n.d., smrhfoundation.com/st-marthas-regional-hospital
36 Stanisław Adamiak and Jan Dohnalik, "The Prohibition of Suicide and Its Theological Rationale in Catholic Moral and Canonical Tradition: Origins and Development," *Journal of Religion and Health* 62, no. 6 (2023).
37 *Rodriguez v. British Columbia (Attorney General)*, [1993] 3 SCR 519, decisions.scc-csc.ca/scc-csc/scc-csc/en/item/1054/index.do.
38 British Columbia Civil Liberties Association (BCCLA), "In Memory of Gloria Taylor," October 9, 2012, bccla.org/2012/10/in-memory-of-gloria/.
39 Douglas Todd, "The Story at the Heart of Friday's Supreme Court Ruling on Assisted Suicide," *Vancouver Sun*, February 4, 2015, vancouversun.com/news/staff-blogs/b-c-woman-chooses-a-dignified-death-in-switzerland.
40 *Carter v. Canada (Attorney General)*, 2015 SCC 5, [2015] 1 SCR 331, decisions.scc-csc.ca/scc-csc/scc-csc/en/item/14637/index.do.
41 Jocelyn Downie, "Alarming Gap in Assisted Dying in Antigonish," *SaltWire*, December 17, 2018, saltwire.com/nova-scotia/opinion-alarming-gap-in-assisted-dying-in-antigonish-268714.
42 The Canadian Press, "NS Catholic Hospital Will Offer Assisted Dying After Policy Change," *CBC News*, September 19, 2019, cbc.ca/news/canada/nova-scotia/catholic-hospital-offering-assisted-dying-policy-change-1.5289820.
43 Andrea Woo, "Family Sues after BC Catholic Hospital Denies MAID Request on Religious Grounds," *Globe and Mail*, June 18, 2024, theglobeandmail.com/canada/article-family-of-woman-forced-to-transfer-from-catholic-hospital-to-another/.
44 *C.V. v. Mount Sinai Hospital*, 2015-20863-I: 2016 HRTO 941, July 18, 2016.
45 Tom Blackwell, "Mount Sinai Hospital's Refusal to Eliminate One Fetus from Twin Pregnancy Triggers Human Rights Battle," *National Post*, July 29, 2016, nationalpost.com/health/mount-sinai-hospitals-refusal-to-eliminate-one-fetus-from-twin-pregnancy-triggers-human-rights-battle-in-toronto.
46 Sinai Health, "Mount Sinai Hospital History," n.d., sinaihealth.ca/about-sinai-health/sinai-health-system-history/mount-sinai-hospital-history/.
47 Peter Wilton, "Days of Shame, Montreal, 1934," *Canadian Medical Association Journal* 169, no. 12 (2003).
48 Rhythm Sachdeva, "Abortion Accessibility in Canada: The Catholic Hospital Conflict," *CTV News*, May 19, 2022, ctvnews.ca/health/article/abortion-accessibility-in-canada-the-catholic-hospital-conflict/.
49 Jenny Yang, "Number of Hospitals in Canada by Province," *Statista Online*, March 5, 2024, statista.com/statistics/440923/total-number-of-hospital-establishments-in-canada-by-province/.
50 Wendy Glauser, "Faith and Access: The Conflict inside Catholic Hospitals," *The Walrus*, February 23, 2022, thewalrus.ca/catholic-hospitals/.
51 St. Francis Xavier University, "Sisters of St. Martha's Gift $500k To StFX To Support Indigenous Students," October 6, 2022, stfx.ca/news/sisters-st-marthas-gift-500k-stfx-support-indigenous-students.
52 Brett Bundale, "Access to Abortion Pill Still an Issue in Nova Scotia: Advocates," *Global News*, November 22, 2018, globalnews.ca/news/4689260/abortion-pill-access-ns/.
53 57th General Assembly of Prince Edward Island, 3rd Session, peildo.ca/islandora/object/leg%3A3295#page/84/mode/2up.

54 LEAF (Women's Legal Education and Action Fund), "*Abortion Access Now PEI v. Government of PEI* Case Summary," *LEAF* (2016), leaf.ca/case_summary/abortion-access-now-pei-v-government-of-pei-2016/.
55 Emily Baron Cadloff, "How PEI Became One of The Most Accessible Places For Women's Health Care In Canada," *Chatelaine,* November 20, 2019, chatelaine.com/health/pei-abortion-access/.
56 Guilbert et al., "Canadian Protocol for the Provision of Medical Abortion Via Telemedicine."

Chapter 6

1 Solarina Ho, "Crisis Pregnancy Centres Criticized for 'Deceptive' Practices," *CTV News,* May 9, 2022, ctvnews.ca/health/article/crisis-pregnancy-centres-criticized-for-deceptive-practices/.
2 Action Canada, "Access at a Glance: Abortion Services in Canada," n.d., actioncanadashr.org/resources/factsheets-guidelines/2019-09-19-access-glance-abortion-services-canada.
3 Ho, "Crisis Pregnancy Centres."
4 Food and Drugs Act R.S.C., 1985, c. F-27, laws-lois.justice.gc.ca/eng/acts/f-27/.
5 David M. Gardner, Barbara Mintzes, and Aleck Ostry, "Direct-to-Consumer Prescription Drug Advertising in Canada: Permission by Default?" *Canadian Medical Association Journal* 169, no. 5 (2003), 425–27.
6 Pregnancy Care Canada, "Abortion, Adoption, Parenting: an Informal Guide for unexpected pregnancy," n.d., issuu.com/pregnancycarecanada/docs/pcc-options-brochure-2020-edition?mode=window.
7 Canada, "What is the Difference between a Registered Charity and a Non-profit Organization?" June 23, 2016, canada.ca/en/revenue-agency/services/charities-giving/about-registered-charities/what-difference-between-a-registered-charity-a-non-profit-organization.html.
8 Joyce Arthur, "Why Anti-Abortion Groups Should Not Be Charities," *Health Insight,* 2023, healthinsight.ca/wellness/sexual-health/why-anti-abortion-groups-should-not-be-charities/.
9 *Everywoman's Health Centre Society (1988) v. MNR (CA),* 1991 CanLII 13581 (FCA), [1992] 2 FC 52, ca.vlex.com/vid/everywoman-s-health-centre-681338721.
10 Charities Registration (Security Information) Act SC 2001, c. 41, s. 113, laws-lois.justice.gc.ca/eng/acts/c-27.55/FullText.html.
11 *Everywoman's Health Centre Society v. MNR.*
12 Everywoman's Health Centre, "Fees," n.d., everywomanshealthcentre.ca/fees/.
13 Shannon Stettner (ed.), *Without Apology: Writings on Abortion in Canada* (Athabasca University Press, 2016), 51.
14 Birthright, "Who is Birthright?" n.d., birthrightwa.org/about-us/.
15 Birthright, "Why Connect With Us?" n.d., birthright.org/why-connect-with-us/.
16 Hannah Heil, "Respect Life Month: Birthright Offers Supplies, Referrals to Pregnant Women," *The Catholic Times,* October 10, 2023, catholictimescolumbus.org/news/hannah-heil/respect-life-month-birthright-offers-supplies-referrals-to-pregnant-women.
17 Birthright of Pittsburgh, "Our Mission," n.d., birthrightpittsburgh.org/about-us/our-mission/.
18 Loretta Ross and Rickie Solinger, *Reproductive Justice an Introduction,* 1st ed. (University of California Press, 2017).
19 Marilyn Bicher, Donna Cherniak, Judith Lermer Crawley, Shirley Pettifer, and Christabelle Sethna, "The Birth Control Handbook and the Montreal Health

20 Press," *RiseUP Feminist Archive,* January 2017, riseupfeministarchive.ca/activism/issues-actions/the-birth-control-handbook-and-the-montreal-health-press/.
20 Mickey Conlon, "Birthright Marks a Half Century of Service," *The Catholic Register,* June 5, 2018.
21 Eugene F. Diamond, "The Morality of Crisis Pregnancy Counseling," *The Linacre Quarterly* 41, no. 3 Article 5 (August 1974), 169.
22 Diamond, "The Morality of Crisis Pregnancy Counseling," 172.
23 Carly Thomsen and Grace Tacherra Morrison, "Abortion as Gender Transgression: Reproductive Justice, Queer Theory, and Anti–Crisis Pregnancy Center Activism," *Signs: Journal of Women in Culture and Society* 45, no. 3 (2020), 703–4.
24 Women's Care Centre, "Contact Us," n.d. womenscarecenter.ca/contact-us/.
25 Viola Pruss, "Fredericton Anti-abortion Group to Rebuild Controversial Downtown Office, Clinic," *CBC News,* April 20, 2017, cbc.ca/news/canada/new-brunswick/hughes-abortion-clinic-fredericton-opponents-rebuilding-fire-1.4076855.
26 Todd Veinotte, "Controversial Women's Centre Opens Next Door to New Brunswick's Only Abortion Clinic," *Global News,* August 1, 2018, globalnews.ca/news/4365826/womens-centre-open-next-to-abortion-clinic/.
27 Aidan Cox, "Clinic 554 to Close, Bringing Clinic-based Abortions to End in Fredericton Area," *CBC News,* January 31, 2024, cbc.ca/news/canada/new-brunswick/clinic-554-fredericton-abortion-1.7100433.
28 Women's Care Center, womenscarecenter.ca/unplanned-pregnancy-support-fredericton-new-brunswick/.
29 Pregnancy Care Canada, "Frequently Asked Questions," n.d., pregnancycarecanada.ca/faq/.
30 Care Net, "Who We Are: A Pro Abundant Life Ministry," n.d., care-net.org/.
31 Heartbeat International, "Welcome to Heartbeat!" n.d., heartbeatinternational.org/about-us.
32 Family Support Centre, "FAQs," n.d., familysupportcentre.ca/faqs.
33 Family Support Centre, "Disclaimer," n.d., familysupportcentre.ca/disclaimer.
34 Joyce Arthur, Annaliese Downey, Angela Katelieva, Olivia Jensen, Katelyn Mitchell, Teale N. Phelps Bondaroff, "Examining the Websites of AntiChoice 'Crisis Pregnancy Centres,'" ARCC (Abortion Rights Coalition of Canada), March 8, 2023, arcc-cdac.ca/media/crisis-pregnancy-centres/cpc-website-review-2023.pdf.
35 ARCC (Abortion Rights Coalition of Canada), "List of Anti-choice Groups in Canada," last updated March 13, 2025, arcc-cdac.ca/media/2020/06/list-anti-choice-groups-province-city.pdf.
36 University of California San Francisco, "The Turnaway Study."
37 Arthur et al. "Examining the Websites."
38 ACOG (American College of Obstetricians and Gynecologists), "Facts Are Important: Medication Abortion 'Reversal' Is Not Supported by Science," n.d., acog.org/advocacy/facts-are-important/medication-abortion-reversal-is-not-supported-by-science.
39 Heartbeat International, "Welcome to Heartbeat!"
40 Annik Mahalia Sorhaindo and Antonella Francheska Lavelanet, "Why Does Abortion Stigma Matter? A Scoping Review and Hybrid Analysis of Qualitative Evidence Illustrating the Role of Stigma in the Quality of Abortion Care," *Social Science & Medicine* 311 (2022).
41 Alice F. Cartwright, Katherine Tumlinson, and Ushma D Upadhyay, "Pregnancy Outcomes after Exposure to Crisis Pregnancy Centers among an Abortion-Seeking Sample Recruited Online," *PloS One* 16, no. 7 (2021), e0255152.

42 Thomsen and Morrison, "Abortion as Gender Transgression."
43 Haiqi Li, "Crisis Pregnancy Centers in Canada and Reproductive Justice Organizations' Responses," *Global Journal of Health Science* 11, no. 2 (2019).
44 Sarah Rudrum, "Student Encounters with a Campus Crisis Pregnancy Centre: Choice, Reproductive Justice and Sexual and Reproductive Health Supports," *Canadian Journal of Sociology* 47, no. 1 (2022).
45 Rudrum, "Student Encounters," 60.
46 *Human Life International in Canada Inc. v. MNR (CA)*, 1998 CanLII 9053 (FCA), [1998] 3 FC 202, ca.vlex.com/vid/life-intl-in-can-681058017.
47 *Alliance for Life v. MNR (CA)*, 1999 CanLII 8152 (FCA), [1999] 3 FC 504, ca.vlex.com/vid/life-v-mnr-681684157.
48 Amanda Connolly, "Canada Summer Jobs Program Will No Longer Fund Anti-abortion, Anti-gay Groups," *Global News,* December 15, 2017, globalnews.ca/news/3914528/canada-summer-jobs-anti-abortion-anti-gay-groups/.
49 Amanda Connolly, "Canada Summer Jobs Attestation Endorsed by 80 Canadian Rights Groups," *Global News,* January 29, 2018, globalnews.ca/news/3993867/canada-summer-job-attestation-endorsed-by-80-canadian-rights-groups/.
50 Liberal Party of Canada, "Protecting Your Sexual and Reproductive Health and Rights," n.d., liberal.ca/our-platform/protecting-your-sexual-and-reproductive-health-and-rights/.
51 Canada, "Promotion of Health and Charitable Registration," n.d. canada.ca/en/revenue-agency/services/charities-giving/charities/policies-guidance/promotion-health-charitable-registration.html.
52 Darren Major, "New Legislation Would Make 'Crisis Pregnancy Centres' Disclose Whether They Provide Abortion Support," *CBC News,* October 29, 2024, cbc.ca/news/politics/abortion-services-charitable-status-1.7366854.
53 Thomsen and Morrison, "Abortion as Gender Transgression."
54 Facebook, "End Fake Clinics," n.d., facebook.com/EndFakeClinics/.
55 Thomsen and Morrison, "Abortion as Gender Transgression."
56 missINFORMED, "Imagining the Next Chapter for Abortion Care in Canada: Pathways to Access and Equity," n.d., missinformed.ca/abortion-care-canada-webinar-registration.
57 Action Canada for Sexual Health & Rights, instagram.com/actioncanadashr/?hl=en.
58 Prince Edward Island, "Sexual Health, Options & Reproductive Services (SHORS)," n.d., princeedwardisland.ca/en/information/health-pei/sexual-health-options-reproductive-services-shors.
59 Corinne H. Rocca, Katrina Kimport, Heather Gould, and Diana G. Foster, "Women's Emotions One Week After Receiving or Being Denied an Abortion in the United States," *Perspectives on Sexual and Reproductive Health* 45, no. 3 (2013).
60 Pathway to Hope, "Offering Hope to Those Facing an Unexpected Pregnancy," n.d., pathwaytohopepcc.org/.
61 Coaching Fathers, "Welcome," n.d., coachingfathers.org/.
62 Clare Heggie, Lin Tong, Aishwarya Heran, Ishika Bhambhani, Shelley McKibbon, and Martha Paynter, "The Role of Doulas and Community Birth Workers in Abortion and Contraception Care: An International Scoping Review," *Contraception* 136 (2024).
63 Martha Paynter, Clare Heggie, Anja McLeod, Melissa Fuller and Mélina Castonguay, "The Role of Doulas in Abortion Care in Canada: A Qualitative Study," *PLOS One* 136 (2024).

64 Clare Heggie, Martha Paynter, and Grisha Cowal, "Doula Practice in Canada: An Environmental Scan," *Canadian Journal of Midwifery Research and Practice* 21, no. 1 (2024).

65 Fiona B. Young, Ozlem Dural, Jocelynn Cook, and Amanda Black, "Trends and Predictors of Unintended Pregnancy in Canada: Results from a National Survey," *Journal of Obstetrics and Gynaecology Canada* 42, no. 5 (2020), 695.

66 Amanda Y. Black, Edith Guilbert, Fareen Hassan, Ismini Chatziheofilou, Julia Lowin, Mark Jeddi, Anna Filonenko, and James Trussell, "The Cost of Unintended Pregnancies in Canada: Estimating Direct Cost, Role of Imperfect Adherence, and the Potential Impact of Increased Use of Long-Acting Reversible Contraceptives," *Journal of Obstetrics and Gynaecology Canada* 37, no. 12 (2015).

67 Amy Metcalfe, Rachel Talavlikar, Beatrice du Prey, and Suzanne C. Tough, "Exploring the Relationship between Socioeconomic Factors, Method of Contraception and Unintended Pregnancy," *Reproductive Health* 13, no. 1 (2016).

Chapter 7

1 Government of Canada, "Guide to the Canadian Charter of Rights and Freedoms," August 2, 2024, canada.ca/en/canadian-heritage/services/how-rights-protected/guide-canadian-charter-rights-freedoms.html#a2e3.

2 *Lobo v. Carleton University*, 2012 ONSC 254.

3 *CBC News*, "Carleton Anti-abortion Group Sues University," February 23, 2011, cbc.ca/news/canada/ottawa/carleton-anti-abortion-group-sues-university-1.1078182.

4 Joyce Arthur, "The Holocaust Has Nothing to Do with Abortion," *Rabble*, April 12, 2017, rabble.ca/columnists/holocaust-has-nothing-do-abortion/.

5 Jacob Serebrin, "Money, Not Free Speech, at Issue in Carleton Pro-life Dispute," *MacLean's*, November 17, 2010, macleans.ca/education/university/money-not-free-speech-is-the-real-issue-in-anti-abortion-group-controversy/.

6 *Wilson v. University of Calgary*, 2014 ABQB 190.

7 *UAlberta Pro-Life v. Governors of the University of Alberta*, 2020 ABCA 1.

8 Hannah Liddle, "Timeline: Protest Encampments," *University Affairs*, May 31, 2024, universityaffairs.ca/features/timeline-encampments/.

9 Matt Scace, "Alberta University Encampment Removals Likely Violated Protestors' Constitutional Rights, Legal Experts Say," *Calgary Herald*, May 11, 2024, calgaryherald.com/news/local-news/alberta-university-encampment-removals-likely-violated-protesters-constitutional-rights-legal-experts-say.

10 Matthew Lapierre and Verity Stevenson, "Quebec Superior Court Judge Rejects McGill Injunction Request to Remove Encampment," *CBC News*, May 15, 2024, cbc.ca/news/canada/montreal/mcgill-injunction-request-1.7203666.

11 Yves Engler, "McGill Admin Battles its Pro-Palestinian Students," *CounterPunch*, November 29, 2024, counterpunch.org/2024/11/29/mcgill-admin-battles-its-pro-palestinian-students/.

12 *CBC News*, "U of T Gets Injunction to Clear Encampment," July 2, 2024, cbc.ca/news/canada/toronto/decision-university-toronto-injunction-encampment-1.7252343.

13 Richard Cuthbertson, "Pro-Palestinian Protestors Leave Dalhousie University Quad, Building," *CBC News*, July 29, 2024, cbc.ca/news/nova-scotia/dalhousie-encampment-trespass-deadline-1.7278475.

14 CCBR (Canadian Centre for Bioethical Reform), "Join the Movement," n.d., endthekilling.ca/.

15 Ad Standards Canada, "Canadian Code of Advertising Standards," July 2019, adstandards.ca/code/the-code-online/.
16 *Canadian Centre for Bioethical Reform v. Grande Prairie (City)*, 2016 ABQB. arcc-cdac.ca/media/2020/06/Canadian-Centre-for-Bio-Ethical-Reform-v-Grande-Prairie-City-2016-ABQB-734.pdf.
17 *Canadian Centre for Bio-Ethical Reform v. City of Peterborough*, 2016 ONSC 1972.
18 Joyce Arthur, "Failures by City of Peterborough Led to Anti-Choice Ads on Buses," Abortion Rights Coalition of Canada, March 27, 2017, arcc-cdac.ca/media/2020/06/Failures-by-City-Peterborough-led-to-anti-choice-ads.pdf.
19 *Lethbridge and District Pro-Life Association v. Lethbridge (City)*, 2020 ABQB 654.
20 Pattison, "Find your voice in Wild Rose Country," n.d., pattisonoutdoor.com/markets/alberta/.
21 *Lethbridge and District Pro-Life Association v. Lethbridge.*
22 *Guelph and Area Right to Life v. City of Guelph*, 2022 ONSC 43.
23 *Association for Reformed Political Action Canada v. Hamilton (City of)*, 2023 ONSC 6443.
24 Lisa Steacy, "BC Community Paper that Refused to Publish Anti-abortion Ad Wins Human Rights Case," *CTV News Vancouver*, November 3, 2023, ctvnews.ca/vancouver/article/bc-community-paper-that-refused-to-publish-anti-abortion-ad-wins-human-rights-case/.
25 Dominika Lirette, "Nelson Ends Banner Dispute by Deciding Not to Hang Any from Non-profits," *CBC News*, May 21, 2019, cbc.ca/news/canada/british-columbia/nelson-bans-banners-1.5144123.
26 Kendall Latimer, "Sask. Group Plans Billboards to Counter Anti-abortion Messages Lining Province's Highways," *CBC News*, August 17, 2022, cbc.ca/news/canada/saskatchewan/sask-abortion-is-health-care-billboards-1.6552460.
27 Kendall Latimer, "Volunteers Say They Won't Be Silenced after 'Abortion is Health Care' Banner Vandalized in Regina," *CBC News*, February 23, 2023, cbc.ca/news/canada/saskatchewan/regina-abortion-is-health-care-banner-vandalized-1.6756205.
28 Latimer, "Sask. Group."
29 Yasmine Ghania, "'Abortion is Healthcare' Billboard Goes Up in Sask. to Counter Anti-abortion Messages," *CBC News*, November 1, 2022, cbc.ca/news/canada/saskatchewan/abortion-is-health-care-billboard-anti-abortion-messages-1.6635516.
30 Saskatchewan, "Population," April 22, 2025, dashboard.saskatchewan.ca/people-community/people/population.
31 Latimer, "Volunteers Say."
32 *CBC News*, "London City Council Votes to Regulate Graphic Anti-abortion Imagery in Public," March 6, 2024, cbc.ca/news/canada/london/london-anti-abortion-sign-graphic-imagery-ban-1.7135233.
33 Calgary, "Bylaw Requirements for Flyers Depicting Graphic Images of Fetuses," n.d., calgary.ca/bylaws/graphic-flyers.html.
34 New Westminster, "Report, Planning and Development, Office of the CAO," December 16, 2024, pub-newwestcity.escribemeetings.com/filestream.ashx?DocumentId=20600.
35 Toronto City Council Agenda Item 2023.EX6.23, July 20, 2023, secure.toronto.ca/council/agenda-item.do?item=2023.EX6.23.
36 Abby O'Brien, "A Toronto Councillor Wants to Change How Anti-abortion Materials Can be Shared," *CTV News Toronto*, June 12, 2023, ctvnews.ca/toronto/article/a-toronto-councillor-wants-to-change-how-anti-abortion-materials-can-be-shared/.

37   Degrassi High 102 — A New Start, Pt. 2., youtube.com/watch?v=wuzFI9u88kA.
38   *Ontario (Attorney-General) v. Dieleman*, 1994 CanLII 7509 (ON SC).
39   Sophie M. Lavoie, "Abortion Conference Brings Together Scholars and Activists in Fredericton," *NB Media Co-op,* June 3, 2024, nbmediacoop.org/2024/06/03/abortion-conference-brings-together-scholars-and-activists-in-fredericton/.
40   Anne Swardson, "Canada Abortion Doctor Shot at Home by Sniper," *Washington Post,* November 9, 1994, washingtonpost.com/archive/politics/1994/11/09/canada-abortion-doctor-shot-at-home-by-sniper/c0a0003c-e4aa-494f-a012-36e842bdd61c/.
41   David Spurgeon, "Abortion Doctor Suffers Second Attack in Six Years," *BMJ* 321, no. 7255 (2000).
42   Larissa Cahute, "Vancouver Abortion Doctor Who Survived Murder Attempts Dies of Illness," *Vancouver Sun,* February 1, 2014, vancouversun.com/news/metro/vancouver-abortion-doctor-who-survived-murder-attempts-dies-of-illness.
43   Eleanor LeBourdais, "Potential for Violence Causing Fear among Canadian Doctors Who Perform Abortions," *Canadian Medical Association Journal* 152, no. 6 (1995).
44   Pam Lowe and Graeme Hayes, "Anti-Abortion Clinic Activism, Civil Inattention and the Problem of Gendered Harassment," *Sociology (Oxford)* 53, no. 2 (2019), 330.
45   *Ontario (Attorney-General) v. Dieleman*, 1994.
46   ARCC, "Safe Access Zone Laws and Court Injunctions in Canada (to Protect Abortion Access)," June 12, 2024 (first compiled June 1, 2017), arcc-cdac.ca/media/2020/06/Bubble-Zones-Court-Injunctions-in-Canada.pdf.
47   Access to Abortion Services Act [RSBC 1996] Chapter 1, bclaws.gov.bc.ca/civix/document/id/lc/statreg/96001_01.
48   *R. v. Lewis*, 1996 CanLII 3559 (BC SC).
49   ARCC, "Safe Access Zone Laws."
50   *Gordon Steven Watson v. Regina* CA029841, and *Donald David Spratt v. Regina* CA029830, ca.vlex.com/vid/r-v-watson-g-680853669.
51   ARCC, "Safe Access Zone Laws."
52   Joseph Brean, "Abortion Protestors Who Thoughts They Found Loophole in 'Bubble Zone' Law Lose BC Appeal," *National Post,* April 29, 2013, nationalpost.com/news/canada/abortion-protesters-who-thought-they-found-loophole-in-bubble-zone-law-lose-b-c-appeal.
53   Brean, "Abortion Protesters."
54   Elizabeth Whitten, "Bubble Zone Gets Royal Assent: NL Becomes Second Canadian Province to Have Bubble Zone Law," *The Overcast,* December 28, 2016, theovercast.ca/bubble-zone-gets-royal-assent-nl-becomes-second-canadian-province-to-have-bubble-zone-law/.
55   Laura Howells, "'Great Relief': Anti-abortion Protestors Respecting New Ban Outside Clinic," *CBC News,* July 14, 2016, cbc.ca/lite/story/1.3677269.
56   Act respecting Health Services and Social Services, CQLR c S-4.2, legisquebec.gouv.qc.ca/en/document/cs/s-4.2.
57   Access to Abortion Services Act SNL2016 Chapter A-1.02, canlii.org/en/nl/laws/stat/snl-2016-c-a-1.02/latest/snl-2016-c-a-1.02.html.
58   Safe Access to Abortion Services Act, 2017, S.O. 2017, c. 19, ontario.ca/laws/statute/17s19.
59   Alison Mah and Kelly Egan, "Protester Tries to Push Legal Boundaries of New Abortion 'Bubble-zone' Law," *Ottawa Citizen,* February 8, 2018,

ottawacitizen.com/news/local-news/protester-tries-to-push-legal-boundaries-of-new-abortion-bubble-zone-law.
60 Kelly Egan, "Priest Charged in Abortion Bubble-zone Flap to Mount 'Free Speech' Defence," *Ottawa Citizen,* October 31, 2018, ottawacitizen.com/news/local-news/priest-charged-in-abortion-bubble-zone-flap-to-mount-free-speech-defence.
61 Egan, "Priest Charged."
62 Egan, "Priest Charged."
63 Catholic Civil Rights League (CCRL), "Crown Drops Charges against Fr. Anthony Van Hee S.J. under the Safe Access to Abortion Services Act," October 28, 2022, ccrl.ca/issues/chargesdropped.
64 Robyn Maynard, *Policing Black Lives: State Violence in Canada from Slavery to the Present* (Fernwood Publishing, 2017).
65 The Canadian Press, "NB Judge Bans Anti-abortion Group from Protesting Outside Bathurst Hospital," *CBC News,* May 29, 2017, cbc.ca/news/canada/new-brunswick/anti-abortion-injunction-bathurst-hospital-vitalite-1.4136390.
66 The Canadian Press, "NB Judge."
67 Meg Cunningham, "Annual 'Pro-Choice Chain' Coming Up as Federal Leaders Promise Improved Abortion Access," *CHMA,* September 10, 2021, chmafm.com/welcome/annual-pro-choice-chain-coming-up-as-federal-leaders-promise-improved-abortion-access/.
68 Kaija Jussinoja, "Pushing for a Bubble Zone Law Outside of Halifax's Women's Choice Clinic," *The Coast,* December 12, 2019, thecoast.ca/news-opinion/pushing-for-a-bubble-zone-law-outside-of-halifaxs-womens-choice-clinic-23028771.
69 An Act to Protect Access to Reproductive Health Care: BILL NO. 242, 2nd Session, 63rd General Assembly Nova Scotia, nslegislature.ca/legc/bills/63rd_2nd/1st_read/b242.htm.
70 Government of Nova Scotia, "State of Emergency Declared in Response to COVID-19, Seven New Cases," Nova Scotia, March 22, 2020, news.novascotia.ca/en/2020/03/22/state-emergency-declared-response-covid-19-seven-new-cases.
71 ARCC (Abortion Rights Coalition of Canada), "Abortion Rights and Healthcare during COVID-19," January 6, 2022, arcc-cdac.ca/covid-19/.
72 Laura O'Connor, "Silent Struggles Amid the Pandemic," *Our Times,* October 27, 2020, ourtimes.ca/article/silent-struggles-amid-the-pandemic.
73 Government of Nova Scotia, "Injunction Granted to Stop Anti-Vaccine, Anti-Lockdown Protests," May 14, 2021, news.novascotia.ca/en/2021/05/14/injunction-granted-stop-anti-vaccine-anti-lockdown-protests.
74 Government of Nova Scotia, "Legislation to Protect Patients, Health-Service Providers, Staff of Healthcare Facilities," October 14, 2021, news.novascotia.ca/en/2021/10/14/legislation-protect-patients-health-service-providers-staff-healthcare-facilities.
75 Act to amend the Criminal Code and the Canada Labour Code: Bill C-3, December 17, 2021, justice.gc.ca/eng/csj-sjc/pl/charter-charte/c3_1.html.
76 Elizabeth Payne, "Ambulances Pelted with Rocks during Protest; Health Workers, Patients, Face Added Stress, Delays," *Ottawa Citizen,* February 1, 2022, ottawacitizen.com/news/local-news/ambulances-pelted-with-rocks-during-protest-health-workers-patients-face-added-stress-delays.
77 Emergencies Act R.S.C., 1985, c. 22 (4th Supp.), laws-lois.justice.gc.ca/eng/acts/e-4.5/page-1.html.
78 Steve Lambert, "Manitoba Introduces Law to Create Protest-free Zones Near Abortion Clinics," *CBC News,* March 7, 2024, cbc.ca/news/canada/manitoba/

abortion-protest-restrictions-manitoba-legislation-1.7137091.
79 The Canadian Press, "Manitoba PCs Say Bill Banning Anti-abortion Protests Near Clinics Should be Expanded," *CBC News,* March 20, 2024, cbc.ca/news/canada/manitoba/manitoba-anti-abortion-protest-bill-1.7150355.
80 Emily Chan, "How Provinces Are Using a Decades-Old Legal Tool to Create Hospital 'Bubble Zones,'" *Canadian Civil Liberties Association,* April 14, 2022, ccla.org/get-informed/talk-rights/how-provinces-are-using-a-decades-old-legal-tool-to-create-hospital-bubble-zones.

Chapter 8

1 "ROSE Clinic (Reproductive Options and Services)," Nova Scotia Health, n.d., nshealth.ca/clinics-programs-and-services/rose-clinic-reproductive-options-and-services.
2 Linepharma International, "Product Monograph Including Patient Medication Information Mifegymiso," Ontario: April 15, 2019, pdf.hres.ca/dpd_pm/00050659.pdf
3 Andrea Carson, Emma Stirling-Cameron, Martha Paynter, Sarah Munro, Wendy V. Norman, Kelley Kilpatrick, Stephanie Begun, and Ruth Martin-Misener, "Barriers and Enablers to Nurse Practitioner Implementation of Medication Abortion in Canada: A Qualitative Study," *PloS One* 18, no. 1 (2023).
4 Lydia Mainey, Catherine O'Mullan, Kerry Reid-Searl, Annabel Taylor, and Kathleen Baird, "The Role of Nurses and Midwives in the Provision of Abortion Care: A Scoping Review," *Journal of Clinical Nursing* 29, no. 9–10 (2020).
5 Regina M. Renner, Madeleine Ennis, Damien Contandriopoulos, Edith Guilbert, Sheila Dunn, Janusz Kaczorowski, Elizabeth K. Darling, Arianne Albert, Claire Styffe, and Wendy V. Norman, "Abortion Services and Providers in Canada in 2019: Results of a National Survey," *CMAJ Open* 10, no. 3 (2022).
6 CART (Contraception and Abortion Research Team), "Planning Canada's Midwifery Abortion Implementation Study, Proceedings of a National Research Planning Meeting: April 13, 2019," med-fom-cart-grac.sites.olt.ubc.ca/files/2018/07/Planning-Canadas-Midwifery-FINAL.pdf.
7 Government of Prince Edward Island, "Midwifery Services," January 30, 2024, princeedwardisland.ca/en/information/health-pei/midwifery-services.
8 Ontario Health, "Ontario Connecting People to More Care from Midwives," News Release, May 3, 2024, news.ontario.ca/en/release/1004529/ontario-connecting-people-to-more-care-from-midwives.
9 Lillian Roy, "Quebec Midwives Will be Able to Prescribe Abortion Pills by the Fall," *CTV News Montreal,* July 22, 2022, ctvnews.ca/montreal/article/quebec-midwives-will-be-able-to-prescribe-abortion-pills-by-the-fall/.
10 Canadian Association of Midwives (CAM), "National Strategy for Midwife-led Abortion Care in Canada," 2024, canadianmidwives.org/sites/canadianmidwives.org/wp-content/uploads/2024/05/CAM_National_Strategy_for_Midwifery-Led_Abortion_Care_May_2024.pdf.
11 BCCNM (British Columbia College of Nurses and Midwives), Section 8: Restricted activities for certified practice, n.d., bccnm.ca/RN/ScopePractice/part4/section8/Pages/Default.aspx.
12 BCCNM, "BCCNM board approves new limits and conditions for RN Certified Practice," October 4, 2022, bccnm.ca/BCCNM/Announcements/Pages/Announcement.aspx?AnnouncementID=384.
13 CNO (College of Nurses of Ontario), "RN Prescribing Medication List," November 6, 2023.

14 Québec, "Do You Need Birth Control? Talk to a Nurse!" *Santé et Services Sociaux Québec*, n.d., publications.msss.gouv.qc.ca/msss/fichiers/2010/10-255-01A.pdf.
15 Canadian Pharmacists Association (CPhA), "Pharmacist Contraceptive Prescribing Across Canada," *CPhA*, July 2023, pharmacists.ca/cpha-ca/assets/File/cpha-on-the-issues/Contraception-Infographic.pdf.
16 Andrea Carson, Martha Paynter, Wendy Norman, Sarah Munro, Josette Rousel, Sheila Dunn and Denise Bryant-Lukosius. "Optimizing the Nurse Role in Abortion Care," *Canadian Journal of Nursing Leadership* 35, no. 1 (2021); Andrea Carson, Emma Stirling Cameron, Martha Paynter, Wendy Norman, Sarah Munro, and Ruth Martin-Misener, "Nurse Practitioners on the 'Leading Edge' of Medication Abortion Approach Care: A Feminist Qualitative Approach," *Journal of Advanced Nursing* 79, no. 2 (2021).
17 Paynter et al., "Nurses Are Key Members."
18 Lindsay Sheinfeld, Grady Arnott, Julie El-Haddad, and Angel M. Foster, "Assessing Abortion Coverage in Nurse Practitioner Programs in Canada: A National Survey of Program Directors," *Contraception* 94, no. 5 (2016).
19 Jessica Liauw, Brigid Dineley, K. Gerster, N. Hill, and D. Costescu, "Abortion Training in Canadian Obstetrics and Gynecology Residency Programs," *Contraception* 94, no. 5 (2016).
20 Daniel T. Myran, Jillian Bardsley, Tania El Hindi, and Kristine Whitehead, "Abortion Education in Canadian Family Medicine Residency Programs," *BMC Medical Education* 18, no. 1 (2018).
21 Daniel T. Myran, Caitlin L. Carew, Jingyang Tang, Helena Whyte, and William A. Fisher, "Medical Students' Intentions to Seek Abortion Training and to Provide Abortion Services in Future Practice," *Journal of Obstetrics and Gynaecology Canada* 37, no. 3 (2015).
22 Tara A. Cessford and Wendy V. Norman, "Making a Case for Abortion Curriculum Reform: A Knowledge-Assessment Survey of Undergraduate Medical Students," *Journal of Obstetrics and Gynaecology Canada* 33, no. 1 (2011).
23 Martha Paynter, Danielle LeBlanc, Lianne Yoshida, Anna Finlayson, Kristen Turtle, Marion Brown, C.J. Blennerhassett, and Laurie Graham, "Implementation of an Interprofessional Health Education Course on Abortion Care," *Teaching and Learning in Nursing* 17, no. 2 (2022).
24 Paynter et al., "Nurses Are Key Members," 21.
25 UBC CPD (University of British Columbia Continuing Professional Development), "The CART Access Project," Vancouver: Faculty of Medicine, n.d., ubccpd.ca/cart-access-project.
26 UBC CPD, "The CART Access Project."
27 CASN, "Entry-to-Practice Abortion Care Competencies."
28 Abortion Rights Coalition of Canada, "Statistics — Abortion in Canada," April 18, 2024, arcc-cdac.ca/media/2020/07/statistics-abortion-in-canada.pdf.
29 Renner et al., "First and Second-Trimester."
30 Renner et al., "First and Second-Trimester."
31 X. Guan, Wendy V. Norman, Edith Guilbert, A. Albert, K. O'Connell White, H.E. Jones, and Regina M. Renner, "Second-Trimester Surgical and Medical Abortion Practice in Canada in 2012: A National Survey," *Contraception* 95, no. 5 (2017).
32 Christabelle Sethna and Marion Doull, "Accidental Tourists: Canadian Women, Abortion Tourism, and Travel," *Women's Studies* 41, no. 4 (2012), 457.
33 W.D. Thomas, "The Badgley Report on the Abortion Law," *Canadian Medical Association Journal* 116, no. 9 (1977).
34 Boulder Abortion Clinic, n.d., drhern.com/.

35 Dupont Clinic, "Our Clinic: Experience Exceptional Abortion care," n.d., dupontclinic.com/?gclid=CjwKCAjwvvmzBhA2EiwAtHVrb1vYptmvd04F71IsN-PYy13km4Zvd0EN6Zt5KWRKoSke4aofrAhuYaRoC-KoQAvD_BwE.
36 Partners in Abortion Care Clinic, "Contact," n.d., partnersclinic.com/contact/.
37 Tanja Armenski, Brendan Sheahan, Duncan Currie and Larry McKeown, "Crossing the Border during the Pandemic: 2020 in Review," *Statistics Canada*, February 23, 2021, publications.gc.ca/collections/collection_2021/statcan/45-28/CS45-28-1-2021-7-eng.pdf.
38 Women's College Hospital, "Bay Centre for Birth Control (BCBC) Referral Form — Second Trimester Abortion," Toronto, n.d., womenscollegehospital.ca/wp-content/uploads/2022/06/F-8109-BCBC-2nd-Trimester-Referral-Form-May-19-2022.pdf.
39 BC Women's Hospital and Health Centre, "Abortion & Contraception," n.d., bcwomens.ca/our-services/gynecology/abortion-contraception.
40 Guttmacher Institute, "State Bans on Abortion Throughout Pregnancy," March 5, 2025, guttmacher.org/state-policy/explore/state-policies-abortion-bans.
41 Andy Blatchford, "Canada is Open to Americans Who May Lose Access to Abortions, But There's a Catch," *Politico*, May 5, 2022, politico.com/news/2022/05/05/canada-americans-access-abortions-00030209.
42 Mitchell Consky, "Canadians Open Their Doors to Americans Seeking Abortions," *CTV News*, June 28, 2022, ctvnews.ca/world/article/canadians-open-their-doors-to-americans-seeking-abortions/.
43 Isaac Maddow-Zimet and Candace Gibson, "Despite Bans, Number of Abortions in the United States Increased in 2023," *Guttmacher Institute*, March 2024, guttmacher.org/2024/03/despite-bans-number-abortions-united-states-increased-2023.
44 US Department of State, "Return to Pre-Pandemic Passport Processing Times," Media Note, Office of the Spokesperson, December 18, 2023, 2021-2025.state.gov/return-to-pre-pandemic-passport-processing-times/.
45 Jean-Frederic Levesque, Mark F. Harris, and Grant Russell, "Patient-Centred Access to Health Care: Conceptualising Access at the Interface of Health Systems and Populations," *International Journal for Equity in Health* 12, no. 1 (2013).
46 Madeleine Ennis, Regina Renner, Bimbola Olure, Stephanie Begun, Wendy V. Norman, Sarah Munro, "Provision of Care to Diverse Populations: Results from the 2019 Canadian Abortion Provider Survey," *BMJ Sexual and Reproductive Health* 50, no. 4 (October 15, 2024).
47 Renner et al., "First and Second-Trimester."
48 Egale, "Northwest Territories Makes History," n.d., egale.ca/egale-in-action/northwest-territories-makes-history/.
49 Human Rights Act SNWT 2002, c.18, canlii.org/en/nt/laws/stat/snwt-2002-c-18/latest/.
50 Canadian Human Rights Act R.S.C., 1985, c. H-6, laws-lois.justice.gc.ca/eng/acts/h-6/.
51 Egale, "Brief on Statistics Canada Sex and Gender Data — Census 2021," October 2022, egale.ca/wp-content/uploads/2022/10/Brief-on-Statistics-Canada-Sex-and-Gender-Data%E2%80%93Census-2021.pdf.
52 Statistics Canada, "Canada is the First Country to Provide Census Data on Transgender and Non-binary People," *The Daily*, April 27, 2022, www150.statcan.gc.ca/n1/daily-quotidien/220427/dq220427b-info-eng.htm.
53 Elias G. Thomas, Bahareh Goodarzi, Hannah Frese, Linda J. Schoonmade, and Maaike E. Muntinga, "Pregnancy Experiences of Transgender and

54 Melisa M. Holmes, Heidi S. Resnick, Dean G. Kilpatrick, and Connie L. Best, "Rape-Related Pregnancy: Estimates and Descriptive Characteristics from a National Sample of Women," *American Journal of Obstetrics and Gynecology* 175, no. 2 (1996).

55 Rachel Dowd, "Transgender People Over Four Times More Likely Than Cisgender People to be Victims of Violent Crime," *UCLA School of Law Williams Institute*, March 23, 2021, williamsinstitute.law.ucla.edu/press/ncvs-trans-press-release/.

56 Heidi Moseson, Laura Fix, Sachiko Ragosta, Hannah Forsberg, Jen Hastings, Ari Stoeffler, Mitchell R. Lunn et al. "Abortion Experiences and Preferences of Transgender, Nonbinary, and Gender-Expansive People in the United States," *American Journal of Obstetrics and Gynecology* 224, no. 4 (2021).

57 Rachel K. Jones, Elizabeth Witwer, Jenna Jerman, "Transgender Abortion Patients and the Provision of Transgender-Specific Care at Non-Hospital Facilities That Provide Abortions," *ContraceptionX* 2 (2020).

58 A.J. Lowik, "Trans-Inclusive Abortion Services: A Manual for Providers on Operationalizing Trans-inclusive Policies and Practices in an Abortion Setting," 2021, optionsforsexualhealth.org/wp-content/uploads/2019/07/FQPN18-Manual-EN-BC-web.pdf.

59 Bloor West Village Women's Clinic, "Abortion and D&C Services in Toronto and the GTA," n.d., bloorwestwomensclinic.com/.

60 Cabbagetown Women's Clinic, cabbagetownwomensclinic.com/.

61 Lowik, "Trans-Inclusive Abortion Services," 18.

62 *Vancouver Rape Relief Society v. Nixon*, 2004 BCCA 516, ca.vlex.com/vid/rape-relief-soc-v-680839725.

63 *Vancouver Rape Relief Society v. Nixon*.

64 Human Rights Code, RSBC 1996, c 210, bclaws.gov.bc.ca/civix/document/id/consol31/consol31/00_96210_01.

65 *Vancouver Rape Relief Society v. Nixon*, 2005 BCCA 601, rapereliefshelter.bc.ca/wp-content/uploads/2021/03/BC-Court-of-Appeal-Reasons-for-Judgement-2005.pdf.

66 BC Human Rights Tribunal, "2016 Updates," bchrt.bc.ca/2016-updates/.

67 *CBC News*, "City of Vancouver to Cut Funding to Women's Group on Basis of Transgender Discrimination," March 19, 2019, cbc.ca/news/canada/british-columbia/city-of-vancouver-to-cut-funding-to-women-s-group-on-basis-of-transgender-discrimination-1.5062688.

68 Vancouver Rape Relief and Women's Shelter, "What We do and Who We Serve," 2021. rapereliefshelter.bc.ca/who-we-serve-and-what-we-do/.

69 Maria Cheng, "Indigenous Women in Canada Forcibly Sterilized Decades after Other Rich Countries Stopped," *Associated Press News*, July 12, 2023, apnews.com/article/canada-indigenous-women-sterilization-apology-reparations-ebcacc0f27b8d4c12d8690718202531d.

70 Cheng, "Indigenous Women in Canada."

71 Holly A. McKenzie et al. "Indigenous Women's Resistance of Colonial Policies, Practices, and Reproductive Coercion," *Qualitative Health Research* 32, no. 7 (2022).

72 Renée Monchalin, Astrid V. Pérez Piñán, Madison Wells, Willow Paul, Danette Jubinville, Kimberly Law, Meagan Chaffey, Harlie Pruder, and Arie Ross, "A Qualitative Study Exploring Access Barriers to Abortion Services among Indigenous Peoples in Canada," *Contraception* 124 (2023).

73 Native Women's Association of Canada (NWAC), "Is A Genocide Taking Place in Canada? Short Answer: Yes," Ottawa, June 19, 2023, nwac.ca/media/2023/06/is-a-genocide-taking-place-in-canada-short-answer-yes.
74 Jane Kirby, "A Broad Vision for Reproductive Justice," *Briarpatch Magazine*, December 21, 2017, briarpatchmagazine.com/articles/view/broad-vision-reproductive-justice.
75 Government of Canada, "Annual Report to Parliament 2020," *Indigenous Services Canada*, November 3, 2020, sac-isc.gc.ca/eng/1602010609492/1602010631711.
76 Renée Monchalin, "Novel Coronavirus, Access to Abortion Services, and Bridging Western and Indigenous Knowledges in a Postpandemic World," *Women's Health Issues* 31, no. 1 (2021).
77 Renée Monchalin, Danette Jubinville, Astrid V. Pérez Piñán, Willow Paul, Madison Wells, Arie Ross, Kimberly Law, Meagan Chaffey, and Harlie Pruder, "'I Would Love for There Not to Be so Many Hoops…': Recommendations to Improve Abortion Service Access and Experiences Made by Indigenous Women and 2SLGTBQIA+ People in Canada," *Sexual and Reproductive Health Matters* 31, no. 1 (2023).
78 Jenna Smith, "Parliamentary Committee Notes: Overrepresentation (Indigenous Offenders)," *Public Safety Canada*, March 9, 2023, publicsafety.gc.ca/cnt/trnsprnc/brfng-mtrls/prlmntry-bndrs/20230720/12-en.aspx.
79 Martha Paynter, Ruth Martin-Misener, Adelina Iftene, and Gail Tomblin Murphy, "The Correctional Services Canada Institutional Mother Child Program: A Look at the Numbers," *The Prison Journal* 102, no. 5 (2022).
80 Jessica Liauw, Jessica Foran, Brigid Dineley, Dustin Costescu, and Fiona G Kouyoumdjian, "The Unmet Contraceptive Need of Incarcerated Women in Ontario," *Journal of Obstetrics and Gynaecology Canada* 38, no. 9 (2016).
81 Martha Paynter and Clare Heggie, "Distance between Institutions of Incarceration and Procedural Abortion Facilities in Canada," *Contraception* 124 (2023).
82 Martha Paynter, Paula Pinzón Hernández, Clare Heggie, Shelley McKibbon, and Sarah Munro, "Abortion and Contraception for Incarcerated People: A Scoping Review," *PloS One* 18, no. 3 (2023).
83 Public Safety Canada, "2021 Corrections and Conditional Release Statistical Overview," *Figure A17*, June 20, 2023, publicsafety.gc.ca/cnt/rsrcs/pblctns/ccrso-2021/index-en.aspx#sec-a17.
84 UN (United Nations), "United Nations Minimum Standards for the Treatment of Prisoners (the Mandela Rules)," *United Nations Office on Drugs and Crime* (2015), unodc.org/documents/justice-and-prison-reform/Nelson_Mandela_Rules-E-ebook.pdf.
85 Beatrice du Prey, Rachel Talavlikar, Rupinder Mangat, Elizabeth A. Freiheit and Neil Drummond, "Induced Abortion and Contraception Use among Immigrant and Canadian-born Women in Calgary, Alta.," *Canadian Family Physician* 60, no. 9 (2014).
86 Susitha Wanigaratne, Mei-ling Wiedmeyer, Hilary K. Brown, Astrid Guttmann, and Marcelo L. Urquia, "Induced Abortion According to Immigrants' Birthplace: A Population-Based Cohort Study," *Reproductive Health* 17, no. 1 (2020).
87 Ellen Wiebe, "Contraceptive Practices and Attitudes among Immigrant and Nonimmigrant Women in Canada," *Canadian Family Physician* 59, no. 10 (2013).
88 Hilary K. Brown, Simon Chen, Astrid Guttmann, Susan M. Havercamp, Susan Parish, Joel G. Ray, Lesley A. Tarasoff, Simone N. Vigod, Adele Carty, and Yona Lunsky, "Rates of Recognized Pregnancy in Women with Disabilities in Ontario, Canada," *American Journal of Obstetrics and Gynecology* 222, no. 2 (2020).

89 Hilary K. Brown, Joel G. Ray, Ning Liu, Yona Lunsky, and Simone N. Vigod, "Rapid Repeat Pregnancy among Women with Intellectual and Developmental Disabilities: A Population-Based Cohort Study," *Canadian Medical Association Journal* 190, no. 32 (2018).
90 Vanessa Balintec, "We're Welcoming Record Numbers of International Students. Here's How They Got Caught Up in the Housing Crisis," *CBC News*, August 28, 2023, cbc.ca/news/canada/international-student-timeline-1.6947913.
91 IRCC (Immigration, Refugees and Citizenship Canada), "SOCI — Canada's Temporary Foreign Worker Programming," Government of Canada, September 13, 2023. canada.ca/en/immigration-refugees-citizenship/corporate/transparency/committees/soci-sept-28-2023/canadas-temporary-foreign-worker-programming.html.
92 Y.Y. Chen, "Canada Health Act at 40," Research Roundtable at the University of Ottawa, June 20, 2024, healthcoalition.ca/what-can-rescue-the-canada-health-act/.
93 Chen, "Canada Health Act at 40."

Chapter 9

1 CIHI, "Induced Abortions."
2 This number does not include the data from free-standing clinics in BC and NL, where data is reported as a category of "24 years of age or younger," without more granularity. In NL, there were no hospital abortion patients aged seventeen or younger; in BC, patients aged seventeen or younger comprised 8.5 percent of all hospital patients twenty-four years of age or younger. Using these proxies, of the 3,381 clinic patients aged twenty-four and younger, 288 may have been under seventeen; this does not change the overall rate of 2 percent in Canada.
3 Claudine Provencher and Nora Galbraith, "Fertility in Canada, 1921 to 2022," Statistics Canada, January 31, 2024, publications.gc.ca/collections/collection_2024/statcan/91f0015m2024001-eng.pdf.
4 Kaylee Ramage, Suzanne Tough, Catherine Scott, Anne-Marie McLaughlin, and Amy Metcalfe, "Trends in Adolescent Rapid Repeat Pregnancy in Canada," *Journal of Obstetrics and Gynaecology Canada* 43, no. 5 (2021).
5 Diana Greene Foster, Heather Gould, and M. Antonia Biggs, "Timing of Pregnancy Discovery among Women Seeking Abortion," *Contraception* 104, no. 6 (2021).
6 Margot Sanger-Katz et al., "Who Gets Abortions in America?"
7 Guttmacher Institute, "Parental Involvement in Minors' Abortions' State Laws and Policies," September 1, 2023, guttmacher.org/state-policy/explore/parental-involvement-minors-abortions.
8 Mollie Dunsmuir, *Abortion: Constitutional and Legal Developments*, Government of Canada — Law and Government Division, November 1998, publications.gc.ca/Collection-R/LoPBdP/CIR/8910-e.htm.
9 Kevin W. Coughlin, "Medical Decision-making in Paediatrics: Infancy to Adolescence," *Canadian Paediatric Society*, Position Statement: April 12, 2018 (reaffirmed January 11, 2024), cps.ca/documents/position/medical-decision-making-in-paediatrics-infancy-to-adolescence.
10 Éducaloi, "Abortion For People Under 18," n.d., educaloi.qc.ca/en/capsules/abortion-for-people-under-18/.
11 Coughlin, "Medical Decision-making."
12 Medical Consent of Minors Act, SNB 1976, c. M-6.1.
13 Government of Canada, "The United Nations Convention on the Rights of the Child: An Overview for Children and Teenagers," November 5, 2021, canada.ca/en/public-health/services/national-child-day/united-nations-convention-rights-of-the-child.html.

14 Alberta Health Services, "Consent to Treatment/Procedures(s) Minors/Mature Minors," October 25, 2010, albertahealthservices.ca/assets/info/hpsp/if-hpsp-phys-consent-summary-sheet-minors-mature-minors.pdf .

15 Government of Manitoba, "Informed Consent Guidelines for Immunization," *Population and Public Health Branch,* approved July 2013; amended September 2023, gov.mb.ca/health/publichealth/cdc/protocol/consentguidelines.pdf.

16 *A.C. v. Manitoba (Director of Child and Family Services)*, 2009 SCC 30, [2009] 2 SCR 181, decisions.scc-csc.ca/scc-csc/scc-csc/en/item/7795/index.do.

17 Child and Family Services Act, CCSM c C80, web2.gov.mb.ca/laws/statutes/ccsm/_pdf.php?cap=c80.

18 Daniel Del Gobbo, "*A.C. v. Manitoba*: Bioethics and the 'Best Interests' of Mature Minors," *The Court,* York University, June 29, 2009, thecourt.ca/ac-v-manitoba-defining-the-best-interests-of-mature-minors/.

19 *A.C. v. Manitoba.*

20 Del Gobbo, "*A.C. v. Manitoba.*"

21 Andrew Jeffrey, "Alberta Legislation on Transgender Youth, Student Pronouns and Sex Education to Become Law," *CBC News,* December 4, 2024, cbc.ca/news/canada/calgary/alberta-legislation-on-transgender-youth-student-pronouns-and-sex-education-set-to-become-law-1.7400669.

22 Hadeel Ibrahim, "Holt Says She'll Change Gender-identity Policy for Schools, Stop Move to Dissolve DEC," *CBC News,* October 23, 2024, cbc.ca/news/canada/new-brunswick/new-brunswick-gender-identity-policy-1.7359786.

23 Jaimie F. Veale, Ryan J. Watson, Tracey Peter, and Elizabeth M. Saewyc, "Mental Health Disparities Among Canadian Transgender Youth," *Journal of Adolescent Health* 60, no. 1 (2017), 48.

24 Giuseppina Di Meglio, Colleen Crowther, and Joanne Simms, "Contraceptive Care for Canadian Youth, Canadian Paediatric Society (CPS) Adolescent Health Committee Position Statement," *Canadian Paediatric Society* (June 12, 2018, reaffirmed January 11, 2024), cps.ca/documents/position/contraceptive-care.

25 Statistics Canada, "Sex at Birth and Gender — 2021 Census Promotional Material," January 3, 2023, statcan.gc.ca/en/census/census-engagement/community-supporter/sex-birth-gender.

26 Kacie M. Kidd, Gina M. Sequeira, Claudia Douglas, Taylor Paglisotti, David J. Inwards-Breland, Elizabeth Miller, and Robert W.S. Coulter, "Prevalence of Gender-Diverse Youth in an Urban School District," *Pediatrics* 147, no. 6 (2021), 1.

27 Ayden I. Scheim, Todd Coleman, Nathan Lachowsky, and Greta R. Bauer, "Health Care Access among Transgender and Nonbinary People in Canada, 2019: A Cross-Sectional Survey," *CMAJ Open* 9, no. 4 (2021).

28 Shane Magee, "NB Judge Rules Against School District in Challenge to Gender-identity Policy," *CBC News,* July 5, 2024, cbc.ca/news/canada/new-brunswick/anglophone-east-decision-713-1.7255292.

29 Jeremy Simes, "Challenge of Sask. School Pronoun Law Can Proceed despite Notwithstanding Clause, Judge Rules," *CBC News,* February 16, 2024, cbc.ca/news/canada/saskatchewan/judge-pronoun-challenge-ruling-1.7117608.

30 Alberta Human Rights Commission, "Protected Grounds," n.d., albertahumanrights.ab.ca/what-are-human-rights/about-human-rights/protected-grounds/.

31 Canadian Human Rights Act, R.S.C., 1985, c. H-6.

32 New Brunswick, "Child Protection," March 2021, gnb.ca/content/dam/gnb/Departments/sd-ds/pdf/Protection/Child/booklet-e.pdf.

33   Government of British Columbia, "Duty to Report," n.d., gov.bc.ca/assets/gov/public-safety-and-emergency-services/public-safety/protecting-children/t15-0191_dutytoreport_pamphlet11x85in2folds.pdf.
34   "Youth Criminal Justice Act," *Youth Justice*, December 2022, ycja.ca/youth-justice/youth-criminal-justice-act.
35   Criminal Code (R.S.C., 1985, c. C-46), PART VIII: Section 273.2.
36   Criminal Code (R.S.C., 1985, c. C-46), Section 273.1 (1).
37   College of Early Childhood Educators, *Racism and Bias in Reporting to Child Welfare*, 2022, college-ece.ca/wp-content/uploads/2022/06/SAPP_Racism_and_Bias_Reporting_to_Child_Welfare_EN-FINAL.pdf .
38   Criminal Code (R.S.C., 1985, c. C-46), Section 155 (1).
39   Statistics Canada, "Family Violence in Canada: A Statistical Profile; Section 2: Police-reported Family Violence against Children and Youth, 2009," November 17, 2015, statcan.gc.ca/n1/pub/85-224-x/2010000/part-partie2-eng.htm.
40   Julie S. Lalonde, "Incest Survivors Need Their #MeToo Moment," *Chatelaine Magazine*, May 31, 2022, chatelaine.com/living/features-living/incest-survivors-need-their-metoo/.
41   Public Safety Canada, "Human Trafficking Isn't What You Think It Is," July 15, 2024, canada.ca/en/public-safety-canada/campaigns/human-trafficking.html.
42   Vancouver Police Department, "Human Trafficking," n.d., vpd.ca/crime-prevention-safety/human-trafficking/.
43   Canadian Centre to End Human Trafficking, "Human Trafficking Trends in Canada," Report: 2019, canadiancentretoendhumantrafficking.ca/wp-content/uploads/2021/10/ENG-Human-Trafficking-Trends-in-Canada-%E2%80%93-2019-20-Report-Final-1.pdf.
44   Public Safety Canada, "About Human Trafficking," February 13, 2024, publicsafety.gc.ca/cnt/cntrng-crm/hmn-trffckng/abt-hmn-trffckng-en.aspx.
45   Public Safety Canada, "About Human Trafficking."
46   Karuna S. Chibber, M. Antonia Biggs, Sarah C. M. Roberts, and Diana Greene Foster, "The Role of Intimate Partners in Women's Reasons for Seeking Abortion," *Women's Health Issues* 24, no. 1 (2014).
47   WAGE (Women and Gender Equality Canada), "Fact sheet: Intimate Partner Violence," July 31, 2024, canada.ca/en/women-gender-equality/gender-based-violence/intimate-partner-violence.html.
48   Leanne Findlay, Evelyne Bougie, Dafna Kohen and Kristyn Frank, "An Exploration of Methods to Estimate the Number of Immigrant Girls and Women at Risk of Female Genital Mutilation or Cutting in Canada," *Analytical Studies: Methods and References* 11, no. 633 (September 6, 2023).

Chapter 10

1   Duke Appiah, Chike C. Nwabuo, Imo A. Ebong, Melissa F. Wellons, and Stephen J. Winters, "Trends in Age at Natural Menopause and Reproductive Life Span Among US Women, 1959–2018," *JAMA* 325, no. 13 (2021).
2   UNFPA (United Nations Population Fund), "By Choice, not by Chance: Family Planning, Human Rights and Development," November 14, 2012.
3   Action Canada for Sexual Health & Rights, "UN Human Rights Body Slams Canada for Failure to Ensure Access to Abortion, Affordable Contraception," November 21, 2016, actioncanadashr.org/about-us/media/2016-11-21-un-human-rights-body-slams-canada-failure-ensure-access-abortion-affordable-contraception.
4   Levesque et al., "Patient-Centred Access to Health Care."

5   Paynter, "Nexplanon, a 3-Year Birth Control Implant."
6   Lawrence B. Finer, "The Harms of Denying a Woman a Wanted Abortion," Advancing New Standards in Reproductive Health, April 16, 2020, ansirh.org/sites/default/files/publications/files/the_harms_of_denying_a_woman_a_wanted_abortion_4-16-2020.pdf.
7   Dominika Śmiałek and Julia Żuławińska, "Period Products Cost Calculator," *Omni Calculator*, 2023, omnicalculator.com/everyday-life/period-products-cost.
8   Employment and Social Development Canada, "Menstrual Products Now Available at No Cost to Employees in Federally Regulated Workplaces," December 15, 2023, canada.ca/en/employment-social-development/news/2023/12/menstrual-products-now-available-at-no-cost-to-employees-in-federally-regulated-workplaces.html.
9   Jill E. Sergison, Lauren Y. Maldonado, Xiaoming Gao, and David Hubacher, "Levonorgestrel Intrauterine System Associated Amenorrhea: A Systematic Review and Metaanalysis," *American Journal of Obstetrics and Gynecology* 220, no. 5 (2019).
10 Alison Edelman, Elizabeth Micks, Makalapua L. Motu'apuaka, Lyndsey S. Benson, and Fiona Stewart, "Continuous or Extended Cycle vs. Cyclic Use of Combined Hormonal Contraceptives for Contraception," *Cochrane Database of Systematic Reviews* 2023, no. 12 (2014), CD004695.
11 Steven G. Morgan and Jamie R. Daw, "Canadian Pharmacare: Looking Back, Looking Forward," *Healthcare Policy* 8, no. 1 (2012).
12 Health Canada, "Canada Health Act Annual Report," Minister of Health, 2014, canada.ca/content/dam/hc-sc/migration/hc-sc/hcs-sss/alt_formats/pdf/pubs/cha-ics/2015-cha-lcs-ar-ra-eng.pdf.
13 American College of Obstetricians and Gynecologists), "Effectiveness of Birth Control Methods," 2024, acog.org/womens-health/infographics/effectiveness-of-birth-control-methods.
14 James Trussell, Anjana M. Lalla, Quan V. Doan, Eileen Reyes, Lionel Pinto, and Joseph Gricar, "Cost Effectiveness of Contraceptives in the United States," *Contraception* 79, no. 1 (2009).
15 Government of British Columbia, "Free Contraceptives," July 30, 2024, www2.gov.bc.ca/gov/content/health/health-drug-coverage/pharmacare-for-bc-residents/what-we-cover/prescription-contraceptives.
16 CART (Contraception Access Research Team), "British Columbia 2015 Sexual Health Indicators," *Canadian Sexual Health Survey*, June 15, 2017. med-fom-cart-grac.sites.olt.ubc.ca/files/2017/08/2015-BC-Sexual-Health-Indicators-CART-CSHS_2017-06-15.pdf.
17 Amanda Y. Black, Edith Guilbert, Fareen Hassan, Ismini Chatziheofilou, Julia Lowin, Mark Jeddi, Anna Filonenko, and James Trussell, "The Cost of Unintended Pregnancies in Canada: Estimating Direct Cost, Role of Imperfect Adherence, and the Potential Impact of Increased Use of Long-Acting Reversible Contraceptives," *Journal of Obstetrics and Gynaecology Canada* 37, no. 12 (2015).
18 Elizabeth Nethery, Laura Schummers, K. Suzanne Maginley, Sheila Dunn, and Wendy V. Norman, "Household Income and Contraceptive Methods Among Female Youth: a Cross-Sectional Study Using the Canadian Community Health Survey (2009–2010 and 2013–2014)," *Canadian Medical Association Journal* 7, no. 4 (2019).
19 CART (Contraception Access Research Team), "Contraception Cost-Effectiveness in British Columbia," University of British Columbia, June 22, 2018. med-fom-cart-grac.sites.olt.ubc.ca/files/2023/02/Contraception-Cost-Effectiveness_CART-Report_2018-06-21.pdf.

20 Government of British Columbia, "Universal Contraception Coverage Starts April 1," March 31, 2023, news.gov.bc.ca/releases/2023HLTH0033-000430.
21 The Canadian Press, "Tens of Thousands of BC Residents Received Free Contraception in Eight Months, Eby Says," *Global News*, December 8, 2023, globalnews.ca/news/10158381/high-uptake-bc-free-contraception/.
22 Wendy V. Norman, "Considerations on Contraception Cost-Effectiveness," University of British Columbia, n.d., mcusercontent.com/353019c4e982ae7e-b8ea53150/files/ad6a308e-fc79-b35c-935a-1d83e4e460d3/Contraception_Cost_Effectiveness_UBC_CART_Analysis_2023_11_26.pdf.
23 Government of British Columbia, "Universal Contraception."
24 Rev Bras Enferm, "Evidence of Intrauterine Device Insertion by Nurses in Primary Health Care: An Integrative Review," *Brazilian Journal of Nursing* 77, no. 1 (2024).
25 Government of Canada, "A Prescription for Canada: Achieving Pharmacare for All," June 2019, canada.ca/en/health-canada/corporate/about-health-canada/public-engagement/external-advisory-bodies/implementation-national-pharmacare/final-report.html.
26 *CBC News*, "Women's Health Advocates Applaud Manitoba's Plan to Subsidize Prescription Birth Control," November 22, 2023, cbc.ca/news/canada/manitoba/manitoba-throne-speech-birth-control-1.7035927.
27 Statutes of Canada: Bill C-64, An Act Respecting Pharmacare, 2024 c. 24, laws.justice.gc.ca/eng/AnnualStatutes/2024_24/FullText.html.
28 Public Health Agency of Canada, "Snapshot of Diabetes in Canada, 2023," canada.ca/en/public-health/services/publications/diseases-conditions/snapshot-diabetes-canada-2023.html.
29 Diabetes Canada, "Diabetes in Canada: 2022 Backgrounder," February 2022, diabetes.ca/DiabetesCanadaWebsite/media/Advocacy-and-Policy/Backgrounder/2022_Backgrounder_Canada_English_1.pdf.
30 Health Canada, "Government of Canada Passes Legislation for a First Phase of National Universal Pharmacare," October 10, 2024, canada.ca/en/health-canada/news/2024/10/government-of-canada-passes-legislation-for-a-first-phase-of-national-universal-pharmacare.html.
31 Diabetes Canada, "Diabetes Canada: Overview of Bill C-64," 2024, diabetes.ca/getattachment/e23899c7-4e92-42b1-92a8-d6435fe5b4bc/Diabetes-Canada-Position-Paper-Final.pdf?lang=en-CA.
32 College of Midwives of Ontario, "Designated Drugs and Substances Regulation," 2024, cmo.on.ca/standards-and-resources/designated-drugs-and-substances-regulation/.
33 *CBC News*, "Nurses in Ontario Will Soon be Able to Prescribe Birth Control."
34 Nursing Specialty Perinatal Course, "Contraceptive Management in Reproductive Health for BCCNM Certification," British Columbia Institute of Technology (BCIT), n.d., bcit.ca/courses/contraceptive-management-in-reproductive-health-for-bccnm-certification-nspn-7720/.
35 British Columbia College of Nurses & Midwives, "Framework for Midwife Certification in Hormonal Contraceptive Therapy," December 2020, bccnm.ca/Documents/education_program_review/RM_Framework_for_Certification_in_Hormonal_Contraceptive_Therapy.pdf.
36 Canadian Press, "Quebec Nurses to Prescribe Birth Control Pills," *CTV News*, January 31, 2007.
37 Enferm, "Evidence of Intrauterine Device Insertion."
38 Allison A. Merz, Alba Gutiérrez-Sacristán, Deborah Bartz, Natalie E. Williams, Ayotomiwa Ojo, Kimberly M. Schaefer, Melody Huang et al. "Population Attitudes

toward Contraceptive Methods over Time on a Social Media Platform," *American Journal of Obstetrics and Gynecology* 224, no. 6 (2021).

39   Anna Schneider-Kamp and Jennifer Takhar, "Interrogating the Pill: Rising Distrust and the Reshaping of Health Risk Perceptions in the Social Media Age," *Social Science & Medicine* 331 (2023).

40   Angela Cooke-Jackson, Valerie Rubinsky, and Jacqueline N. Gunning, "'Wish I Would Have Known That before I Started Using It': Contraceptive Messages and Information Seeking among Young Women," *Health Communication* 38, no. 4 (2023).

41   Rachel E. Stoddard, Andrea Pelletier, Emily N. Sundquist, Maetal E. Haas-Kogan, Bina Kassamali, Melody Huang, Natasha R. Johnson, and Deborah Bartz, "Popular Contraception Videos on TikTok: An Assessment of Content Topics," *Contraception* 129 (2024).

42   EPF (European Parliamentary Forum for Sexual and Reproductive Rights), "Contraception Policy Atlas Canada," *Action Canada for Sexual and Rights*, July 2023, actioncanadashr.org/sites/default/files/2023-09/CCInfoCAN_A3_EN_2023_SEP20_0.pdf.

Chapter 11

1   WHO (World Health Organization), "Basic Documents: Forty-Ninth Edition," May 31, 2020, apps.who.int/gb/bd/pdf_files/BD_49th-en.pdf.

2   Repertory of Practice of United Nations Organs, "Charter of the United Nations: Chapter IX- International Economic and Social Co-Operation," March 23, 2022, legal.un.org/repertory/art57.shtml; World Health Organization, *Constitution*, in force April 7, 1948, who.int/about/governance/constitution.

3   Government of Canada, "Canada and the World Health Organization," n.d., international.gc.ca/world-monde/international_relations-relations_internationales/multilateral-multilateraux/who-fao.aspx?lang=eng.

4   Canada's Human Rights Commitments, "Universal Declaration of Human Rights," n.d., humanrightscommitments.ca/universal-declaration-of-human-rights.

5   UN (United Nations), "Universal Declaration of Human Rights," un.org/sites/un2.un.org/files/2021/03/udhr.pdf.

6   UNHR (United Nations Human Rights), "International Covenant on Civil and Political Rights," December 16, 1966, ohchr.org/en/instruments-mechanisms/instruments/international-covenant-civil-and-political-rights.

7   UNHR (United Nations Human Rights), "International Covenant on Economic, Social and Cultural Rights," December 16, 1966, ohchr.org/en/instruments-mechanisms/instruments/international-covenant-economic-social-and-cultural-rights.

8   Government of Canada, "Canadian Human Rights Act," August 31, 2021, laws-lois.justice.gc.ca/eng/acts/h-6/FullText.html.

9   UNHR (United Nations Human Rights), "Convention on the Elimination of All Forms of Discrimination Against Women," December 18, 1979, ohchr.org/en/instruments-mechanisms/instruments/convention-elimination-all-forms-discrimination-against-women.

10 CEDAW (Committee on the Elimination of Discrimination Against Women), "Convention on the Elimination of All Forms of Discrimination Against Women," November 25, 2016, documents.un.org/doc/undoc/gen/n16/402/03/pdf/n1640203.pdf.

11 UN (United Nations), "Economic and Social Council," March 31, 2015,

docstore.ohchr.org/SelfServices/FilesHandler.ashx?enc=4slQ6QSmlBEDzFE-ovLCuW4yzVsFh%2Fjl1u%2Ft0KVExfQShAk52qzbciaq4MKqmsZiQLU-dE8HnJ%2Bz%2BHA3TZVUOFxRAuj4E3LcrqFcgjDwjLTOyQDnlreLGWDrS-bl8QniQw8.

12 Action Canada for Sexual Health and Rights, "Action Canada Submission to 57th CESCR for Canada's Review," February 1, 2016, actioncanadashr.org/resources/policy-briefs-submissions/2016-02-12-action-canada-submission-57th-cescr-canadas-review.

13 Economic and Social Council, "List of Issues in Relation to the Sixth Periodic Report of Canada," United Nations, February 4, 2016, documents.un.org/doc/undoc/gen/g16/025/55/pdf/g1602555.pdf.

14 Economic and Social Council, "Concluding Observations on the Sixth Periodic Report of Canada," United Nations, March 23, 2016, docstore.ohchr.org/SelfServices/FilesHandler.ashx?enc=4slQ6QSmlBEDzFEovLCuW4yzVsF-h%2Fjl1u%2Ft0KVExfQT6EfAENdSjJTaz3raPv3QWT3Y59q3zadXvBYMpLN-W5%2FsveoBdxLZoVN%2Fzz31c7YEgqRm0DpoVivqHo2yN5iIam.

15 *Christian Medical and Dental Society of Canada v. College of Physicians and Surgeons of Ontario*, 2019 ONCA 393.

16 Canadian Labour Congress, "Canada's Unions: Workers have Waited Long Enough to Pass Bill C-64, An Act Respecting Pharmacare," June 18, 2024, canadianlabour.ca/canadas-unions-workers-have-waited-long-enough-to-pass-bill-c-64-an-act-respecting-pharmacare/.

17 Cadloff, "How PEI Became."

18 UNHR (United Nations Human Rights), "Management Plan 2022–2023," ohchr.org/sites/default/files/2022-05/OMP-2022-2023.pdf.

19 International Covenant on Civil and Political Rights, "Views Adopted by the Committee Under Article 5 (4) of the Optional Protocol, Concerning Communication No. 2348/2014," United Nations, August 30, 2018.

20 *Toussaint v. Attorney General of Canada*, "Amended Statement of Claim," October 14, 2020, 6, socialrights.ca/2020/amended%20statment%20of%20claim%20Toussaint.pdf.

21 Aditya Rao and Tracy Glynn, "Remembering Nell Toussaint's Struggle for Medicare for All, Regardless of Immigration Status," Canadian Health Coalition, January 9, 2024, healthcoalition.ca/remembering-nell-toussaints-struggle-for-medicare-for-all-regardless-of-immigration-status/.

22 *Toussaint v. Attorney General of Canada*, "Amended Statement of Claim," 8.

23 *Toussaint v. Canada (Attorney General)*, (2011) 420 N.R. 364 (FCA), ca.vlex.com/vid/toussaint-v-can-g-680873977.

24 Supreme Court of Canada, Appeal Decision, *Toussaint v. Attorney General of Canada*, Applications for Leave, Case 34446, April 5, 2012, decisions.scc-csc.ca/scc-csc/scc-l-csc-a/en/item/11057/index.do?iframe=true.

25 United Nations Committee on Civil and Political Rights, "Views Adopted by the Committee under Article 5 (4) of the Optional Protocol, Concerning Communication No. 2348/2014," August 30, 2018, docstore.ohchr.org/SelfServices/FilesHandler.ashx?enc=l%2bjL3%2bEPYDfJe12uMVWt1WCD-KQD2SrBeBP7%2ffbuCHeETLOag8w8Ijs8qyDVQxMPCQz%2b%2brF2Tcnbc-B67614xEFEiLsKwB%2f8UArQWmzt1TCt0%3d.

26 *Toussaint v. Canada (Attorney General)*, 2022 ONSC 4747, canlii.org/en/on/onsc/doc/2022/2022onsc4747/2022onsc4747.html.

27 *Toussaint v. Canada (Attorney General)*, 2022 ONSC 4747, Section 134.

28 Martha Jackman, "The Housing Tell: Toussaint's Ground-Breaking Victory for Human Rights in Canada," *National Right to Housing Network,* September 28, 2022, housingrights.ca/tousssaint-victory-2022/.
29 Government of Ontario, "March 31, 2023 is the End Date for the Temporary Physician and Hospital Services for Uninsured Persons (PHSUP) Pandemic Response Funding," Health Insurance Branch, March 29, 2023, ontario.ca/document/ohip-infobulletins-2023/bulletin-230305-physician-and-hospital-services-uninsured-persons#section-0.
30 Liam Casey, "Other Programs Can Help Uninsured, Ontario Health Minister Says as Coverage to End," *Global News,* March 27, 2023, globalnews.ca/news/9581234/other-programs-can-help-uninsured-ontario-health-minister-says-as-coverage-to-end/.
31 Maan Alhmidi, "Ontario Doctors Blast Province for Ending Health Care for Uninsured Residents," *Global News,* March 25, 2023, globalnews.ca/news/9578660/ontario-doctors-blast-province-ending-health-care-uninsured-residents/.

Conclusion

1 Dorothy Shaw and Wendy V. Norman, "When There Are No Abortion Laws: A Case Study of Canada," *Best Practice & Research: Clinical Obstetrics & Gynaecology* 62 (2020).
2 Leger360, "Abortion Rights in Canada," Report, May 17, 2024, leger360.com/abortion-rights-in-canada/.

INDEX

2SLGBTQIA+ communities,
    health care exclusion, 111, 140, 159
    struggles for gender-affirming care, 154–6

abortion,
    commonness of, 12, 16–17, 22, 60, 67, 177
    democratization of, 85, 128
    as health care, 8, 22, 28, 34, 48, 90
    misperceptions/myths about, 7, 18–21, 27, 60, 147
    policies on induced, 33, 55, 63, 89
    popular depictions of, 12, 116–18
    as public good, 7–8
    secrecy around, 12, 73, 95, 108, 122, 151
    sex-selective, 46–7
Abortion to Abolition: Reproductive Health and Justice in Canada, 4, 7, 29
Abortion Caravan, 32
Abortion Care Canada (formerly National Abortion Federation Canada), 3–4, 85
    work for mifepristone access, 66, 75, 80
abortion clinics, 132
    bubble zones around, 123–9, 178
    crisis pregnancy centres versus, 9, 28, 100–1, 105–6
    feminist organizing in support of, 32, 45, 109
    free-standing, *see* free-standing/private clinics
    funding for, 28, 37–40, 44, 175–6
    gender-inclusive name changes to, 6, 131, 142–3
    medication abortion prescribing at, 64, 70
    restrictions/bans on, 138–9
    revenue loss of, 71, 76, 103
    safety/security concerns for, 20, 73–4, 111–12, 121–2, 178
    workforce surveys of, 68–9, 73, 79
    see also Morgentaler abortion clinics
Abortion Rights Coalition of Canada (ARCC), 73, 85, 91, 107
    work against abortion ads, 26–7, 117
Action Canada for Sexual Health and Rights, 3, 34, 110, 139
    paying for patient mifepristone, 79–80
    work to increase abortion access, 168, 171
ADH (stillbirth legal case), 55–6
Ad Standards Canada,
    Code stipulations/violations, 26–8, 116–19
    pharmaceutical claims and, 101–2
age of majority, provincial differences in, 20, 151–3
Alberta, 96, 120, 142, 144
    abortion access in, 4–6, 32, 147, 151
    age of medical consent impacts in, 151, 153, 155
    anti-abortion organizing in, 106, 114–16, 118
    coverage/leave for abortion/pregnancy loss, 52, 76
    demand for abortion in, 4, 32, 103, 146
    gender-affirming treatment in, 155–6
    gestational duration limits in, 52
    Health Services, 5, 52
    ProChoice YQL, 3–6
    referrals for abortion services in, 5–6, 32
    see also Calgary; Edmonton
anesthesia use, 16, 65, 103
anti-abortion movement, 56, 66
    40 Days for Life campaigns, 126–7

advertising, 26–8, 110, 116–20
bubble zones to counter, 123–9, 178
crisis pregnancy centres and, 100–4, 107–9
graphic image use by, 114–15, 120, 129
injunctions against, 121–7
messaging of, 17–18, 86, 109, 120
myths/misinformation circulation by, 12, 114, 178
politicians, 43, 45
protests/demonstrations by, 113, 121–9
university/student groups, 113–16, 128–9
violence/harassment by, 20, 73–4, 121–2, 128–9
"We Need a Law" campaigns, 26–8, 45–8, 116
see also crisis pregnancy centres
anti-choice organizations/lobby, 1, 107, 109, 116
Arthur, Joyce, 26, 85–6, 107
aspiration, vacuum, see vacuum aspiration
Association for Reformed Political Action (ARPA, Hamilton), 119
Atlantic Canada, abortion access in, 46, 51–2
autonomy,
bodily, 2, 22–3, 45, 179
child/youth, 2, 20, 152–4
constitutional/legal affirmation of, 5, 45, 152–4
nurse practitioner, 88
patient, 6, 19–20, 82, 111
reproductive, 4, 41, 82, 154
undermining, 6, 105

Baddeley, Sarah, 26
Badgley committee/report, 33–4, 137, 150–1
Bathurst (New Brunswick), Chaleur Hospital, 38, 126–7, 131–2
Baulieu, Etienne-Emile, 65, 74
belief-based denial of care,
access delays and inequalities due to, 86, 99
institutional, 93–4, 99
interdisciplinary teams and, 87
use of term, 9, 85
Bill C-3 (criminalizing intimidation of health workers/patients): 127–8

Bill C-43 (criminalizing abortion): 43
Bill C-64 (creation of pharmacare program): 166–7, 172–3
Bill C-150 (decriminalizing homosexuality, sale of contraception), 31
Bill C-233 (criminalizing abortion): 46
Bill C-311 (criminalizing those who harm pregnant people): 47
birth control, 104
counselling, 5, 161
coverage/payment for, 67, 75, 150, 162, 179
implanted, 67, 80, 82, 133
NP/pharmacist prescribing of, 167–8, 178
pills, see birth control pills
prescription, 14, 40, 67, 82–3, 167
provision/access to all, 32, 168, 179–80
see also contraception; IUDs
birth control pills, 65, 67, 86, 163–4, 179
Birthright, 103–5
Blackmer, Jeff, 90
Black people, 6, 111, 140
blood work, 87
coverage/fees for, 21, 35, 47, 74–5
physician review of, 19, 78
streamlining abortion process and, 98, 131, 150
telemedicine and, 77–80
Borowski, Joseph (legal case), 45
Bourne, Aleck, 30–1
Britain, 65
early court case on abortion provision, 30–1
historical criminalization of abortion, 29–30
mifepristone approval, 66
British Columbia,
age of majority/medical consent in, 151–2
anti-abortion organizing in, 106, 120, 123
emergency contraception use, 14
gestational duration caps in, 52
hormonal contraception coverage, 75, 164, 168, 171
legal cases/legislation on abortion, 58, 123, 151
MAiD legal cases in, 93–4
pharmacare coverage in, 10
see also Vancouver

Calgary, 4, 112, 114–16, 120, 141
Calgary Birth Control Association, 32
Campus Pro-Life (CPL, University of Calgary), 114–15
Canada Health Act (CHA), 176
   Canada's "abortion law," 34, 41
   development of, 34
   Medicare standards/principles in, 31, 34–6, 76, 147, 163
   medication/legal abortion coverage/funding, 36–40, 103
   regulation of abortion, 27, 34, 48
Canada Health Transfer, 35, 37–8
Canadian Association of Schools of Nursing (CASN), 72, 135
Canadian Centre for Bioethical Reform (CCBR) anti-abortion ads, 115–19
Canadian Charter of Rights and Freedoms,
   abortion access impacts, 8, 34, 113, 176
   ad campaigns and, 117–19
   anti-abortion protests, 123, 128, 178
   provincial court differences in interpreting, 113–16
   Section 1 (reasonable limits), 92, 113, 123
   Section 2 (religion/expression/assembly/association), 9, 28, 92–9, 113–19, 123, 178
   Section 7 (life, liberty, security of person), 5–6, 27, 43, 55, 93–4, 154, 174–5
   Section 9 (arbitrary detention), 114
   Section 12 (freedom from cruel/unusual punishment), 98
   Section 15 (equality rights), 39, 92, 94, 98, 114, 154, 174
   student group anti-abortion images and, 113–16
Canadian Civil Liberties Association, 38, 128, 156, 175
Canadian Code of Advertising Standards, 26–8, 116–19
Canadian Medical Association (CMA), 27
   Code of Ethics and Professionalism, 88–91
   Journal (CMAJ), 42, 89–90
Canadian Nursing Association (CNA), Code of Ethics, 88
Canadian Pharmacists' Association (CPhA), 81

Care Net (CPC conglomerate), 106–7
Carter, Kay, 94
Chabot, Frederique, 34, 41
charities, registered,
   abortion-supportive, 80, 102–3
   crisis pregnancy centres as, 9, 102–3, 107, 109–10, 178
   policies regulating, 9, 102–3, 109–10, 112
Charlottetown, 97, 172
Chen, Y.Y, 147–8
clinicians, 101, 121
   increasing medication abortion competence, 80, 98, 111
   legislative limitations placed on, 25–6, 54
   mifepristone coverage/stocking, 74, 80–1
competence,
   clinicians' contraception, 61, 80, 105
   concerns about prescriber, 80, 98–9
   need for education to increase, 72, 98–9, 135–6
   NP/RN/midwife abortion care, 72, 88, 132–3, 135–6
conscientious objection/objectors, 74, 81
   alternate conceptions of, 85
   anti-war history into health services, 85–6
   Canadian Medical Association on, 88–91
   Charter rights and, 92–4, 97–9
   institution-based, 93–7
   MAiD cases, 86, 93–5
   mainstream concept of, 86–7, 171–2
   province-wide, 97–8
   referrals and, 87, 90–2, 172
   variability in policies on, 90–2, 98
consent, 2
   informed, 151, 168
   parental, *see* parental consent
   patient, 20, 67–8, 94
   provincial variation on age of, 19–20, 151–4, 157, 179
   to sexual activity, 10, 140, 157
   TAC/hospital requirements, 34, 151–4
   youth ability to, 10, 140, 151, 156, 159
contraception,
   approval process for new, 66–7, 83
   Canadian inequities in access to, 161–3, 171, 176

conscientious objection and, 86, 92–3, 95
coverage of hormonal, 75, 164–5, 168, 171
decriminalization of, 30–1, 104, 161
disinformation about, 167–8
emergency, *see* emergency contraception
implant (Nexplanon), 67, 80, 133, 162, 164
IUD, *see* IUDs
long-acting, reversible (LARC), 14, 161, 164–5, 167
marginalized communities and, 144–6, 158, 168, 171–2
mifepristone as, 82–3
NP/RN/pharmacist/midwife prescribing of, 81–3, 133–5, 162, 167
pharmacare/public health coverage for, 10, 33, 56, 163–5, 168–73, 179–80
tiers of, 163–4
uptake post-abortion, 80, 112, 131, 150, 165
youth and, 149–50, 155
Contraception and Abortion Research Team (CART-GRAC), 3, 63, 135
abortion workforce survey, 68–9, 73, 79
Canadian Community Health Survey, 164–5
on practitioner adoption of mife, 68, 70, 72
contraceptive pill, *see* birth control pills
counselling,
absence of, 5, 103, 134, 171
contraception, 161, 167
CPC/anti-abortion, 100, 104, 107–10, 121
nurses providing, 132, 134–5
pre-abortion, 90–1, 103, 132
COVID-19 pandemic,
abortion demand amid, 37, 127
anti-vaccine convoy protests, 127–8
care impacts of, 90, 127, 137
medication abortion prescribing, 40, 79
telemedicine increases amid, 40, 77–9, 127
tightening of companion/safety rules in, 20, 127–8
uninsured persons funding in, 175–6

Criminal Code,
anti-abortion legislative amendments (actual/proposed), 46–7
consent/incest/female genital cutting, sections on, 157–9
decriminalization of abortion, 5, 27, 41–5, 104, 150–1
evolution of, 30–1
MAiD cases and, 93–4
R. v. Bedford decision impacts on, 27
R v. Morgentaler decision impacts on, 5, 27, 41–5
Section 223 (definition of a child), 47, 53, 57–8
Section 241b (assistance in suicide), 93–4
Section 251 (abortion) (now repealed), 5, 27, 31, 41–5, 89, 150
Section 342 (concealing body of child), 53–6, 58
Section 432.2 (intimidating health professionals), 127–8
stillbirths and, 53, 57–8
therapeutic abortion committees and, 31, 33, 150–1
criminalization, abortion,
British, 29–31
MAiD cases and, 94
Morgentaler decision impacts, 27, 42–3
provider fear/risk of, 6–7, 25, 46–7
provincial post-Confederation, 4, 30, 43
stillbirths and, 53–6, 58
various countries, 48
see also decriminalization of abortion
crisis pregnancy centres (CPCs),
abortion clinics/providers versus, 28, 99–100, 110–11
ads/marketing for, 7, 9, 101–2, 110–11
charitable status of, 9, 102–3, 109–10, 178
fake care by, 110–13
freedom of expression disputes, 116
interest in, 104, 108, 111–12
misleading/delaying abortion seekers, 9, 28, 105–9, 112, 150
see also Birthright
curricula, health professional, 134–6, 146
C.V. (fetal reduction case), 95–6

Daigle, Chantal (legal case), 45–6, 137
Dalhousie University, 28, 116, 134

data, 96, 177
  abortion rates, 12, 17, 69–70, 103
  abortion training/education, 134, 140, 167–8
  on complications, 18, 61
  contraception, 162–5, 167–8
  crisis pregnancy centre, 107–8
  gestational duration, 136–8
  health service funding, 35, 37, 39–40, 103
  marginalized communities, 145–7, 158–9
  medication abortion, 17, 61, 63–5, 68–71, 81–2
  patient/abortion seeker, 16–18, 70, 108, 111–12
  procedural abortion, 15, 17, 71, 76
  provider workforce, 19, 58, 68–70, 73, 81, 140
  stillbirth, 50
  telemedicine, 40, 78–9
  therapeutic abortion committee, 33–4
  transgender/nonbinary people, 141–2, 154–6
  unintended pregnancy, 112, 145, 162, 164–5
  youth abortion seeker, 149–50, 164–5, 215n2
decriminalization of abortion,
  access issues despite, 5–7, 33, 97, 112, 147
  Canada's complete, 1–5, 8, 24, 177
  Canadian timing of, 31, 104, 154, 161
  geographic barriers despite, 21, 171–2
  inaccessibility of medication abortion despite, 59, 64
  increased demand after, 103
  international recommendations toward, 28, 179–80
  therapeutic abortion committees and, 41, 91, 150
  in various countries, 1, 25
  see also criminalization, abortion
Degrassi High abortion episode, 121
Desrosiers, Jacques, ROSE Clinic named for, 3, 44, 131
Diamond, Eugene, 104–5
dilatation and curettage (D&C), 13, 42, 63
direct-to-consumer prescription drug advertising, 81, 101
disabilities, people with, 46
  Charter provisions to protect, 114, 140–1, 170
  systemic discrimination facing, 10, 88, 94, 147–8, 159, 176
Dobson, Cynthia (legal case), 46
doctor(s), 25, 65, 118
  abortion now not requiring, 18, 72, 87, 98, 128–33
  abortions performed/prescribed by, 3–4, 17, 59–60, 67–70, 95–6, 136
  assistance in dying, 94–5
  belief-based denial of care, 62, 85–93, 104–7, 171–2
  bubble-zone legislation for, 123–5, 127
  Canada Health Act on, 34–6, 38
  (de)criminalization of, 25, 27, 30–1, 42–5, 94
  family, *see* family doctors
  fees/funding for, 21, 35–40, 52, 76–8, 103, 175–6
  therapeutic abortion committee consultation, 18–19, 31–4, 52, 130, 150, 178
  treatment of uninsured patients, 176
  violence/protest against, 121–5, 129
doulas,
  abortion, 20, 60, 111–12, 178
  birth/labour, 17, 134
Downie, Jocelyn, 89–91, 94–5

ectopic pregnancy, 63, 78–9
Edmonton, 1, 141
Ella, *see* ulipristal acetate
emergency contraception, 165
  mifepristone versus, 60–1, 83
  misconceptions about, 14
  see also ulipristal acetate
End Fake Clinics student group, 110
Erdman, Joanna, 67, 83, 121–2
escorts, patient, 2
  harassment of, 74
  police/prison, 128, 145
  policies on, 20, 132

Fainman, Jack, 74, 122
family doctors, 7
  abortions performed/prescribed by, 16, 19, 68–70, 76, 177
  contraception and, 163, 165
  need for greater abortion training, 7, 134
  patient relationships with, 90–2, 153

female genital mutilation/cutting, 159–60
feminists, 42
    criticism of, 7, 109, 144
    movement/work of, 32, 45, 65
    support for, 2, 25
fetuses, 100
    Criminal Code provisions on, 53–4, 56, 58, 89, 150
    fathers' interest/rights over, 45–6, 137
    graphic anti-choice images of, 116–18, 120
    historical legislation on, 29, 32
    legal status of, 45–7, 54–7, 137
    stillbirth and, 49–51, 54–6, 137
    termination/reduction of, 13, 17, 25, 52–4, 87, 95–6
first trimester,
    abortion rates in, 17, 118, 136
    lower risks in, 32, 72
    medication abortion provision in, 19, 70–1, 78
    primary care physician abortion provision, 19
    procedural abortion process in, 15–16, 134
    self-referrals in, 19, 91
Food and Drugs Act, 81–2, 101–2
Food and Drug Administration (US),
    approval of mifepristone, 13, 66
    OTC oral contraception approval, 83, 86
France,
    abortion legislation in, 1, 4–5, 21, 24–5
    availability of abortion drugs, 13, 64–6, 74, 82
    Canada on abortion versus, 1, 24–5, 48
Fredericton (New Brunswick), 141
    Clinic 554: 38, 44, 105–6
    private-pay/free-standing clinic, 126, 131
free-standing/private clinics, 136
    as anti-abortion protest targets, 124–6
    funding/fees for, 36–9, 44, 71, 76, 131
    gestational duration/age restrictions, 52, 215n2
    provincial variability/lack of, 40, 42, 126
funding, 144
    abortion access inequities and, 6, 76, 176, 179
    contraception, 33, 80, 175
    of crisis pregnancy centres, 109
    of free-standing clinics, 37–40, 44–5, 71, 131
    lack of abortion, 5, 37, 39–40
    medication abortion, 3–5, 37–8, 75, 120
    need for improved, 6, 21, 110, 179
    university, 115–16

Gallant, Brian, 130–1
gender affirming care, 2, 7, 155–6
gender-inclusive care,
    abortion provision, 6, 131, 140–3, 148
    Vancouver Rape Relief Society (VRRS) case, 143–4
genocide,
    Indigenous, 7, 144
    university group activism and, 114–16
Genocide Awareness Projects (GAP), 114–15
geography,
    barriers to abortion access due to, 20–1, 108, 120, 136, 145, 172
    medication abortion and, 59, 72, 80, 83–4
    telemedicine abortion access despite, 9, 80
gestational duration, 118
    abortion access limitations based on, 13, 22, 29, 32–4, 136
    Canada's no legal restrictions on, 5, 17, 25
    challenges in determining, 26, 54–5, 78–9
    complicated care in later, 13, 16, 18–19
    definition(s) of, 17, 54
    expanding capacities for, 6, 10, 68, 130, 136–8, 178
    legal cases related to, 29, 32, 55–6, 89
    provincial differences in capacity for, 25, 51–2, 97
    right to abortion based on, 1, 89
    stillbirth and, 50–2, 55
gestational limits,
    crisis pregnancy centres delaying care past, 106, 108
    medication abortion, 21, 71
    varying abortion access, 5–6, 26–8, 43, 48, 148–9
Gomperts, Rebecca, 82

Guelph and Area Right to Life, 119
Guilbert, Edith, 70, 78-9

Halappanavar, Savita, 26
Halifax, 26, 141
   complexity of health care institutions in, 54, 131
   Morgentaler clinic in, 44, 71, 126
   out-of-province student coverage in, 36, 76
   ROSE Clinic in, *see* Reproductive Options and Services (ROSE) Clinic
   student activism in, 116, 127
Health Canada, 135
   abortion drug approvals, 13, 65-6, 71-2, 132
   contraception approval, 61, 67
   Food and Drugs Act enforcement, 101-2
   limitations on mifepristone use, 9, 15, 67-9, 78
   methotrexate use, 63-4
   new medication approval process, 66-7
Heartbeat International (CPC conglomerate), 106-7
Holt, Susan, 75, 155-6
   abandoning Regulation 84-20: 38, 44, 131
homosexuality, decriminalization of, 31, 154
hospitals, 6, 88
   abortion in, 15-16, 36, 42, 71, 136-8
   admissions due to complications, 17-18, 56-7, 61-2
   bubble zones around, 122, 124-7
   conscientious objection by, 96-7
   demand for abortion in, 101, 103
   denial of funding for abortions outside, 38-40, 44-5
   gestational duration and use of, 52, 54, 120
   public funding of, 28-9, 35-6, 75-6, 163
   referrals to, 19, 90, 103, 120, 132
   religious-affiliated, 93-7
   removing barriers to, 20-1, 130-1, 142, 171-2
   therapeutic abortion committees in, 31-4, 41, 150
   uninsured fees/funding for using, 21, 38, 74, 175-6
   youth abortion experiences in, 150-1, 153
Human Life International (CPC), 109

incarceration, 7
   health professional risk of, 25-6, 30, 43, 46
   impacts on health, 47-8, 140
   of pregnant people, 10, 47, 145-6, 148
incest, 28, 157-8, 160
Indigenous people, 166
   specific needs of, 10, 111, 140, 144-5, 148
   systemic violence/oppression facing, 6, 140, 144, 157-9
   women's experiences, 21, 144-5
Interim Federal Health Benefit Program (IFHP) case, 173-5
international students, 147-8, 167
IUDs (intrauterine devices), 78, 133
   copper, 14, 61, 164
   effectiveness of, 14, 164, 167
   insertion of, 80, 98
   Mirena, 61, 162

Kinew, Wab, 128, 166
Kopp, James, 74

legislation, abortion, 30, 110, 170
   federal versus provincial, 34-40, 44, 59
   France, *see* France
   Ireland, 25-6
   South Africa, 24-5, 91
   United States, *see* United States
   Yugoslavia, 24
legislation, bubble-zone, 123-5, 127-8
legislation, gender diversity, 154-6
legislation, MAiD, 93-5
legislation, midwifery, 58, 88, 132-3
Lemay, Gloria, 56-8
Lethbridge and District Pro-Life Association (DPLA), 118-19
Levesque, Jean-Frederic, health care model, 139-40, 161, 168
Levkovic, Ivana (legal case), 55-6
levonorgestrel,
   emergency contraception (Plan B), 14, 61
   Mirena IUD, 61, 162

Lobo v. Carleton University, 114
Lowik, A.J., 142–3

Manitoba, 45, 51, 147
  age of majority/medical consent cases in, 151, 153–4
  anti-abortion protest/violence in, 122, 128
  contraception coverage/prescribing in, 10, 75, 81, 133, 166–8, 171
  crisis pregnancy centres in, 106
  Regulation 46/93 (Jane Doe case) in, 39
  see also Winnipeg
Marleau Letter, 37–8
medical assistance in dying (MAiD), 63–4, 86, 93–5
Medical Care Act (1966), 31, 35
Medicare, 64
  abortion coverage through, 21, 36, 52, 75–7, 150
  approving out-of-province/country care, 6, 76–7
  Canada Health Act governing, 34, 36, 38
  contraception lack of coverage through, 163, 179
  expansion of services covered by, 31, 166, 179
  lack of coverage under, 21, 40, 74, 79, 139, 147–8, 172–3
medication abortion, 64, 81, 172
  approval/benefits of, 3, 65, 83–5, 128–9, 139–40, 177
  barriers to access, 68–70, 73, 142, 146, 150
  commonness of/clinics offering, 22, 97–8, 131
  competence/need for education, 98–9, 110, 136
  concept of, 8, 13, 60, 82
  costs of/billing for, 21, 74–7
  declining clinic use with 71–2
  health workforce prescribing, 4–5, 68–9, 73, 79, 87, 95
  "medical" abortion versus, 13
  Medicare coverage of, 36–8, 40, 120, 167
  "mystery shopping" experiment, 70–1
  NP/RN/midwife prescribing of, 10, 19, 69, 72, 98, 132–3
  OTC medications to mitigate, 14–15
  procedural abortion versus, 4–5, 13, 18, 74
  safety/effectiveness of, 18, 59–63, 71, 82
  side effects/risks, 14, 17–18, 62–3, 79
  similarities to miscarriage, 14–15, 18, 60–2, 65
  telemedicine and, 77–80
  typical process of, 14–15, 60, 72–4, 110
  see also methotrexate; Mifegymiso; mifepristone; misoprostol
Mendocino, Marco, 31, 139
methotrexate, 63–4
midwives, 17, 140, 152
  contraception prescribing by, 161–2, 165–7
  legal cases involving, 56–7
  medication abortion prescribing by, 19, 59–60, 72, 98–9, 177–8
  prohibition of lay, 57–8, 88
  registration/regulation/training of, 58, 87–8, 132–4
Mifegymiso, 74, 102
  initial regulatory requirements, 13, 67–8
Mifeprex, 66, 71
mifepristone,
  activism to support, 2, 38, 66, 75, 80–2, 97, 131–2
  barriers to prescribing, 6, 67–9, 81, 98
  benefits of, 13, 21–2, 59, 83–4, 92, 101
  as contraception, 14, 60, 82–3
  delays in approval for, 13, 65–7, 177
  function/approval of, 14–15, 37–40, 82, 103
  limits on use, 15, 21, 63, 71, 76–7, 172–3
  misconceptions about, 14, 67–8
  NP/RN/midwife prescribing, 4, 59–60, 69–73, 83, 132–3, 177–8
  pharmacist stocking/prescribing, 81, 83, 87, 178
  provincial support for, 9–10, 36, 69, 148
  public funding for, 4, 36, 40, 74–7, 120, 167
  safety/effectiveness of, 61–4, 67–8, 72–3
  telemedicine and 77–8
  trials and RU-486 approval in France, 65–6, 82

use in abortion process, 13–15, 60, 63, 71–3
miscarriage, 2, 29, 112
　fetal status/stillbirth and, 53–6, 137
　lack of definition of, 9
　medication abortion similarities to, 14–15, 18, 60–2, 65
　pill-induced, 8, 68
misINFORMED youth campaign 110
misoprostol, 103
　development/function of, 13, 64
　distribution of, 82, 102
　use in abortion process, 14–15, 22, 60–3, 67–8
Moncton, 106, 142
　abortion clinics in, 38, 127, 130–2, 138
Montreal, 96, 141
　later gestational care in, 17, 97
　Morgentaler clinic in, 37, 41–2, 70
Morgentaler, Henry,
　legal battles and support for, 2, 8, 41–5, 122
　as revolutionary abortion provider, 37, 41, 44, 65
　study on safety of clinic abortions, 42
　see also R. v. Morgentaler
Morgentaler abortion clinics,
　closing/reopening of, 38–9, 44, 71
　fees at, 37–9, 44
　firebombing of, 73, 121, 129
　protests at, 122, 124–6
　running of, 2, 36–7, 41–2, 70–1, 105
Morgentaler Amendment, 41–2
Morrison, Grace T., 105, 108
Mulroney, Brian, 43

National Abortion Federation (NAF) Canada, see Abortion Care Canada
Nelson Right to Life Society (NRLS), 119
New Brunswick, 50, 58, 148
　abortion access in, 2–4, 40, 75, 120, 138, 167
　age of majority/medical consent in, 20, 151–2
　anti-abortion legislation/protest in, 44, 126–7
　crisis pregnancy centres in, 105–6
　gender-affirming policies/care in, 154–6
　NP prescribing in, 132
　Regulation 84-20 in, 37–8, 131
　therapeutic abortion committees in, 18–19, 130, 172, 178
　see also Bathurst; Fredericton; Moncton
newcomers, 159
　health care coverage for, 10, 77, 140, 146–8
Newfoundland, 58, 168
　abortion clinic coverage/access, 37–8, 147, 172
　age of majority/medical consent in, 151, 153
　Athena Centre in, 37, 40, 124–5
　see also St. John's
Nexplanon (contraceptive implant), 67, 80, 133, 164
Nixon, Kimberly, 143–4
nonbinary people, 141–2, 155–6
Norman, Wendy, 62, 66, 68, 134, 164
Northwest Territories, 148
　absence of free-standing abortion clinics, 40, 126
　age of majority/medical consent in, 151–2
　provincial human rights code, 141, 143
Nova Scotia, 30, 53
　abortion access in, 87, 99, 120, 131
　age of majority/medical consent in, 151–2
　anti-abortion movement in, 106, 108, 127
　Canada Health Act/Medicare coverage in, 35–6, 76–7
　conscientious objection in, 87, 91, 93–4
　demand for abortion in, 4, 97, 138, 147
　lack of free-standing clinics in, 40, 44
　St. Francis Xavier University, 97
　St. Martha's Regional Hospital, 93–7
　see also Halifax
Nunavut, 147, 149, 151
　no free-standing abortion clinics in, 40, 126
nurse practitioners,
　abortion care competency training, 72, 134–5
　counselling provision, 132, 134–5
　medication abortion prescribing, 10, 19, 69–70, 72, 98, 132–3

obstetrician-gynecologists, 46, 65, 78
  lack of access to, 47
  performing procedural abortion, 71–2, 76, 134, 136
  violence against 64, 74
Omnibus Bill (1969),
  contraception decriminalization, 31, 104, 161
  partial abortion decriminalization, 31, 41, 91, 104, 150, 154
O'Neill, Sam, 95
Ontario, 30, 58, 116, 149
  abortion access in, 39, 52, 64, 99
  age of majority/medical consent in, 151–2
  anti-abortion campaigns/protests in, 28, 106, 114, 117–20, 125–6
  bubble-zone legislation in, 122, 125–6
  College of Physicians and Surgeons of, 92, 172
  conscientious objection in, 87, 92, 172
  Medicare portability in, 35–6, 76
  newcomer/non-status Medicare/abortion coverage, 146–7, 174–6
  RN/midwife/pharmacist prescribing in, 81, 83, 98, 133, 167
  SHORE Centre, 64, 99
  stillbirth case in, 55
  violence against abortion providers in, 42, 69, 74, 122
  see also Ottawa; Toronto
Ontario v. Dieleman, 122–3
Ontario Health Insurance Plan (OHIP), 52, 76–7, 174
Ottawa, 32, 128, 141
  anti-abortion activism in, 92, 114, 125–6

Palestine, university protest encampments for, 115–16
parental consent, 30, 50
  Canadian abortion not requiring, 5, 19, 25, 150, 159
  gender diversity and, 154–5
  US requiring, 150
people of colour, 111, 140, 146
  facing state violence, 6, 157–8
pharmacare,
  coverage of contraception, 10, 165
  legislation, 166–7, 172
  need for universal, 40, 163, 168

pharmacies/pharmacists,
  bubble-zone legislation for, 125–7
  dispensing/other fees, 75–6
  ethical guidelines for, 81, 87–8, 90
  medication abortion provision, 36, 75–7, 80–1, 177
  prescribing contraception, 81, 83, 133, 162–3, 167, 178
  purchasing emergency contraception at, 14, 81
  role in abortion care, 60–1, 68, 81, 125–6
Physician and Hospital Services for Uninsured Persons (PHSUP) funding, 175–6
physicians, see doctor(s)
Plan B, see levonorgestrel
Planned Parenthood, 2, 92
poverty,
  CPCs espousing work to counter, 102, 104
  gestational duration and, 17, 22
  lack of abortion/contraceptive access and, 6, 91, 102, 162, 171–2
  period, 162–3
pregnancy loss, 2
  employment leave for, 52–3
  legal classifications of, 54, 58
  stigmatization of, 51
primary care, 61
  abortion as part of, 3, 19, 67–71, 126, 177
  conscientious objection in, 85, 92, 99
  medication abortion prescribing in, 9, 38, 70–5
  referrals through, 19, 131–2
  surveys of workforce, 4, 19, 68–71, 73, 98
  virtual care in, 40
Prince Edward Island, 138
  lack of abortion access on, 2, 10, 45, 71, 97–8, 131
  Sexual Health and Options for Reproductive Services (SHORS), 98, 111, 131–2, 142, 172
  see also Charlottetown
prisoners, see incarceration
procedural abortion,
  barriers to accessing, 40, 59, 62, 72, 146
  concept of, 13

conscientious objection in, 80, 95
demand for, 4–5, 15, 17, 71, 138
medication abortion versus, 13, 18, 20–2, 70–2
payment/coverage for, 21, 37–8, 40, 74–6
process, 15–16, 20
ranging provincial demand/facilities for, 4, 72, 120, 127, 130–1, 172
safety/effectiveness of, 18–19, 64
self-referral facilities for, 4, 98, 131–2
various terms for, 13, 16
workforce providing, 19–20, 68–72, 76, 136
ProChoice YQL, provider database/hotline, 3–6
products of conception, 51
abortion removal of, 15–16, 60
retained, 62

Quebec, 30, 50, 97, 116, 125
abortion provision in, 52, 68–70, 136
age of majority/medical consent in, 151–2
College of Physicians on abortion provision, 69–70
Daigle trial in, 45–6, 137
fees/coverage for abortion in, 21, 39–40, 77, 148
Morgentaler trial in, 41–2
NP/midwives prescribing in, 19, 69–72, 87–8, 132–3, 167
see also Montreal

Rebick, Judy, 42
referrals,
activism to simplify, 10, 32, 67, 79
conscientious objection/lack of, 85–92, 96, 99, 105, 178
hospital, 19, 67, 96
primary care provider required, 19, 67, 103, 131–2, 172
restrictions on, 79, 103, 120
self-, 4, 19, 99, 103, 120, 130–1
Regina, 106, 156
abortion provision in, 19, 96, 120, 131
billboards around, 120
registered nurses, 87
abortion care competency training, 72, 132, 135

contraception training/education, 83, 133, 167
religion, 6, 143
abortion seeking no matter, 16
Charter-protected right to freedom of, 92–3, 99, 113–14, 123
conscientious objection and, 85–6, 93–4, 97–8, 178
human rights/WHO/UN policies on, 141, 143, 169–70, 174
institutional affiliation with, 93–4, 97, 102
provider obligations despite, 88, 91–2, 97, 140–1, 153, 172–3
religious organizations,
community ads/promotion by, 7, 105, 108
crisis pregnancy centres funded by, 9, 29, 100–2
opposition to abortion, 31, 74, 102
reproduction,
assisted, 50
right to bodily autonomy on, 24, 144
straightforwardness about, 2, 56
reproductive justice, 108, 116
abortion as part of, 7–8
expansive theory of, 31, 104, 144, 179
Reproductive Options and Services (ROSE) Clinic,
naming of, 3, 44, 131, 142
patient access/experiences, 4, 12, 54, 132
R v. Morgentaler, 171, 177
Charter right to bodily autonomy, 5, 27, 42–3, 34, 176
historic impact of, 5, 44, 59, 89, 121, 151
policy changes due to, 42–5, 89
Roe v. Wade decision versus, 5, 43
Rodgers, Sanda, 89–90
Rodriguez, Sue, 93–4
Roe v. Wade, 86
Canadian responses to, 83, 104, 178
restrictions on abortion access, 32–3, 43, 137–8
R v. Morgentaler decision versus, 5, 43
Romalis, Gary, 64–5, 73–4, 122
Ross, Loretta J. (*Reproductive Justice*), 108
R. v. Sullivan and Lemay, 56–7
RU-486, *see* mifepristone
Rudrum, Sarah, 108
Ryan, Rolanda, 37, 124–5

Saskatchewan, 96
  abortion access in, 19, 40, 51, 126, 131
  age of majority/medical consent in, 151–2
  anti-abortion activism in, 106, 120
  Medicare coverage in, 147, 167
  mifepristone coverage in, 75, 120
  lack of gender-affirming care in, 154–6
  stillbirths in, 50, 55
  see also Regina; Saskatoon
Saskatoon, 19, 120, 132
Saxe, Dianne, 120
Schummers, Laura, 18, 63
second trimester,
  abortion rates in, 17, 19, 136–7
  barriers to abortion access in, 32, 136
  extension of care into, 137–8
  fees for abortion in, 39–40
sexual assault, 2, 28, 157
  increased vulnerability to, 142, 159–60
shame, 151, 173
  abortion as power, not, 2, 22
  anti-abortion ads creating, 26
  religious institutions/CPCs fuelling, 6–7, 106, 111, 178
Short, Hugh, 74, 122
Smith, Danielle, 6, 155–6
social media, youth use of, 110, 150, 159, 167
Society of Obstetricians and Gynaecologists of Canada (SOGC), 46–7, 78
Solinger, Rickie (*Reproductive Justice*), 108
South Africa, 24–5, 91
spontaneous abortion, *see* miscarriage
Spratt, Donald, 123–5
sterilization, 95, 163
  Indigenous women's forced, 7, 144
stigmatization, abortion,
  anti-abortion ads/violence and, 26, 74, 120
  belief-based denial of care and, 86, 97
  gestational duration and, 6, 17, 138
  hindering access, 8, 108, 146
  measures to reduce, 59–60, 74
  misinformation/lack of training and, 2, 7, 12, 22–3, 73, 151
  pregnancy loss/stillbirth and, 51, 58
  provincial health care funding and, 5
stillbirth,
  abortion versus spontaneous, 51
  Criminal Code provisions, 53–8
  employment insurance/unpaid leave and, 52–3
  gestational duration and, 49–52, 54–6, 137
  impacts of varying definitions of, 49–52, 58
  legal cases of, 50, 55–6
  rates of, 50
  required registration of, 49–52, 58
  stigmatization of, 51, 58
St. John's, 172
  Athena Health Centre in, 37, 40, 124–5
students, 116, 155
  abortion access for, 36, 97
  abortion education for medical/health, 3, 134–6
  anti-abortion organizing, 108, 113–14
  coverage in other provinces, 36
  international, 77, 147–8
  pro-abortion support, 82, 104, 110, 114–15, 127
Sullivan, Mary, 56–7
Summerhill, Louise, 103–4
Supreme Court of Canada,
  on abortion law, 42–3, 45–6, 137
  age of majority/medical consent cases, 153–4
  Canada v. Bedford, 27
  medical assistance in dying (MAiD) cases, 86, 93–5
  R v. Morgentaler, see R v. Morgentaler
  R. v. Sullivan and Lemay, see R. v. Sullivan and Lemay
  stillbirth cases, 55–6
  Toussaint IFHP case, 173–5
surgical abortion, *see* procedural abortion
Sweden, 86
  mifepristone approval in, 66, 71

Taylor, Gloria, 94
telemedicine,
  abortion access via, 9, 77–80
  blood work and, 77–80
  clinical practice guide to support, 78
  COVID-19 increases in, 40, 77–9, 127
  shift to, 77–8, 84
  statistics on use of, 40, 78–9
therapeutic abortion committees (TACs),
  Badgley report on, 33–4, 150–1
  consent requirements, 34

Criminal Code cases and, 31, 33, 150–1
decriminalization of abortion and, 41, 91, 150
doctor consultation process, 18–19, 31–4, 52, 130, 150, 178
ending of, 18–19
in hospitals, 31–4, 41, 150
inequities caused by, 33–4
provincial use of, 18–19, 130, 172, 178
statistics on, 33–4
third trimester,
abortion access in, 32, 96, 136–7
abortion rates in, 17, 177–8
medication abortion process in, 17
Thomsen, Carly, 105, 108
Toronto, 36, 116
abortion access in, 17, 40, 76, 95–6, 138
anti-abortion protests in, 120–2, 125, 128–9
Birthright, 103–4
Cabbagetown Women's Clinic, 40, 52
midwife medication abortion provision, 98, 133
Morgentaler clinic in, 42, 73, 121, 125, 129
Mt. Sinai Hospital, 95–6, 138
trans/nonbinary people in, 141–3
Toussaint, Nell, 173–6
trafficking, human, 158, 160, 174
trans people,
abortion care, 17, 141–3
demographics, 141–2, 155
health care/services for, 2, 7, 154–6
legal cases involving, 143–4
youth, 154–6
see also gender-inclusive care; nonbinary people
Trudeau, Pierre, 34, 41
Omnibus Bill, see Omnibus Bill
Trudeau, Justin, 109–10, 128, 166
Turnaway Study, 22, 158–9

UAlberta Pro-Life (UAPL), 115–16
ulipristal acetate (Ella), 14, 61
ultrasounds, 87, 98, 100, 150
calls for banning "entertainment," 47
fees for, 74–5, 77–9
telemedicine and, 77–80
use in abortion, 16, 19, 54, 67–8, 77–9, 131

Unfinished Revolution conference, 71
United Nations, 169
contraception access as human right, 161, 168
Convention/Committee on the Elimination of All Forms of Discrimination against Women (CEDAW), 161, 170–2
Convention on the Rights of the Child, 152–3
Human Rights Commissioner/Committee, 173–5
International Covenant on Civil and Political Rights (ICCPR), 10, 170, 174
International Covenant on Economic, Social and Cultural Rights (ICESCR), 10, 170–2
minimum standards for treatment of prisoners, 146
United States, 50
abortion drug approvals, 13, 61
abortion safety in, 18, 78
abortion seekers in, 16, 80, 108, 150, 157
Aid Access, 82–3
anti-abortion movement in, 73–4, 103, 108, 122
anti-war movement in, 85–6
anxiety about abortion restrictions in, 1, 64, 83, 138–9, 178
Canadians seeking abortion in, 32–3, 96, 137–8
contraception approval in, 66–7, 83
Dobbs v. Jackson Women's Health Organization, 1, 24, 48, 70, 120, 138–9
FDA, see Food and Drug Administration
mifepristone (Mifeprex) approval in, 66, 71
Roe v. Wade, see *Roe v. Wade*
Turnaway Study, 22, 158–9
trans/nonbinary people in, 142, 155–6

vacuum aspiration, 12, 15–16, 42, 87
Vancouver,
abortion access in, 17, 138, 142
anti-abortion ads/protests/violence in, 73–4, 118, 122–5
belief-based denial of care in, 95–6

Elizabeth Bagshaw Clinic, 65, 124
Everywoman's Health Centre, 102–3, 123–4
St. Paul's Hospital, 57, 95–6
trans/nonbinary people in, 141, 143–4
Willow Clinic, 63–4
Vancouver Rape Relief Society (VRRS) case, 143–4
Van Hee, Anthony, 126
violence, 116
   abortion care as mitigating, 91, 102, 162
   anti-abortion, 17, 20, 47, 69, 73–4, 121–2
   anti-trans/gender-diverse, 91, 143–4
   bubble-zone legislation to counter, 123–9, 178
   gendered, 157–60, 179
   intimate partner, 15, 20, 22, 157–60
   racialized people facing state, 6, 126, 157–8
   sexual, 7, 156–60
   youth facing familial, 153, 156–60, 166
Von Dehn, Cecilia "Sissy," 124–5
Voudaris, Stephanie, 56

Wagantall, Cathay, 46–7
Wiebe, Ellen, 63–6
Wilson, Bertha, 43
Wilson v. the University of Calgary, 114–15
Winnipeg,
   abortion access legal case in, 39–40
   anti-abortion movement/violence in, 74, 106, 122
waiting periods, mandatory,
   absence of Canadian, 5, 25, 147–8
   Irish, 25–6
   justification for, 148
"We Need a Law" campaigns, 26–8, 45–8, 116
Winter, Cyril, 125–6
Women on Waves/Women on Web, 82
Women's Legal Education and Action Fund (LEAF), 3, 26
   abortion court case work/lobbying, 57, 75, 124
World Health Organization, 169
   abortion care recommendations, 28, 50, 59, 72
   mifepristone as essential medicine, 61, 66

Yukon, 58, 91
   abortion/contraception access in, 75, 103, 148, 168
   age of majority/medical consent in, 151–2
youth, 148
   abortion-seeking experiences, 140, 149–50, 154–7, 169–60
   age of majority/medical consent legislation, 20, 151–2
   "best interests of the child" legal principle, 152–3
   contraception access/use, 150, 165, 167
   crisis pregnancy centre targeting of, 101, 109–10
   duty to report harm to, 156–8, 160
   fertility rates among, 149
   intersecting discrimination/disadvantages facing, 149–50, 152–60, 179
   social media, use of, 110, 150, 159, 167
   transgender, 154–6

Introduction

The River Spey is one of the classic open canoe journeys in the UK. That said, it is increasingly popular with touring kayaks, and if broken down into day trips is very enjoyable in whitewater river kayaks and inflatable canoes. The Spey has stretches of flat water and lochs, gentle moving water and exciting grade 2 rapids. It can be paddled as a complete journey or, if using the agreed access and egress points, can be broken down into superb day paddles. The Spey starts its journey high in the mountains at Loch Spey, and flows and tumbles its way down to the Spey Dam and then across a flatter area passing Laggan village, and down past Lochain Uvie where we start the river description. It then flows down to the sea passing many villages and beautiful rural spots on the way.

There are usually many wonderful wildlife sightings when on the river, ranging from ospreys to dippers, otters and salmon. The wild flowers on the riverbank in summer make a beautiful display, and the fishing huts particularly in the mid to lower sections of the river are manicured to perfection, showing a great diversity in river usage throughout.

The journey down the River Spey from Lochain Uvie to Spey Bay is 135 kilometers and passes over three OS 1:50,000 map sheets, 35 Kingussie and the Monadhliath Mountains, 36 Grantown and Aviemore, and 28 Elgin, Dufftown and surrounding area. It is a stunning journey to complete and should be a must on every paddler's tick list.

The author

Nancy is a passionate paddler who is most at home in her canoe. She is also regularly found in a sea kayak and occasionally in a white water kayak. Multi-day journeys are her favourite personal adventure, especially if they are spent on the water with her family and friends.

She has spent her career working in the outdoors and currently works for half her time as an instructor for Glenmore Lodge, the National Outdoor Training Centre, where you will find her delivering a range of paddlesport and mountaineering courses. In addition to this Nancy works for other organisations and occasionally runs bespoke guided or training course for groups. She holds a range of high level outdoor qualifications including the BCU Level 5 Canoe Coach award and enjoys most other outdoor sports.

Nancy visited the Aviemore area as a child and has many happy memories of her holidays here. In her late teens she returned to work as a ski instructor, then moved to the west coast of Scotland before returning to live near Aviemore in 2002. She has been paddling on the River Spey since 1990, when she was introduced to its beauty on a staff training trip from Lowport Outdoor Education Centre. Since then she has paddled regularly in the area and all around Scotland.

Nancy Chambers paddling on Loch Spey. Photo | Nick March.

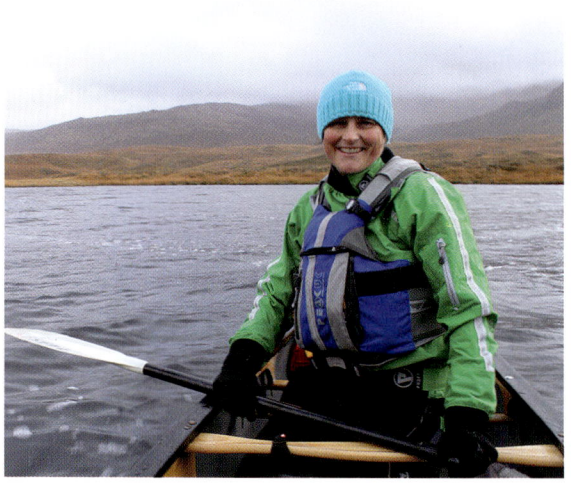

Acknowledgements

There are lots of people to thank for their help during the writing and photo taking for this book. Doug Cooper for helping with the initial idea. Dave Craig for being a great font of knowledge on the river. Franco and Vicky at Pesda Press. Donald Macpherson for helping with photos and information about writing a book. Alison Faulconbridge for helping with the photos and just being great craic on the river. Tom and Kate Oxtoby for being models for photos and reading my writing prior to sending it to Franco. Karl and Carol Atherton for suggestions on the upper section. The many landowners and ghillies that I have chatted to on and about the river. The many folks I have paddled with over the years on the Spey who have increased the enthusiasm that I have for the river, and who have been models for the pictures. The biggest thanks need to go to my family, Nick, Olly and Eddy, who have helped and supported me by giving me the time to complete the project, being willing models on the river, and taking some photos as well. If I have missed someone out apologies and many thanks for your help.

All photos taken by Nancy Chambers unless acknowledged in the caption.

Important notice – disclaimer

Canoeing and kayaking whether in a loch, river or sea environment has its inherent risks as do all adventurous activities. This guidebook highlights some considerations to take into account when planning your own river journey.

While we have included a range of factors to consider, you will need to plan your own journey and within that ensure there is scope to be adaptable to local tides, weather conditions and ever changing river hazards. This requires knowing your own abilities, then applying your own risk assessment to the conditions that you may encounter. The varying environmental conditions within the river and its lochs means that every day good judgement is required to decide whether to paddle or not.

The information within this book has been well researched, however neither the author, nor Pesda Press can be held responsible for any decision of whether to paddle or not and any consequences arising from that decision.

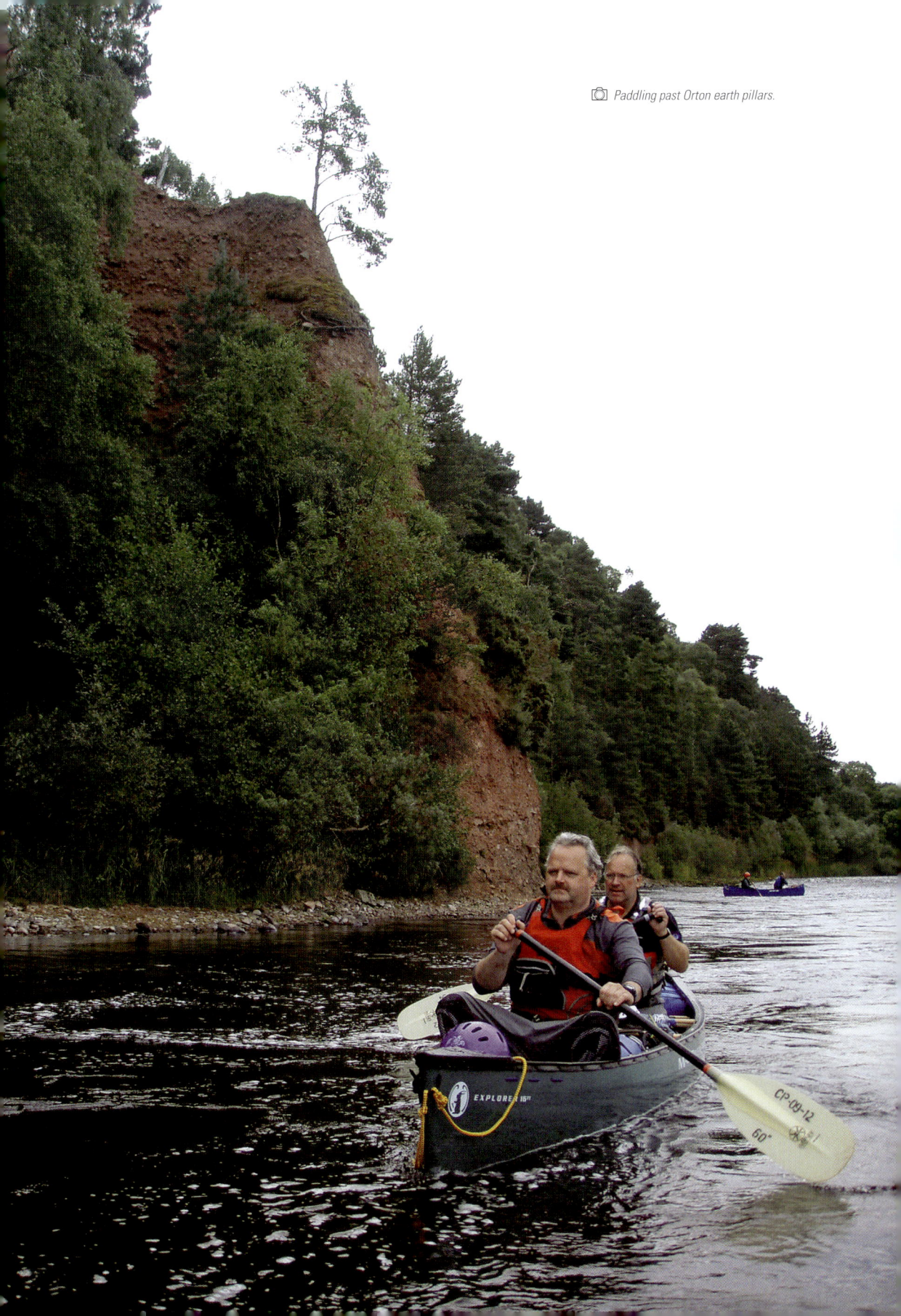
Paddling past Orton earth pillars.

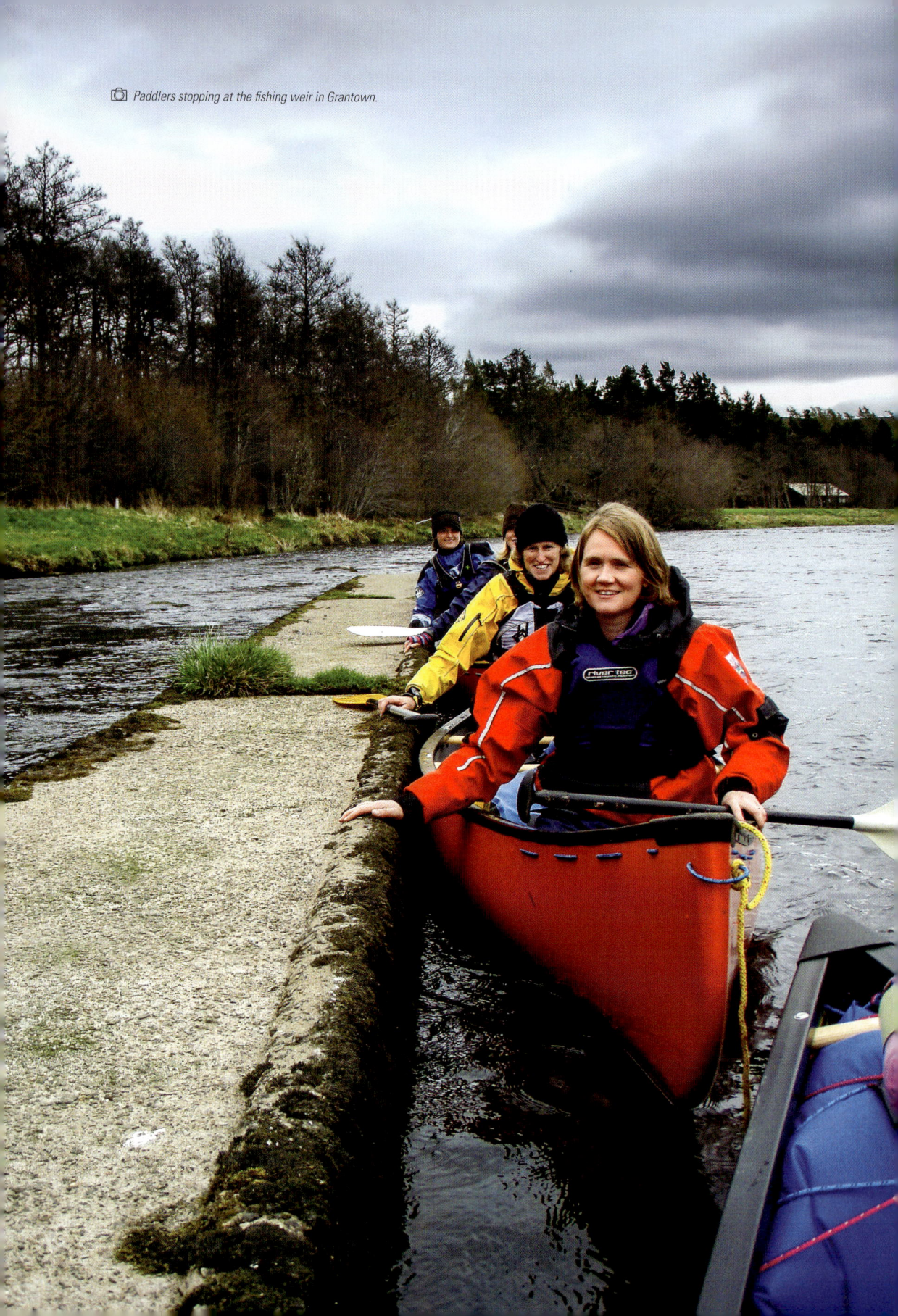
Paddlers stopping at the fishing weir in Grantown.

Planning your River Journey

Whether it's a one-day trip with novices, or a multi-day adventure with experienced paddlers, thorough planning can make all the difference to your paddling adventure. Carrying the right kit, knowing the best campsites and checking the weather forecast will help make your river journey an enjoyable experience, for everyone!

Ability and group

When you are planning your journey down the River Spey you first of all need to think about your own ability and that of the group that you are going with. If you are planning to do the whole river as novices and have limited experience, you should consider joining a guided or instructional group to complete the journey. There are some sections of the river where there is little flow and the rapids are easy to negotiate, so if you are less experienced you can have a great day out on these sections without a guide or instructor. If you are happy paddling on grade 2 moving water then a fully self-guided trip may be appropriate for you.

If you go with the guided option, a suitably qualified guide or instructor will make the journey a memorable experience for you. They should know all the best campsites, know the best places to play on the river, and in the event of a mishap be able to sort it out, including dealing with any capsizes, changes to plans, shuttles and so on. They may also organise your boat, paddles, equipment and food for the journey, allowing you to just turn up and enjoy the river.

If you are organising your own group a suggested maximum number of boats in one group would be six or seven, although a more manageable group size would be three or

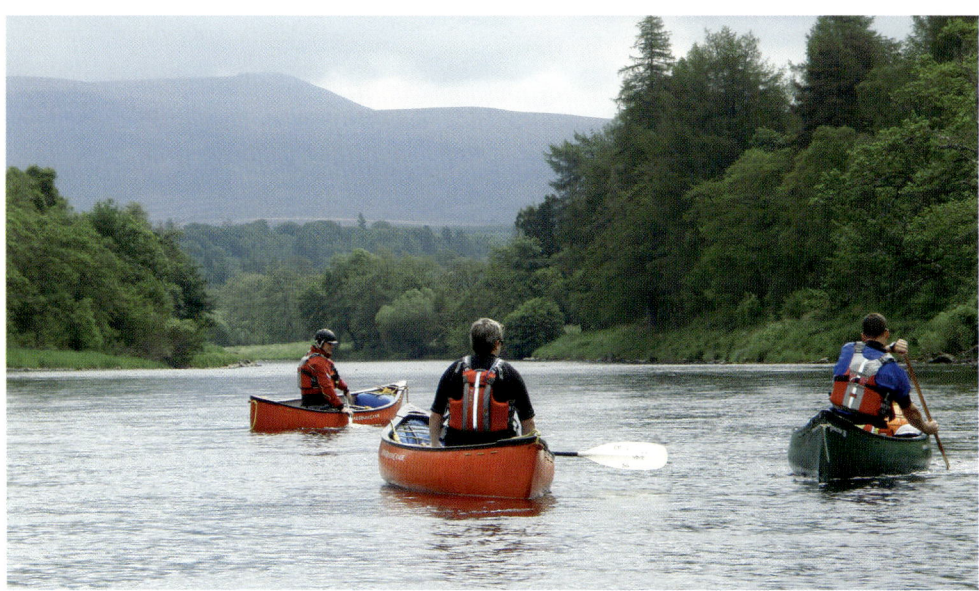
Group leaving the access point at Ballindalloch.

four boats. Some people don't like paddling in groups, and for them solo paddling (or paddling a single tandem boat) is the preferred option. If you choose to paddle with just one boat, then you must be aware of the additional risks involved. If you are paddling on your own and you capsize, then your only option is to self-rescue, which is a reasonably advanced skill and requires a good level of knowledge and skill base. If you are leading a group of friends on the river in the BCU scheme, the minimum level of skill and experience suggested would be a 4 Star Leader in your chosen craft. It is essential that at least one member of the group knows what to do in the event of an emergency on the river, and has the appropriate safety equipment with them to deal with a pinned or capsized boat and crew, and they should really explain this to the rest of the group prior to departing on the river.

Completing the descent of the River Spey can be done as either day trips with a shuttle for each section, which means that you can paddle a light boat, or you can set off for the full journey with all of your camping and paddling equipment. This latter option means that you will have to carry everything in your boat, which makes it much heavier and potentially less manoeuvrable. This is a skill in itself, and if you have not paddled a fully laden boat before it is worth practising your river skills (breaking in and out and ferry gliding) with all of your kit in the boat prior to your trip.

Shuttles

At some point you will have to move yourself and your boat around. If you can organise enough cars to be in the area, it will take you just under 2 hours to drive to Spey Bay from Newtonmore. You are asked not to leave cars overnight at the car park at Tugnet, but you can leave your vehicle in the campsite at the Spey Bay Golf Club if you are going to camp there after your trip. Contact them directly to arrange leaving your vehicle there on 01343 820424.

There are a number of operators who provide shuttles if doing the whole river; all offer a shuttle service with a minibus and trailer:

Johnny's Taxis 01479 851375

Explore Highland info@explorehighland.com or 0780 807 1810

Boots N Paddles info@canoehirescotland.co.uk or 0845 612 5567

If completing your shuttle by public transport, you need to walk from Spey Bay to Garmouth over the viaduct. From Garmouth you can get a bus to Elgin (there are a few buses direct from Spey Bay, but more from Garmouth). You can then get either a bus or train to Inverness. From Inverness you can get either a bus or train to Aviemore, Kingussie or Newtonmore; depending on connections it will take around 4 to 6 hours.

An idea for a novel shuttle service, if you are paddling from Aviemore to Broomhill with one or two boats, is to ask the Strathspey Steam Railway on 01479 810725 in advance if they will carry your boat back to Aviemore in the guard's van. If they have space they are usually very accommodating.

Equipment and packing

The classic craft of those completing a descent of the River Spey is a canoe, because you can fit a large amount of equipment into the boat with ease. Many people are now using touring kayaks, and certainly for day trips a whitewater river kayak is suitable. There has also been an increase in the number of inflatable canoes (duckies) that are paddling on the river. Whichever craft you choose make sure that it is river worthy and that you have a repair kit for it before you go.

Packing a canoe

Once you have decided what to take with you, it is important to be able to keep it all dry and to fit it all into your craft. Barrels and dry bags are the usual way of doing this. There are a variety of sizes of both available. If you use barrels you would normally be able to take two or three barrels per boat. Two 60 litre barrels will usually fit into most 16 foot boats side by

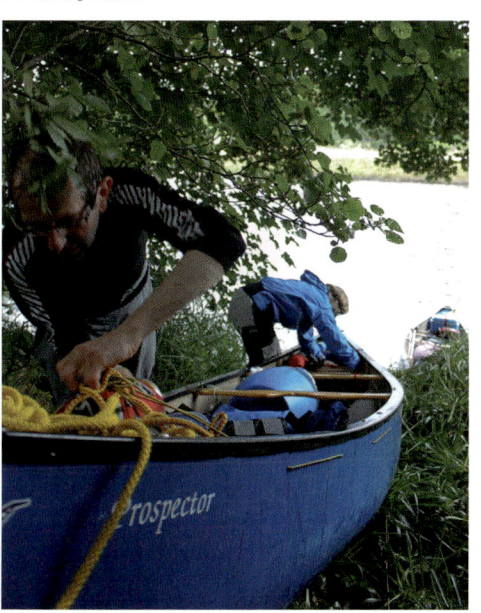
Packing a canoe.

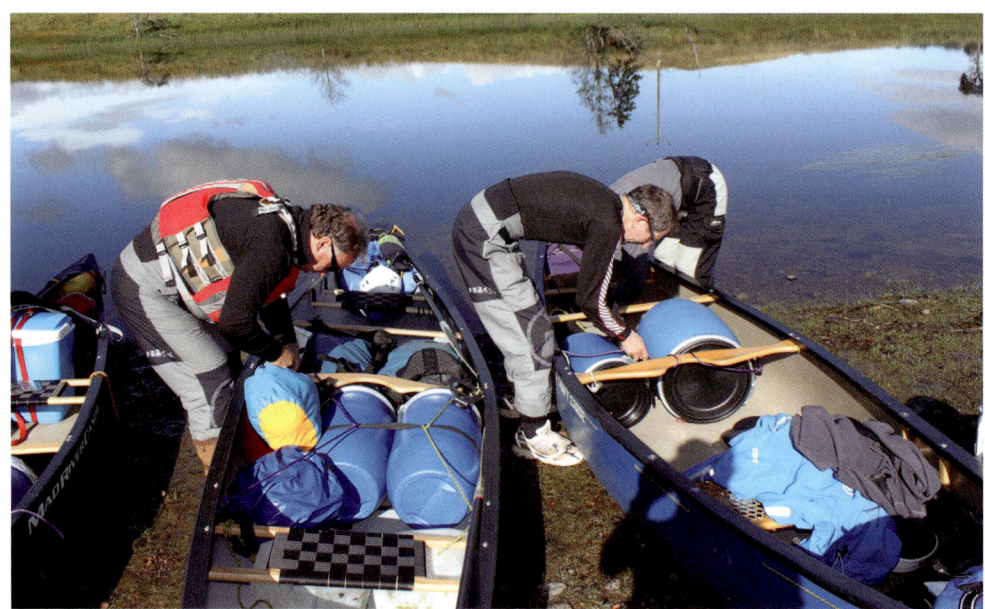
Preparing for the journey ahead.

side, and you can often fit in a third, smaller, 30 litre barrel in front of that.

If you are using dry bags, ensure they are closed properly, and it is worth double bagging items that you need to keep dry, such as your sleeping bag. There are a number of good dry bag rucksacks and carry bags on the market at the moment. Again two of these will normally fit into a 16 foot canoe. You can then have your day bag with essentials in it easily accessible on top or in front of you.

In a tandem canoe, if taking three barrels you will usually choose to have one barrel each for personal kit, and one for communal kit and food.

Once you have got all your kit into your barrels or bags you need to decide how to tie them into your boat. My preferred method is to tie them in so they won't move in the boat as there is no loose line to get tangled up in should you capsize. The down side to this is that if you have to rescue the boat it makes it very heavy to lift, despite reducing the volume of water that you can get into the boat. Using this method means that in all cases the bags or barrels stay with the boat if there is a problem. I usually keep my day bag on a loose line, which is the other method of tying equipment in. The pros to this method are that you can move kit around more easily, and if you capsize you can just empty the water out of the boat and then bring the barrels or bags back in board. The down side is that there is rope floating around in the boat/water which could cause an entanglement. If you use this method make sure you tie a releasable knot so you can get rid of the bags if necessary. There are others who advocate not tying in bags at

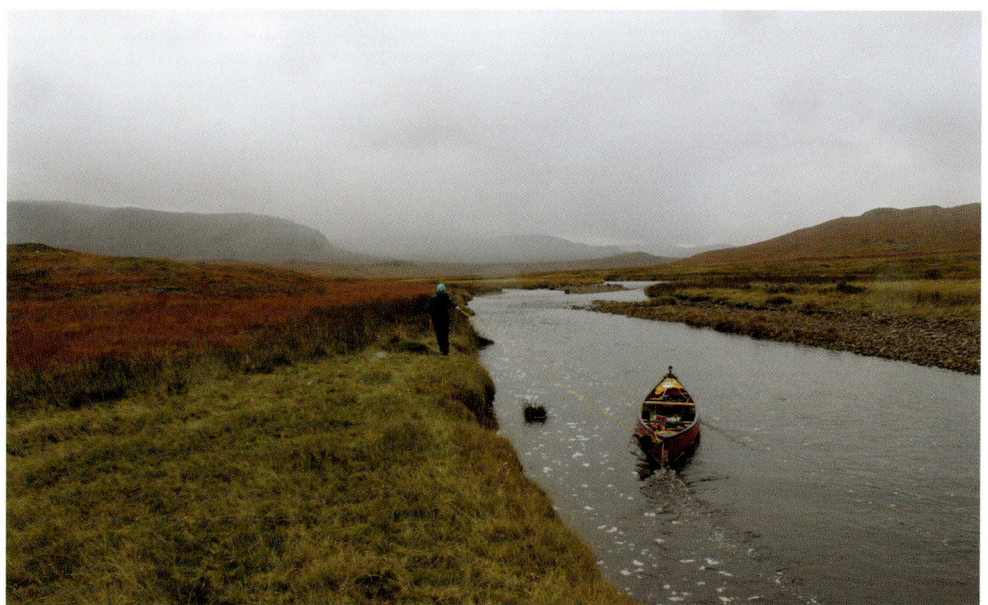
Tracking on the Upper River Spey. Photo | Nick March.

all so there are no entanglement issues. If you choose not to tie your bags in at all, then please be very aware that your kit can get lost if you capsize, and you may need it, especially if it is the communal barrel with tent, stove and food in it.

Packing a touring kayak

In a touring kayak you have slightly less space than in a canoe, so you might have to be a bit more ruthless with your packing list, but you usually have plenty of space to pack a few non-essentials in the hatches as well.

Each touring kayak will have a number of dry hatches for you to pack kit into. I always make sure that any kit that must stay dry is properly sealed in a dry bag. When you are packing your touring kayak, you need to think about the trim of your boat. Normally you want the bow of your boat to be slightly lighter than the stern. So I will often put heavier items such as food, tent and stove in the rear hatch and pack additional, softer stuff such as clothes around it. The bow hatch usually contains lighter items such as sleeping mat, sleeping bag, and clothes.

There will be some items that you will need regularly, and you might want to put some smaller ones in your buoyancy aid pocket or in the cockpit of your boat. If you are carrying water rather than filtering it, I normally carry this in the cockpit as well to keep the trim more neutral, and to avoid any unnoticed leakages onto clothes or other important items. Please be aware that any items that are free in the cockpit may float away if you capsize. You should also check your hatches before the trip to ensure that they are watertight.

Suggested paddling kit list

Paddling kit
- Boat with airbags
- Paddle
- Spare paddle
- Bailer and sponge
- Painter and swim lines (canoe)
- Sail and poles (canoe)
- Spray deck (kayak only)
- Day bag or rucksack for use as a day bag

Personal equipment
- Buoyancy aid with whistle and river knife
- Paddling clothes and good footwear
- Helmet
- Knee pads or kneeling mats (for canoes)

Camping equipment
Personal
- Clothes, shoes, hat and gloves
- Toiletries and towel, including any personal medication
- Sleeping bag and mat
- Lunch bag, water bottle and flask (in day bag/easy access)
- Plate, mug, knife, fork and spoon
- Sun cream and midge repellent (in day bag/easy access)

Shared
- Tent
- Stove, fuel, lighter and cooking pots
- Water carrier and optional filter/purifier (if planning to use river water to drink)
- Toilet paper, trowel and zip lock bags
- Rubbish bags

Day bag/easy access items
- Map and compass and GPS if carried
- Mobile phone (although you may wish to carry this in your buoyancy aid)
- Lunch and snack food
- Flask/water bottle
- First aid kit
- Group shelter and survival bag
- Spare clothes in the event of capsize/feeling cold
- Sun cream, sun hat and sunglasses

Safety equipment
- Rescue kit (slings, karabiners, pulleys, prussics, etc) within easy access in the boat or on your person in a bum bag
- Throw bag
- First aid kit
- Map, compass and GPS (in day bag/easy access)
- Group shelter and survival bag (in day bag/easy access)
- Boat repair kit (duck tape, patches, two-part plumber's putty, spare bolts, adjustable spanner and screwdrivers or multi tool, lashing cord, cable ties, Aquasure or Freesole glue for airbag repairs)
- Mobile phone in a waterproof case, with enough charge for the length of journey you are planning (in day bag/easy access)
- Torch and spare batteries
- Radio/weather app on your phone (for weather reports)

Weather and river levels

When we are journeying on the river it is very important for us to know what the weather will be doing and consequently what the river levels will be like. River levels can change very quickly if there is heavy rain in the area of one or more of the main tributaries. This can turn the River Spey from a gentle river into a raging torrent without eddies and with large tree debris. Check your forecast before you go and keep your eye on the actual weather as you are out on the river.

Weather forecasts

The River Spey gets predominantly south-westerly winds. This is great as the river generally runs in a north-easterly direction so you often get the wind following you. It also means that the majority of the rain has already fallen on the West Coast and we are in the rain shadow here in the North East. However a large portion of the river's catchment area is to the west of us, or in the Cairngorms itself, and this can mean that the river levels can go up very quickly if there is a large amount of rainfall in the mountains. You can get weather forecasts that will tell you about the wind direction, rainfall and temperature from many sources. The internet is an amazing source of information and can localise forecasts for the different villages on the river. Try www.xcweather.co.uk, www.bbc.co.uk/weather, www.metoffice.gov.uk and www.mwis.org.uk as starting points.

Garva bridge in lowish water. Photo | Nick March.

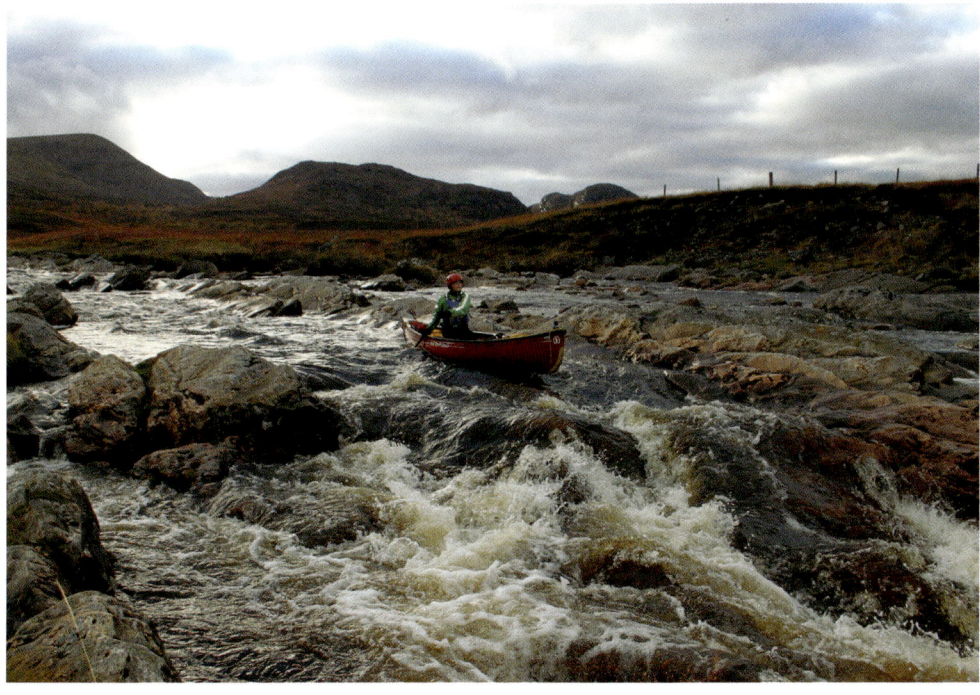

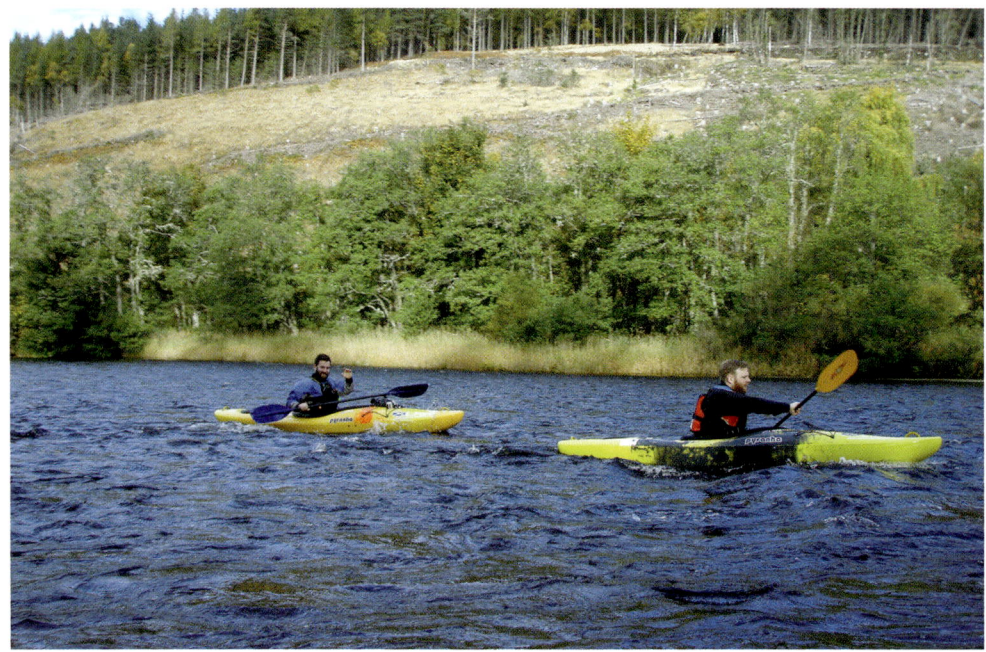
Touring kayaks near Ballindalloch.

If you do not have access to a computer or smartphone then you can get information in a more traditional way through the radio. BBC Radio Scotland has good weather information in its 'out of doors' forecast Monday to Friday 1904hrs, Saturday 0704hrs and 2204hrs and Sunday 0704hrs and 2004hrs.

River levels

To get river levels there is a great website for paddlers called www.wheresthewater.com. This has a reading for the River Spey at Boat o' Brig. To get an indicator of what is happening above Aviemore then also have a look at the River Feshie levels. The Feshie is one of the main tributaries and can be a good indicator to the River Spey rising and falling. If there has been a lot of rain in the Cairngorms then it arrives into the river from the Feshie, the Druie, the Nethy and the Avon. If there has been a lot of rain on the west or in the Monadhliath then it arrives higher up from the Calder and from the Dulnain. Lower down the river you get a lot of water coming in from the Fiddich. Other good sources of information are www.fishpal.com, search for the River Spey where you can get river data all the way down, although on this site it is not interpreted for paddlers. Both of these websites get their information from the Scottish Environment Protection Agency (SEPA) which collects river level data on a daily basis.

If the calibration on the www.wheresthewater.com website is used, anything above a low level is a great fun run. On a medium to high level, or above, think carefully about whether you should get on the river, as there are few eddies and you can often get large tree debris coming down the river with you. If you have a capsize you can travel a long way down the river when you are sorting out a rescue, which can result in boats and people being a long distance apart.

In the summer the river will often be sitting at a low or scrape level but it is still possible to paddle the whole journey. However you may have to start further down the river at Loch Insh, which is a good holding point for the water, or even further down at Aviemore.

Autumn colours on the Spey.

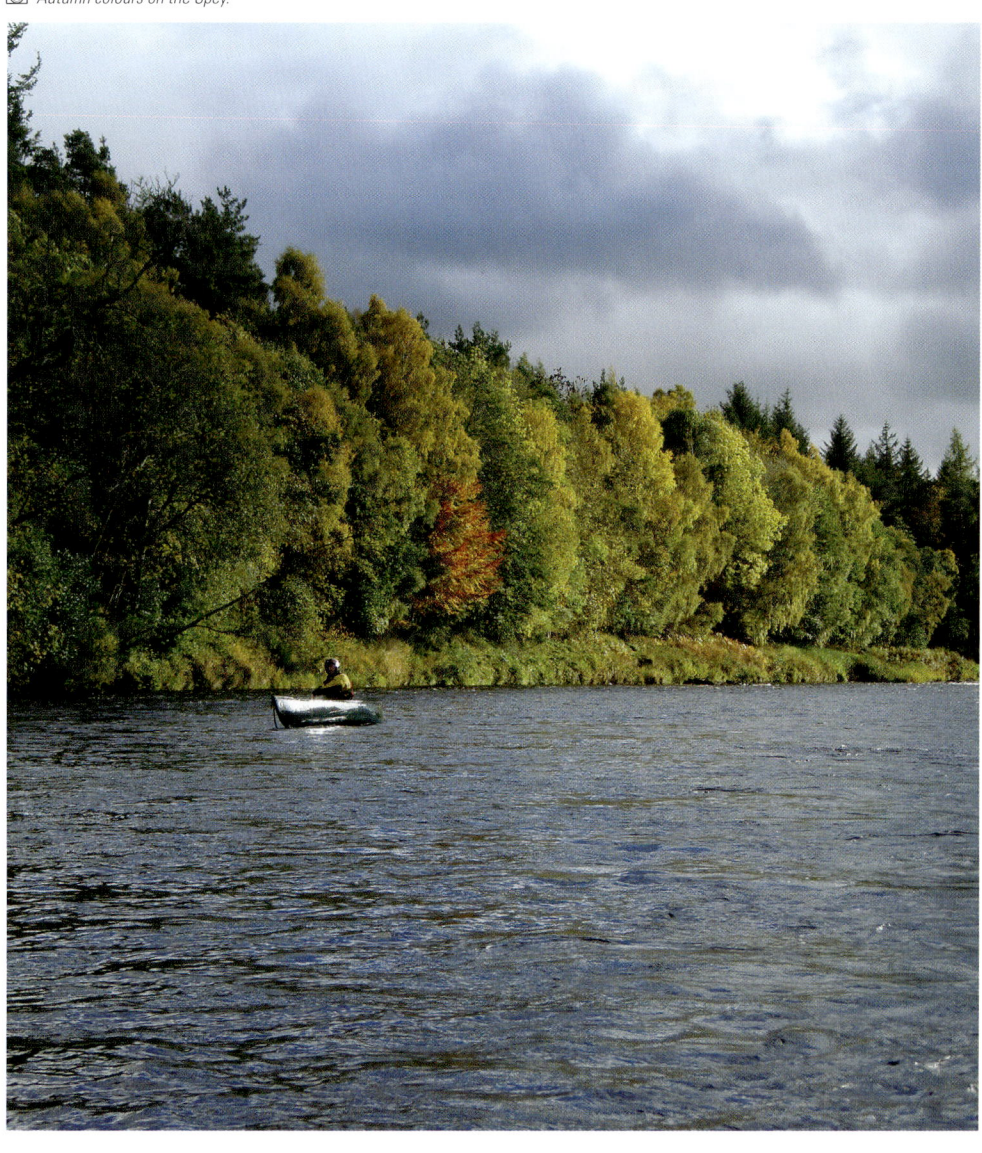

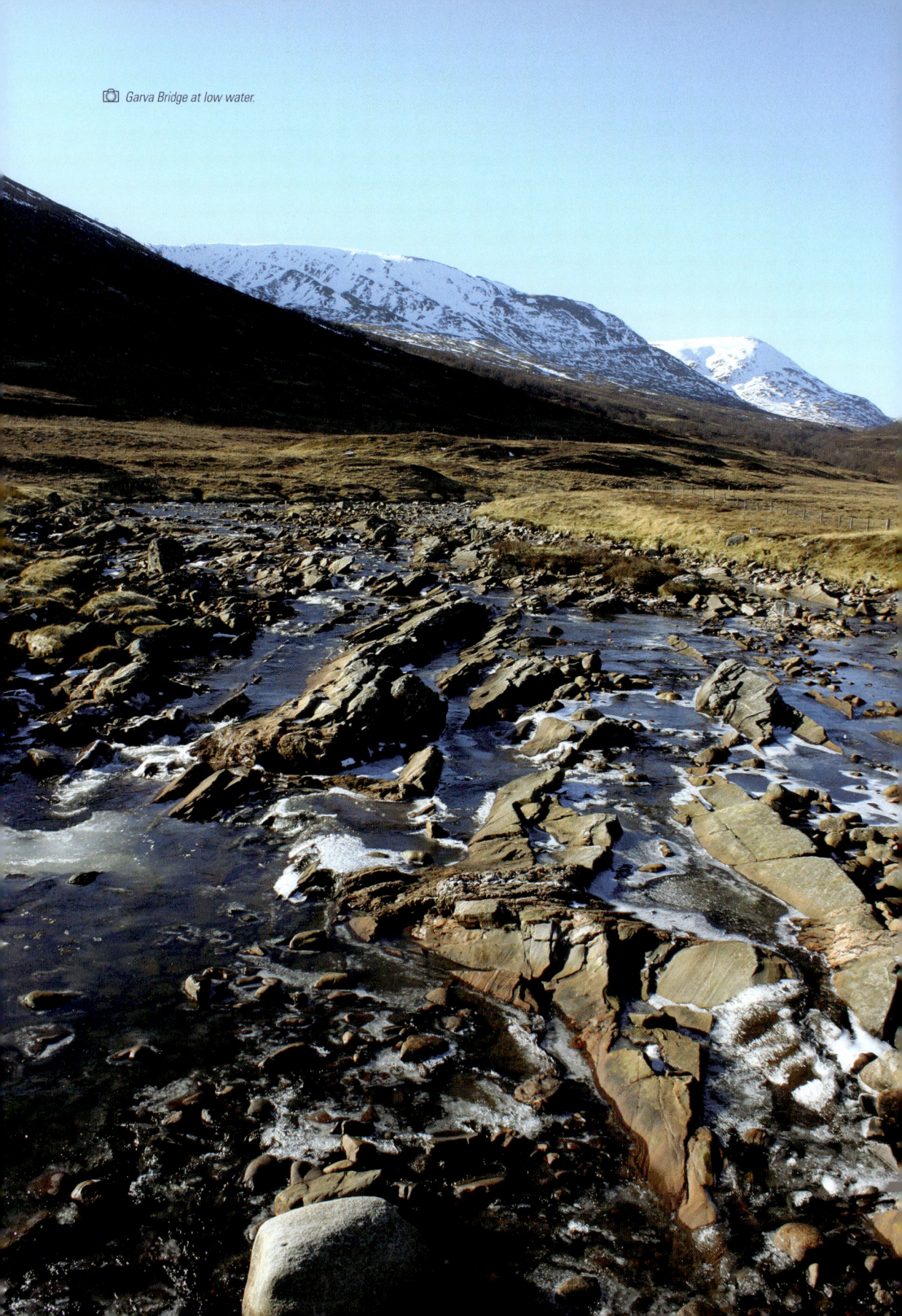
Garva Bridge at low water.

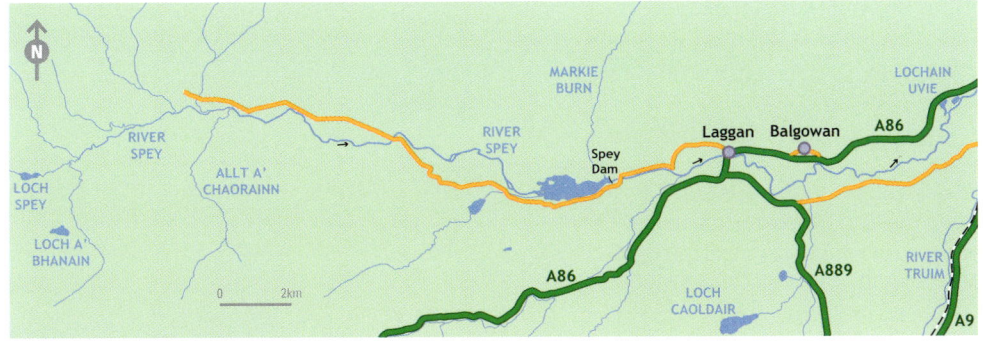

Upper River

The Upper River
Loch Spey to Lochain Uvie

The upper part of the river, above the more usual Lochain Uvie start, is best paddled in medium to high water. There are some rapids up to grade 3 on the section to the Spey Dam. At higher levels these can get up to grade 4 around Garva Bridge (the first major rapid starts at the corner of the forest plantation at NN 503 946). From Spey Dam down is grade 1(+).

The River Spey is a majestic river sweeping gracefully from its source in the Monadhliath Mountains, passing gently through the plains of Strathspey, and then picking up speed as it tumbles down to Spey Bay in Moray. It is a famous river in many rights from the salmon fishing, whisky distilling and paddling, to the interesting and rare wildlife sights that you see when travelling through on a journey down the Spey.

Loch Spey, high in the Monadhliath Mountains, is usually recognised to be the source of the Spey, although you could pick any of the many mountain burns that tumble down into the loch itself as being the true source. The river has been paddled from Loch Spey, however it takes a long walk with your boat and a lot of water to make it a viable option. There is a track leading to Glen Roy from Laggan that follows the river. As you travel along this track in a north-easterly direction from Loch Spey you see the river gaining in width and volume, as more small burns collect together and feed it. The river, more burn here, twists back and forth until it gains a little more maturity. There are some smaller rapids to contend with, and then some bigger ones (around grade 3) near Garva Bridge. The river

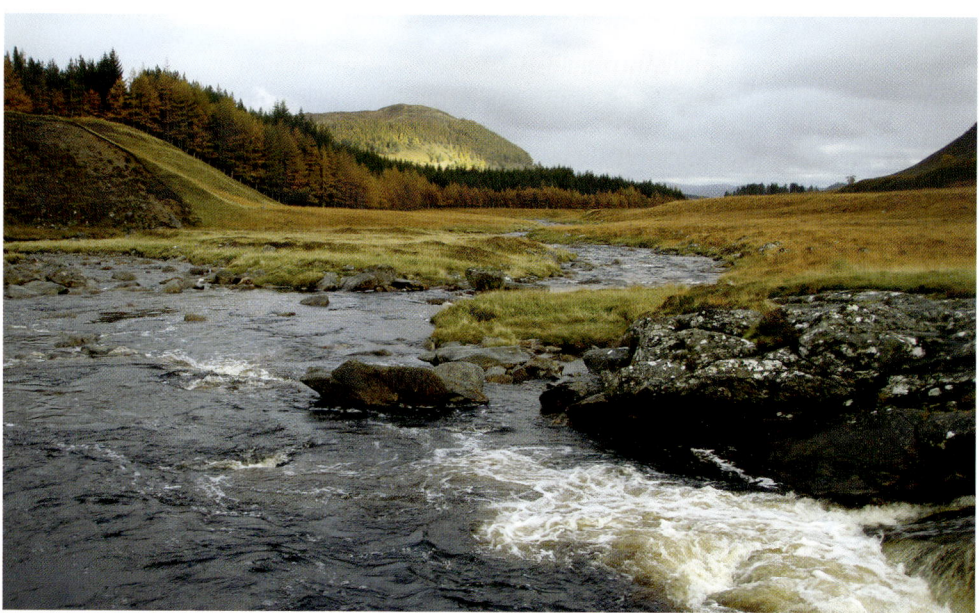
Grade 3 section on the upper river.

continues flowing through farmland down to the loch just above Spey Dam, where the water has been dammed to form a small loch in the beautiful mountainous surroundings. Water from here is piped away and diverted to the aluminium works in Fort William. It generally takes a lot of rain to open the Spey Dam to any significant amount. Passing round the dam you are into a more open section of river where it needs to be raining quite hard to keep the water flowing deep enough to paddle. Here the river takes on a wider outlook, with the tree-lined banks camouflaging the mountains that surround you. As you travel down towards Laggan village you get into a flatter section of river with the banks built up around you to reduce flooding. There have been recent flooding problems with the A86 near Laggan (on the drive between Aviemore and Fort William). There are many suggested solutions to this problem, but currently the main road has been limited to a single track road while they devise a permanent solution. In the winter months, it is not unusual to be driving with a big expanse of water either side of you when the river has flooded. To the north of Laggan Bridge is the first recognised access point on the river (NN 615 942), on the river right below the road bridge. This leads you in normal summer levels into a tree-lined, gravel-banked maze, where you often have to jump out of your boat to wade down sections, or pull across gravel banks before you get into the flow of the river. The banks here are raised up to try to alleviate flooding from the farmlands of the strath. Beyond this initial section the river deepens and you can paddle generally unhindered. As you meander down through the area you get some fine views of the Monadhliath Mountains and down towards the Glen Feshie hills with the Cairngorms in the distance. Once you start seeing the dark, imposing crags at Creag Dhubh on your left, you know that you are getting towards the more normal put-in points on the river. Even so, don't expect to see many other paddlers as far up as this, as most folks will choose to start at Newtonmore, Loch Insh or Aviemore, depending on how many days they have to spend on the river. See the suggested itineraries. Lochain Uvie near Creag Dhubh is the next put-in point here, and you will often share a car park with climbers intent on getting in some of the hard Creag Dhubh routes. If you are a keen hill walker, you can also walk from here to the top of Creag Dhubh to get a superb panorama taking in most of the strath towards Laggan, and with views northwards towards Aviemore. There is a herd of wild goats in this area that is worth looking out for as they clamber precariously about putting us humans to shame.

Between here and the sea the river has many major tributaries, the first being the Calder, followed by the Tromie, Feshie, Druie, Dulnain, Avon and several smaller rivers and burns as well, all of which have their sources in the major hills that surround the Spey. The fact that there is so much potential for water to run into the Spey is one of the reasons that it is so popular as a paddling river, as it is very rare that the river is too low to paddle.

Heading down river near Loch Spey. Photo | Nick March.

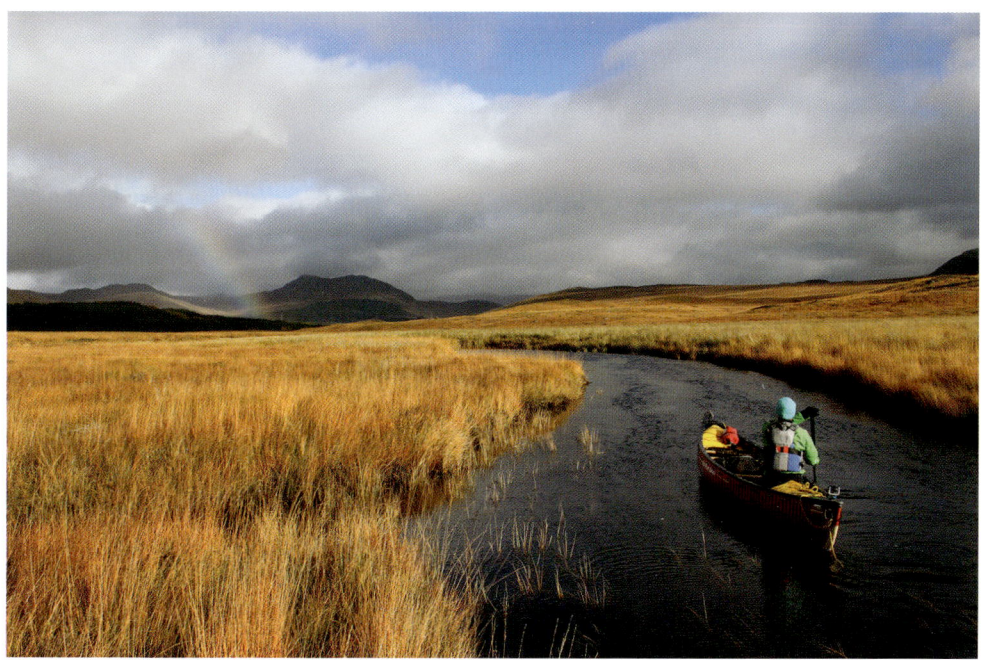

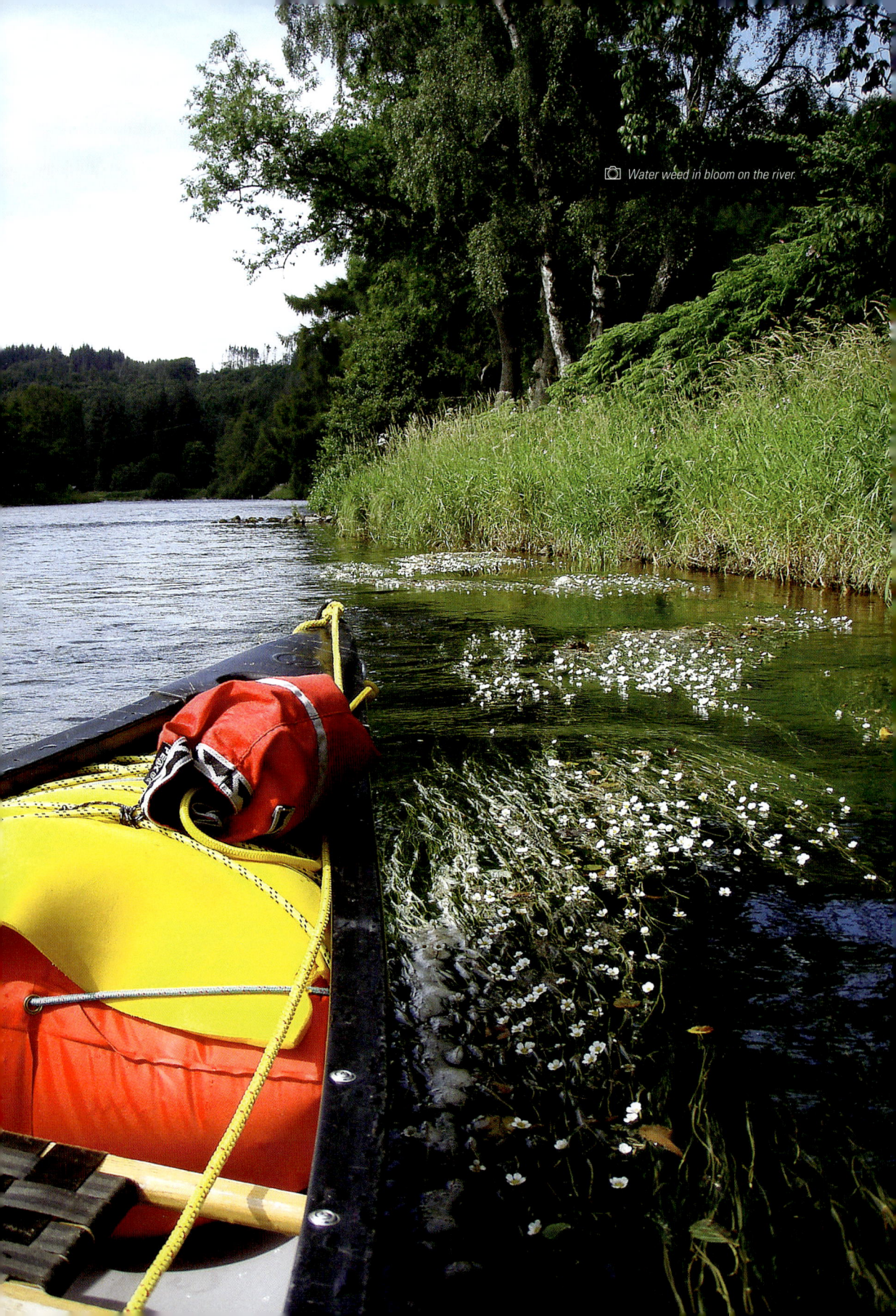
Water weed in bloom on the river.

Suggested Itineraries

This obviously depends on how far you would like to paddle in a day, but most folks can paddle between 20 and 30km per day without too many problems; the fitter you are the further you can go in a day. You may choose to paddle more or less depending on whether you want to explore the area further or want to have your head down and paddle hard. I have used three of the main starting points for the journey as being Lochain Uvie, Loch Insh and Aviemore. In higher water conditions the flow rate will be faster and you will find it easier travelling bigger distances.

From Lochain Uvie to Spey Bay is 135km, from Kincraig church to Spey Bay is 111km, and from Aviemore to Spey Bay is nearly 100km.

Most of these itineraries start and finish near recognised campsites; however, it is possible to wild camp near the river in many places. Please use sustainable practices if you are going to wild camp.

Suggestions for a 5-day trip

Option 1

Day	From	To	Distance (km)
1	Lochain Uvie	Kincraig church	24.0
2	Kincraig church	Boat of Balliefurth	32.4
3	Boat of Balliefurth	Cragganmore	27.0
4	Cragganmore	Craigellachie	22.4
5	Craigellachie	Spey Bay	29.2

Option 2

Day	From	To	Distance (km)
1	Kincraig church	Aviemore	11.3
2	Aviemore	Boat of Balliefurth	21.1
3	Boat of Balliefurth	Cragganmore	27.0
4	Cragganmore	Craigellachie	22.4
5	Craigellachie	Spey Bay	29.2

Suggestions for a 4-day trip

Option 1

Day	From	To	Distance (km)
1	Lochain Uvie	Aviemore	35.3
2	Aviemore	Cromdale	30.6
3	Cromdale	Craigellachie	39.9
4	Craigellachie	Spey Bay	29.2

Option 2

Day	From	To	Distance (km)
1	Aviemore	Boat of Balliefurth	21.1
2	Boat of Balliefurth	Cragganmore	27.0
3	Cragganmore	Craigellachie	22.4
4	Craigellachie	Spey Bay	29.2

Option 3

Day	From	To	Distance (km)
1	Kingcraig church	Boat of Balliefurth	32.4
2	Boat of Balliefurth	Cragganmore	27.0
3	Cragganmore	Craigellachie	22.4
4	Craigellachie	Spey Bay	29.2

Suggestions for a 3-day trip

Option 1

Day	From	To	Distance (km)
1	Lochain Uvie	Aviemore	35.3
2	Aviemore	Blacksboat	51.6
3	Blacksboat	Spey Bay	48.1

Option 2

Day	From	To	Distance (km)
1	Aviemore	Grantown	24.6
2	Grantown	Aberlour	41.6
3	Aberlour	Spey Bay	33.5

Option 3

Day	From	To	Distance (km)
1	Kingcraig Church	Grantown	35.9
2	Grantown	Aberlour	41.6
3	Aberlour	Spey Bay	33.5

Distances

Distances between the agreed access points are here if you wish to make up your own itineraries.

Lochain Uvie to Newtonmore	4.8km
Newtonmore to Kingussie	7.2km
Kingussie to Kincraig church	12.0km
Kincraig church to Aviemore	11.3km
Aviemore to Boat of Garten	11.3km
Boat of Garten to Broomhill	6.8km
Broomhill to Boat of Balliefurth	3.0km
Boat of Balliefurth to Grantown	3.5km
Grantown to Cromdale	6.0km
Cromdale to Advie Bridge	11.5km
Advie Bridge to Cragganmore	6.0km
Cragganmore to Blacksboat Bridge	3.5km
Blacksboat Bridge to Knockando	4.0km
Knockando to Carron Bridge	5.3km
Carron Bridge to Aberlour	5.3km
Aberlour to Craigellachie	4.3km
Craigellachie to Boat o' Brig	12.4km
Boat o' Brig to Fochabers	9.4km
Fochabers to Spey Bay	7.4km
Total	**135km**

Looking towards Loch Spey.

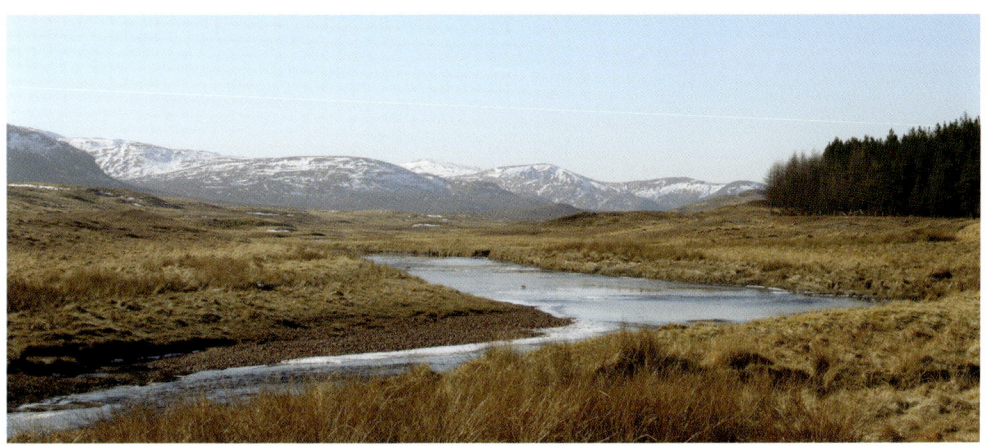

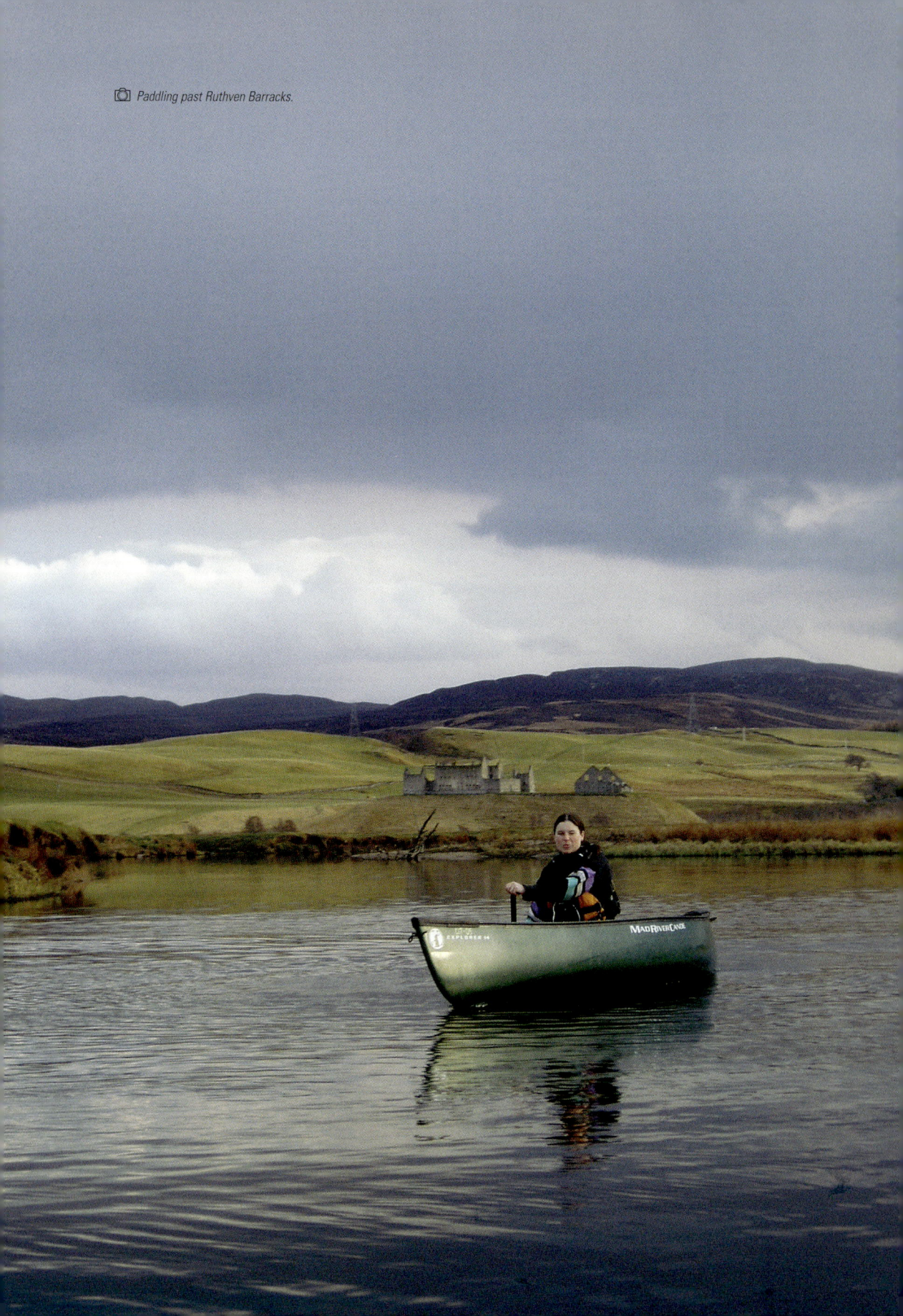
Paddling past Ruthven Barracks.

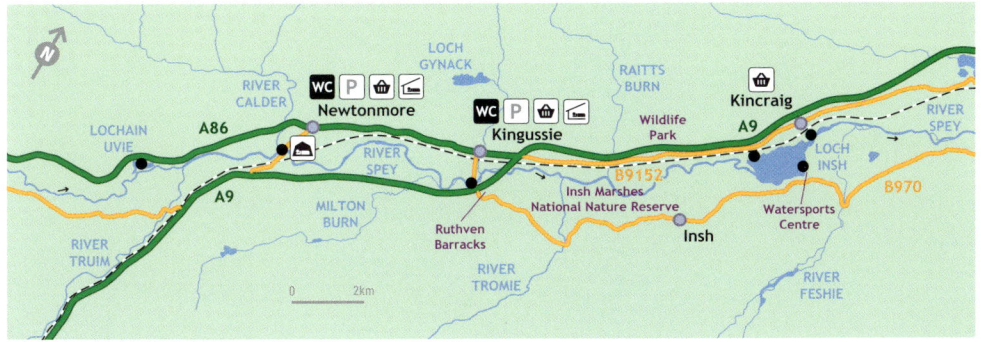

Section 1

Lochain Uvie to Loch Insh

Distance 24km
Start Lochain Uvie, NN 674 957
Finish Kincraig Church car park, NH 838 045
Difficulty Flat water to grade 1 rapids

Agreed access points

Lochain Uvie, NN 674 957 – park in the lay-by at the bottom of the Creag Dhubh crags, access the larger of the two lochs via a small gate (please close this after you). There is a small connecting burn between the lochain and the river where there is a pipe tunnel. If you decide to go through it you must be very aware of the consequences of getting stuck; you can portage round the tunnel on the bank.
Newtonmore, NN 709 980 – access on the river right just below Spey Bridge. If you stay in the Spey Bridge Campsite you may be able to access the river from the campsite.

In Newtonmore please do not leave vehicles and trailers in the lorry park at the Chef's Grill without asking permission.
Kingussie, NN 759 997 – access on the river right below the bridge on the road going to the Ruthven Barracks. Use the gate on the upstream side of the river.
SW Loch Insh, NH 822 043 – use the lay-by opposite the gate lodge and get to the loch by going under the arch by the railway.
Loch Insh Water Sports Centre, NH 837 045 – if you agree launching and landing with them.
Kincraig Church car park, NH 838 045.

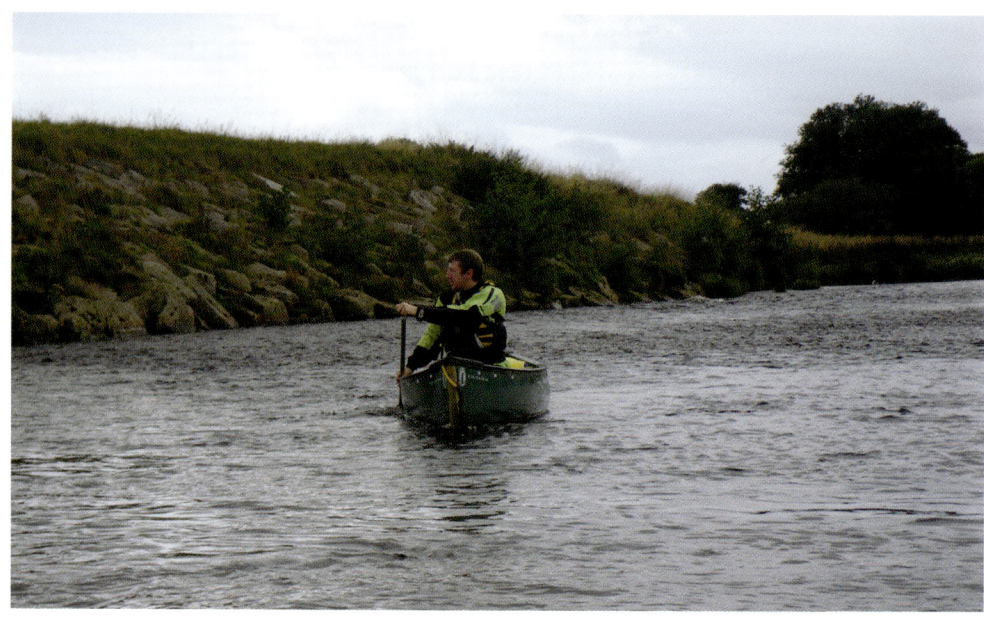
Gentle grade 1 after Kingussie.

Nearby attractions

The following attractions are on or just off your route: Ruthven Barracks; Insh Marshes National Nature Reserve; Highland Folk Museum, Newtonmore, Kincraig village shop; Highland Wildlife Park; Loch Insh Water Sports Centre.

Accommodation

The following campsites and hostels are within easy walking distance of the river: Spey Bridge Caravan and Camping Park, Newtonmore; Newtonmore Hostel; Strathspey Mountain Hostel, Newtonmore; Happy Days Hostel, Kingussie; Loch Insh Water Sports Centre, lodges and sometimes camping.

For B&B and hotel accommodation contact the tourist information centre in Aviemore 01479 810930 or Kingussie 01540 661000.

Description

Starting at the lay-by under the Creag Dhubh crags, there is a small gate across the road; use this to access the loch. Make sure that you close any gates that you use. Paddle through the lily pads on the loch and in the far corner there is a small channel with a tunnel that runs into the river. If you decide to portage across to the other loch there is another channel that also runs into the river. From the first loch, if you decide to go through the tunnel to the river rather than portage around it, please be aware of the width and height of you and your boat, and the consequences of getting stuck for whatever reason.

The river here is flat or very slow moving until you see Invertruim House in the distance on the right-hand side of the river. This marks the start of the small grade 1 rapids. The first rapid on a bend turning left is quite congested with trees and islands, and you need to take a bit of care negotiating these in higher water. Thereafter the rapids are all grade 1 riffles, but they keep the interest going for you. The River Truim comes in from the right and this can cause a few waves in bigger water. As you travel further down this section you start to see some really great views down to the Glen Feshie hills and beyond towards Braeriach. The river has some really pleasant easy grade 1 rapids from now onwards and has an open aspect to it. Just before you go under the bridges at Newtonmore you will get a rapid where the River Calder joins the Spey and in bigger water conditions this can have a few good waves; in lower water you need to watch out for the shallow rocks under you. Going under the road bridge at Newtonmore you are at another agreed access point. This one is on the right-hand side of the river just below Spey Bridge. If you are using the campsite you can ask to launch from the campsite on the left-hand side of the river. Many folk choose to start from here if the upper section is too low. Directly following the road bridge there is a railway bridge, and you often see the trains making their way north and south with passengers waving at you as you pass.

From here the river gets a little more congested with fallen trees and tree roots and the rapids, although still grade 1 in technical difficulty, can be a section that you need to take more care on, particularly in higher water levels. There has been some recent clearing of the tree root debris to create a passable channel in the river.

The river flows down past the Newtonmore golf course and if you have an old map you will see a braided section of the river. This has now been cut off and has formed two smaller lochs alongside the river; a good example of an oxbow lake.

Marking the end of Newtonmore is the Allt na Fèithe Buidhe entering from the left, and the railway is again visible. The river then flows onto a more gentle section; this has flood prevention works on the left of the river changing the view of the hills that you get. On the right-hand side as you near Inverton there is a very steep wooded hillside; this is a good marker that you are halfway between Newtonmore and Kingussie. The last few kilometres into Kingussie are fairly gentle with the odd easy

Craig Dubh crags.

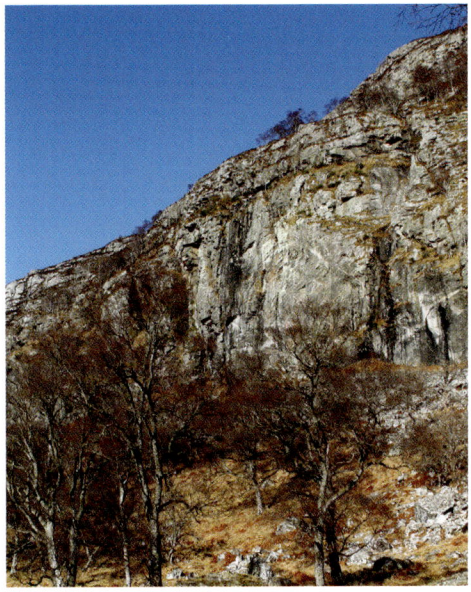

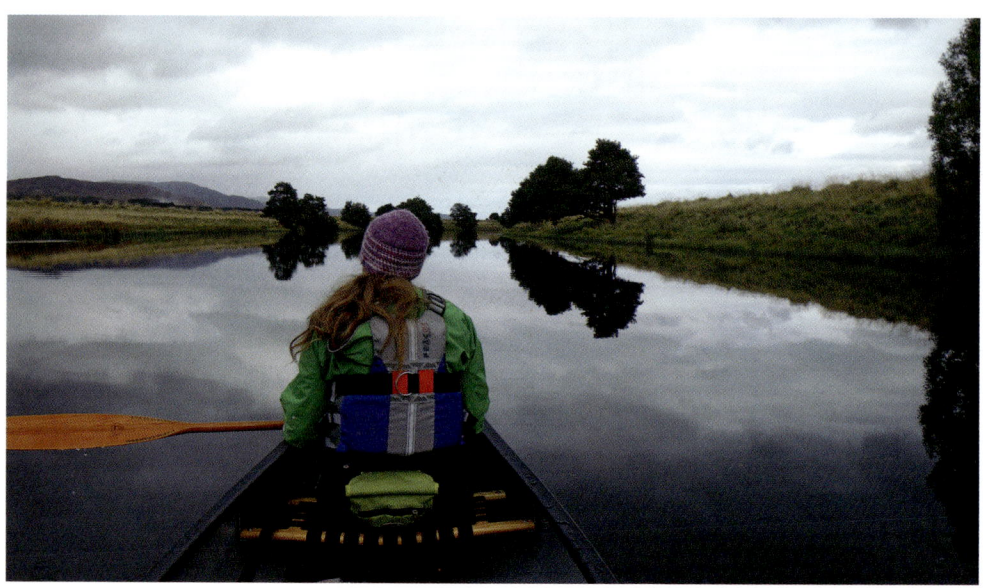
Calm water after Kingussie. Photo | Alison Falconbridge.

rapid helping you along. There is another agreed access point just under the bridge on the B970 which runs from Kingussie to Ruthven Barracks and beyond to Insh. This is on the river right; use the gate on the upstream side of the road.

The Ruthven Barracks is a very prominent ruin in a commanding position. It was built between 1719 and 1721, directly after the Jacobite rising in 1715. It is built on the site of an old castle; the first recorded one dating from 1229. The Barracks are well worth an excursion off the river. They are in the condition that they were when they were destroyed in 1746 when another Jacobite uprising set fire to them. Ruthven Barracks are currently maintained by Historic Scotland.

Directly below the bridge in Kingussie there is a gentle rapid that can sweep you into the trees on the left if you don't anticipate it; it is however easy to stay on the right of the river and avoid the trees. From here, continue paddling and you pass under the bridge carrying the busy A9 and onto the slower flowing section with only a few small rapids that goes through the Insh Marshes National Nature Reserve. Insh Marshes is one of the most important wetlands in Europe. It is managed by the RSPB and, depending on the time of year, you may see birdlife such as lapwings, redshanks, snipe, curlews, whooper swans and greylag geese. Between here and Loch Insh you have a wonderful opportunity to observe the birdlife that the reserve is famed for. If you want to explore the marshes rather than just paddling through them, there are marked paths accessible 1km beyond Ruthven Barracks. In higher water conditions it is not unusual to see this whole area under water, and if you choose to paddle you can pass over fields and fences.

When you reach Loch Insh the first of the access points is in the south-west corner of the loch in a lay-by opposite a gate lodge; go under the railway via an arched bridge. The second of the agreed access points is at Loch Insh Water Sports Centre in the north-east corner of the loch (you may be charged to access and egress here, speak to the water sports office when you park). There is a good café at the centre, the cakes come recommended, and they will also sometimes provide camping). The third access point is at Kincraig Church, river right below the church. Please park considerately in the lay-by opposite the church and close the gate when you are through.

As you paddle out of the river mouth coming from Kingussie, paddling the 2km across the loch is usually a joy with the prevailing wind on your back. You may even get the opportunity to get an improvised sail up here to make the most of the winds.

If you paddle to Kincraig Church, the left side of the island (as you look from the Kingussie end of the loch) usually has the deepest water in it and can be paddled at all levels. There is an osprey nest on the north side of the island, and it is recommended that you are quiet when paddling around the island when the birds are likely to be in the area and nesting (usually March to October). Please do not get out on the island around the nesting area.

Kincraig Church is a small community church which, if you are visiting on a Sunday, will usually have a good number of cars in the car park. If you require any provisions it is a short walk over the bridge to the village shop, and there are local pubs in Kincraig for refreshments and evening meals.

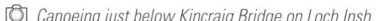
Canoeing just below Kincraig Bridge on Loch Insh.

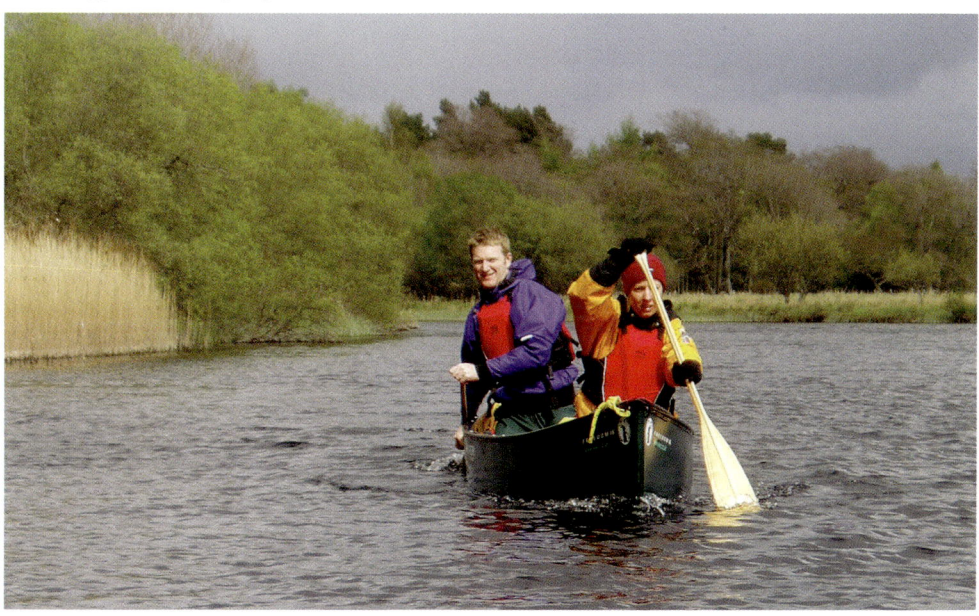

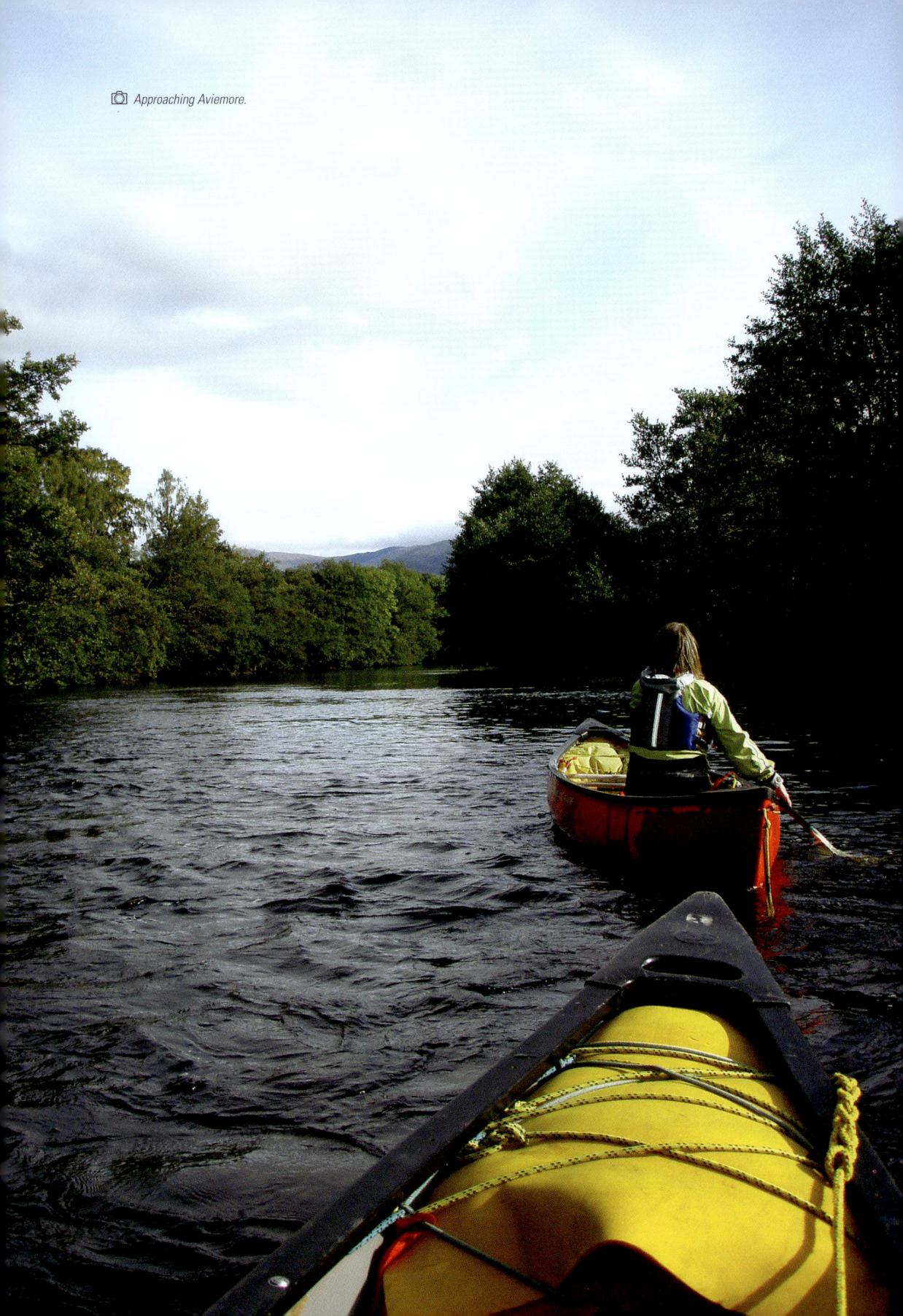
Approaching Aviemore.

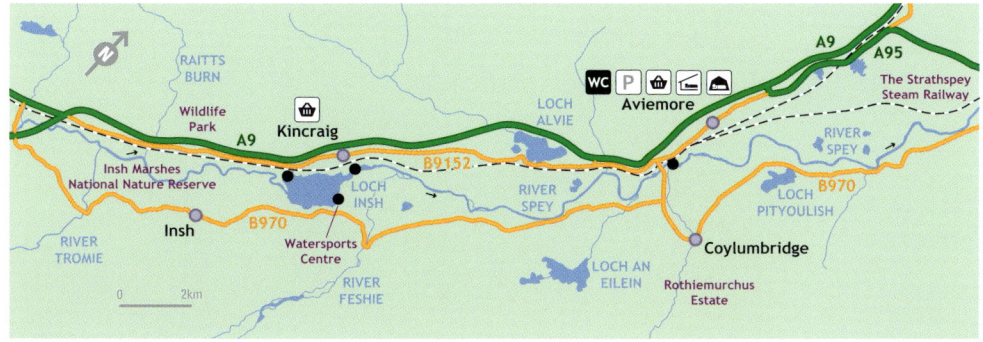

Section 2

Loch Insh to Aviemore

Distance 11.5km
Start Kincraig church car park, NH 838 045
Finish Aviemore Old Bridge Inn riverside car park, NH 894 118
Difficulty Flat water to grade 1 rapids

Agreed access points

Kincraig Church car park, NH 838 045.
Loch Insh Water Sports Centre, NH 837 045 – if you agree launching and landing with them.
South-west Loch Insh, NH 822 043 – use the lay-by opposite the gate lodge. Reach the loch by going under the arch by the railway.
Aviemore Old Bridge Inn riverside car park, NH 894 118.

Nearby attractions

The following attractions are on or just off your route: Kincraig village shop, Highland Wildlife Park, Loch Insh Water Sports Centre, Rothiemurchus Estate, Aviemore village centre.

Accommodation

The following campsites and hostels are within easy walking distance of the river: Loch Insh Water Sports Centre, lodges and sometimes camping; Dalraddy Holiday Park, nr. Aviemore; High Range Touring Caravan and Camping Park, Aviemore; Rothiemurchus Camp and Caravan Park, Coylumbridge; Aviemore Bunkhouse; Aviemore Youth Hostel.

If you fancy staying somewhere quirky try Inshriach House, www.canopyandstars.co.uk. They have a wood-fired sauna and hot tub on the river, and bespoke camping options including a yurt, bothy, beermoth and shepherd's hut, all within easy access to the river.

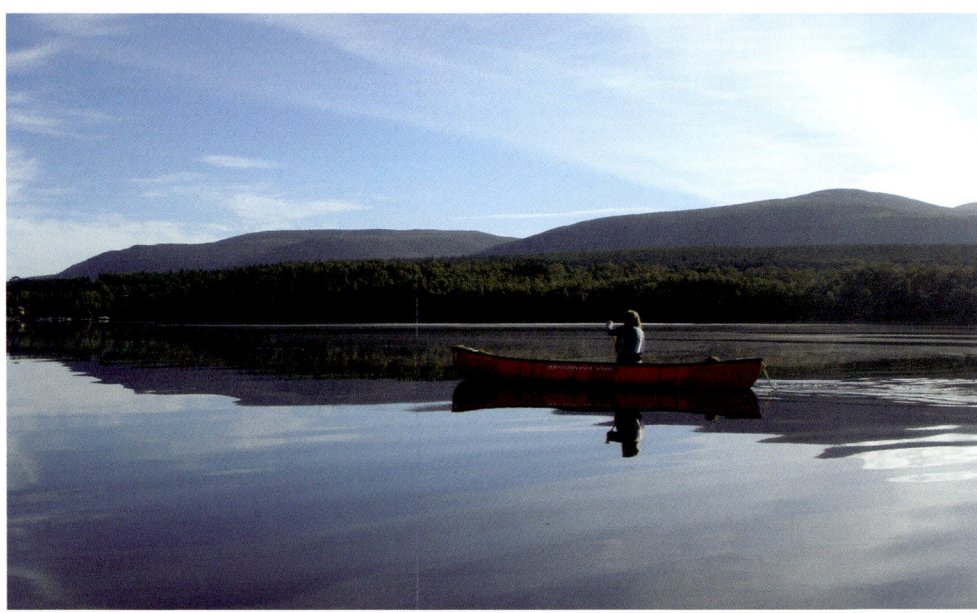
Sunny and calm Loch Insh.

B&B and hotel information for Kincraig and Aviemore can be found through the tourist information centre in Aviemore 01479 810930 or Kingussie 01540 661000.

Description

Starting from Kincraig Church, you can paddle out into the loch, keeping a careful eye out for the ospreys that often nest on the island. From April until October you are asked to stay off the island to allow them to nest quietly. If you have a pair of binoculars with you it's a great place to watch them soar majestically around the area. If you are lucky, you might even catch a glimpse of them catching a fish or feeding their young in the nest.

The predominant south-westerly winds will often push you across the loch and down into the mouth of the river. As you leave the loch glance at the bridge pillars; they were designed and built at the end of the 19th century and are a lasting legacy to the era, especially considering how high the water flow can go down the River Spey. After the bridge, you can paddle either side of the island. Following the island you come to a bend in the river and this is the start of the flowing section. If you are new to paddling, these first bits of moving water are great places to practise some of the river skills that you will require during your journey; breaking in, breaking out and ferry gliding your boat.

Some gentle flowing water will take you over gravel banks and down towards the confluence of the River Feshie, and the first real grade 1 rapid on this section of river. You can paddle either side of the large gravel island. The main flow usually goes down the left-hand channel. This often has a slightly submerged tree in it and is quite a narrow channel, so if you choose to go this way make sure that you can paddle your boat well enough to avoid the hazards. If you go down the right-hand channel, in low water you may have to walk your boat down the first section where it is shallow. It then deepens and flows past another channel of the Feshie and sometimes some other tree hazards, straight down until the two channels meet again. This junction is a common place to find a number of fishermen. Below this rapid on the left-hand side you can see the riverbank slowly collapsing down the sheer gravel and sandbanks, and the red tin-roofed house situated on top that is getting ever closer to toppling into the river itself. There is another lovely, long, easy rapid with a gravel bank on the right-hand side and a few tree stumps mid-river. This is a really nice place to stop and admire the Glen Feshie hills before you start concentrating on the main bulk of the Cairngorms in front of you.

From here there are a few easy rapids all in gently flowing water until you get to a sharp bend at NH 865 070. There are some pylon lines crossing the river prior to this point, so these are good landmarks to identify the area. This marks another tree hazard, and is sometimes best walked around depending on water levels. You should now start to see Kinrara House and the Duke of Gordon's Monument built in 1836 to commemorate the last Duke of Gordon, which is a prominent landmark on the top of the hill to the left of the river.

When you are under the monument there is another potential tree hazard at NH 884 087. The river continues meandering through the countryside with the Craigellachie hills dominating the landscape in front of you, with the steep grind of the Burma Road etched into its surface; it is a must for fit mountain bikers in the area. To the right you see the solid bulk of the Cairngorm Mountains with the deep cleft of the Lairig Ghru splitting Braeriach from the more commonly visited Cairn Lochain and Cairngorm Mountain area.

You might start to hear the gentle hum of the A9 at this point and see the large pylon lines running alongside the river for a few hundred metres. Don't worry, you quickly turn away from them again, and loop around passing some of the large estate houses of Rothiemurchus, taking you back to that sense of wilderness. As you follow the river you are now getting nearer to Aviemore, and when you travel underneath the large pylon line you know you are almost there. Just a quick rapid with a sharp left-hand bend in it, and you will start to see the new road bridge leading to the ski area, quickly followed by the old bridge, which is now a walking and cycling route.

There is easy access and good parking just after this bridge on the river left in the car park opposite The Old Bridge Inn and the Aviemore Bunkhouse.

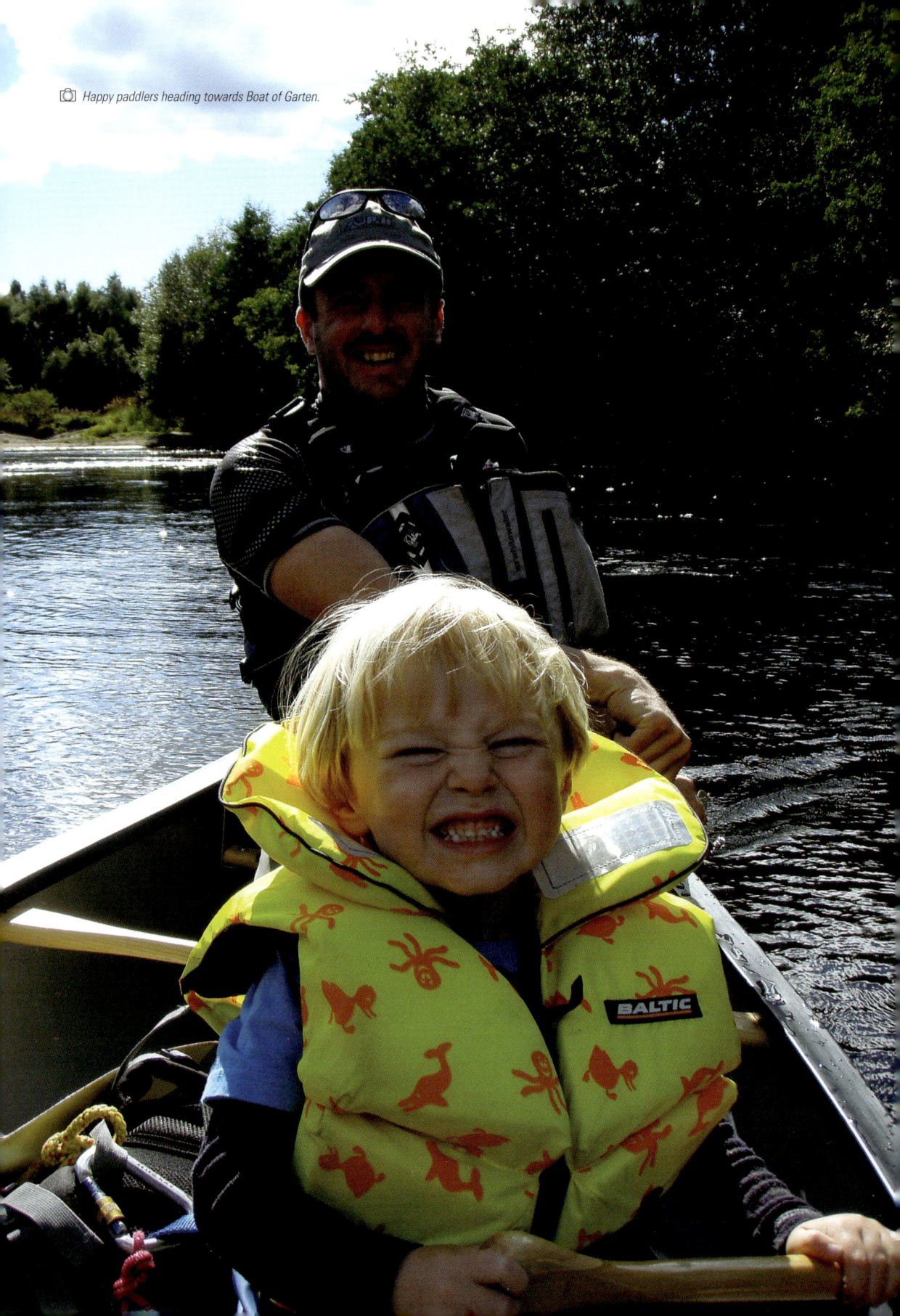
Happy paddlers heading towards Boat of Garten.

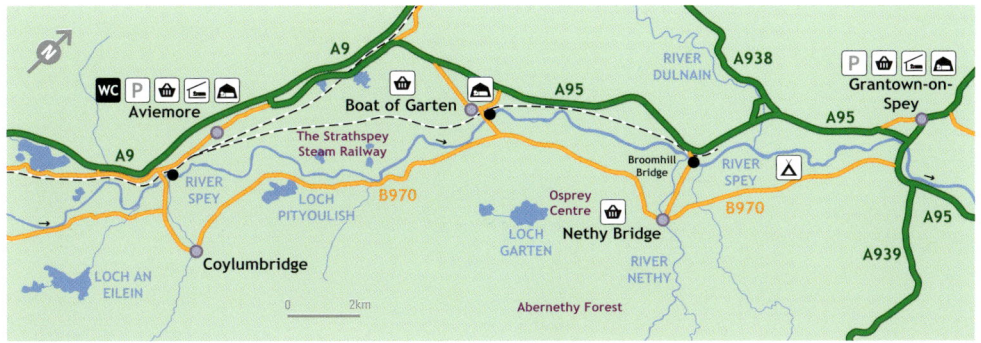

Section 3

Aviemore to Boat of Balliefurth

Distance 21km
Start Old Bridge Inn riverside car park, NH 894 118
Finish Broomhill Bridge, NH 996 224
Difficulty Flat water to grade 1(+) rapids

Agreed access points

Old Bridge Inn riverside car park, NH 894 118. Boat of Garten, parking at the lay-by near to the bridge. Access under the bridge on the left-hand, downstream side, NH 946 191. Broomhill Bridge, parking on the downstream side of the bridge, NH 996 224 – make sure you don't block any access to the river. Access the river on the left under the bridge.

Nearby attractions

The following attractions are on or just off your route: Aviemore village centre, Boat of Garten village, Loch Garten Osprey Centre, The Strathspey Steam Railway, Speyside Wildlife, Nethybridge village.

Accommodation

The following campsites and hostels are within easy walking distance of the river: Aviemore as before, Boat of Garten Caravan and Camping Park, Fraoch Lodge Hostel, Nethy Station Bunkhouse, and Boat of Balliefurth Campsite (marked with a small sign on a pylon saying "Camping this side"). B&B and hotel information for Aviemore and Boat of Garten can be found through the tourist information centre in Aviemore 01479 810930 or Grantown 01479 872242.

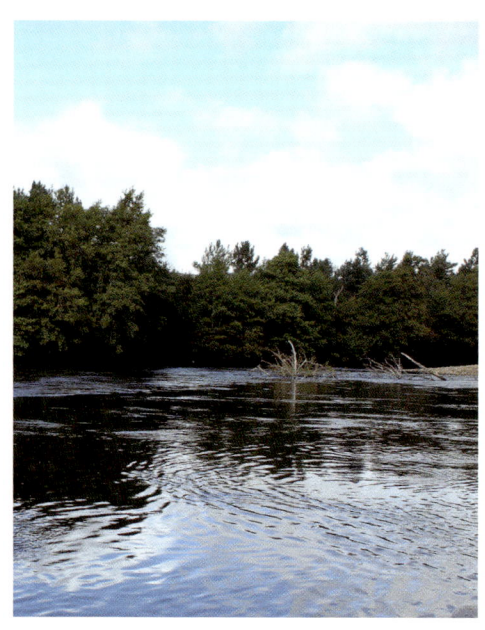
Tree debris just after Aviemore.

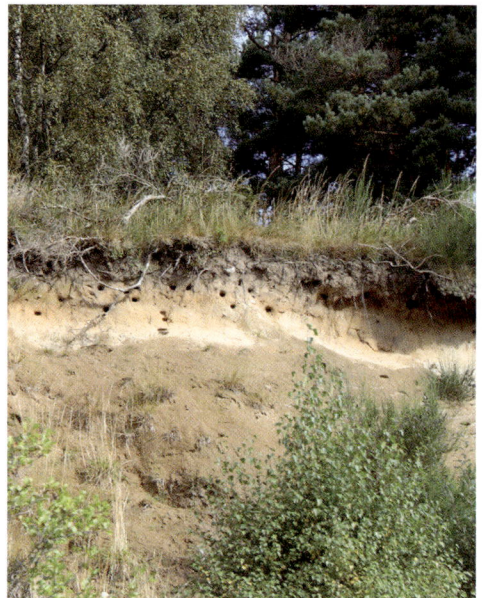
Sand martin holes.

Description

Leaving the car park at the Old Bridge Inn you are immediately into a section of small rapids that have lots of tree hazards which you need to be very careful of, particularly in bigger water flow conditions.

The River Druie, which you pass on the river right just as you get in, was one of the many smaller tributaries used by loggers in the 17th and 18th centuries.

After you pass the confluence of the River Druie on the right there is a sharp right-hand bend. Although this rapid is an easy one there are usually some tree hazards in the way and the flow can often take you towards the trees, first on the left and then the steep, sandy banking at the bottom of the rapid on the right. Once round the corner there are several more rapids that are similar in nature, many with tree hazards in the river and overhanging trees on the banks where the water flow is taking you. You need to be very aware of them. Staying in the middle of the flow is a good, safe bet here, making decisions to go right or left as you need to. As you pass the steep, sandy banks of the river here, keep a lookout for the small tell-tale holes in the sandbanks which are signs of the sand martin, and which you will see on a regular basis as you are travelling down the river.

Once you have passed the Dalfaber golf course on the left you are onto a much flatter section of river with some lovely scenery surrounding you. Make the most of the Cairngorms and look to the right-hand side of the river every now and then as the hills below you are starting to diminish in size. The Kincardine hills including Meall a' Bhuachaille now form the main skyline on the right-hand side of the river. On the left you have some flatter farmland, and then the smaller hills around Carrbridge come into view.

Just after Kinchurdy Farm, which is on the left-hand side, you will see on the right-hand side of the river, camouflaged into the hillside, a small bungalow with a turf roof, followed by a steep banking with a number of sandy holes in it. If you are travelling here near dusk keep a good lookout for badgers in this area. Highland Badgers will offer you trips out to spot badgers if you are interested.

The start of the rapids is marked by a right-hand bend (NH 937 175) just before you come into Boat of Garten. The run into Boat of Garten has a few rapids that are around grade 1 standard and are generally easy to read from the river. On the right-hand bank you might be able to spot some of the fishing huts for the area. If you are a keen fisherperson you can buy permits for the local area from the Boat of Garten post office.

As you approach Boat of Garten you can see the open fields on the sides of the river and in front of you is a bridge; in 1898 this replaced the ferry that transported people across the river.

Access to the village can be gained just underneath the bridge on the downstream side, and after a short walk uphill into the village you will find: the post office which serves tea, coffee and freshly baked produce; Anderson's restaurant; The Boat Hotel; Dow's Stores; the

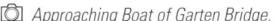
Approaching Boat of Garten Bridge.

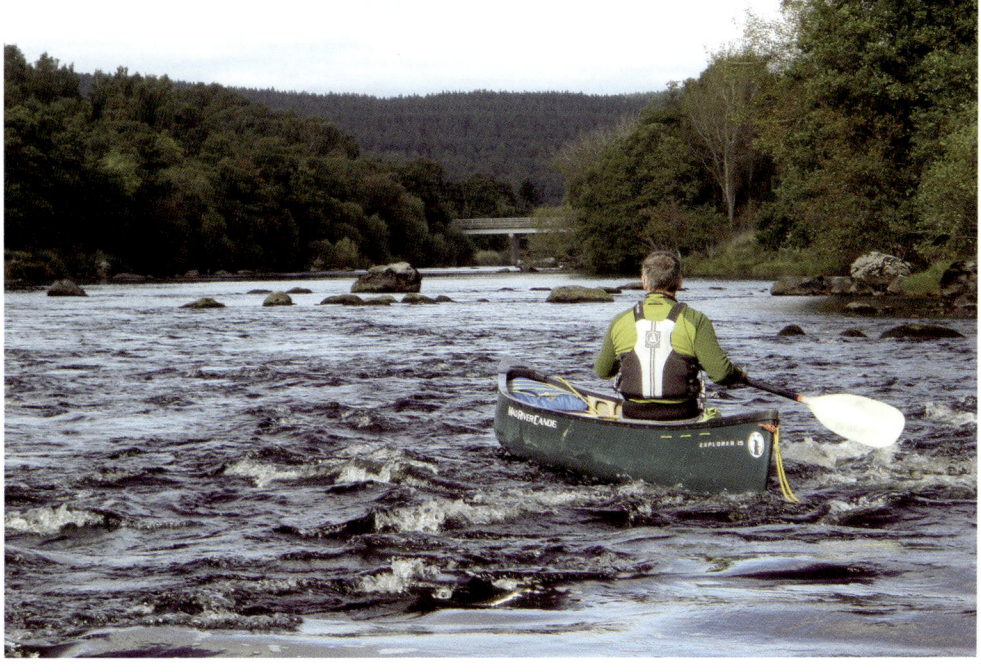

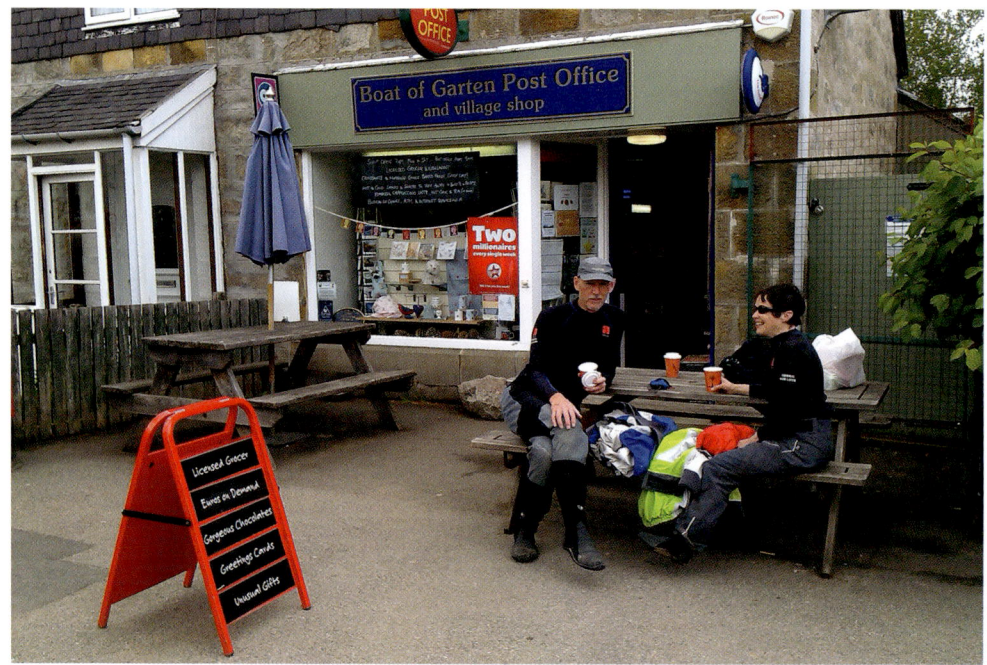

Boat of Garten Post Office. Photo | Donald Macpherson.

Boat of Garten Caravan and Camping Park; and Fraoch Lodge Hostel.

Putting back onto the water under the bridge the gentle flow takes you off downstream again. In low summer levels watch out for the shallow, gravelly areas on the right-hand side of the main river channel. This next section has a lovely slow flow and generally flat water, where the water meanders along and allows you to paddle through the plains between Boat of Garten and Broomhill, and you usually have to paddle quite a lot compared to the rest of the river. This is the main flat-water section on the river. If the wind is behind you then you may even be able to get a sail up and be blown along the river.

The Strathspey Steam Railway which runs from Aviemore to Broomhill is a good feature to look out for on this section of river, and you get a really good view of any trains running along it with usually a cheery wave from the driver and passengers. As you travel along you will find some old stone bridge pillars in the river. This used to be the crossing for the Strathspey branch of the railway going off to Nethybridge, Grantown, and then onto the North Moray Coast. You can still find the old stations dotted along the Speyside Way if you walk or bike along it.

The first rapid on this section that you will come across is just under the bridge at Broomhill. This rapid can be a little awkward as the flow goes into the bridge pillars at an angle. To get through the pillars safely you need to aim across the flow; generally the middle channel is the easiest. Have a look if you are concerned before you paddle through as it can change with different water levels. You can sometimes in higher water use a small channel on river left missing out the main flow altogether. This is the normal take-out unless you are going on to the campsite just downstream.

After the rapid under the bridge you are back onto easy, just-moving water. As you are paddling along you will see a dense area of forest on the right and following this, a field (again on the right). There are some electricity cables which cross the river at this point and this marks the basic campsite at Boat of Balliefurth (Ronnie and Adelaide Macpherson run this). It is a field with access to a loo. There is an area for a campfire and Ronnie sometimes has some wood that you can use on it, ask first though. To get to their house to pay for the camping, follow the dirt road away from the river and the first house you come across on the left is theirs; it has some beautiful views of the river. They usually have a sign up on the electricity pylon when you land giving their phone number and directions to get to their house. Please don't camp on the opposite bank and use the facilities without paying, they charge very little (currently £3 per person per night).

On the left-hand side of the river in the fields there are three sets of standing stones called Tom Nan Carragh, which is an atmospheric place to explore at sunset. It is thought that it is of Pictish or Druidical origin and appears to be aligned on significant astronomical events.

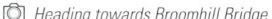 *Heading towards Broomhill Bridge.*

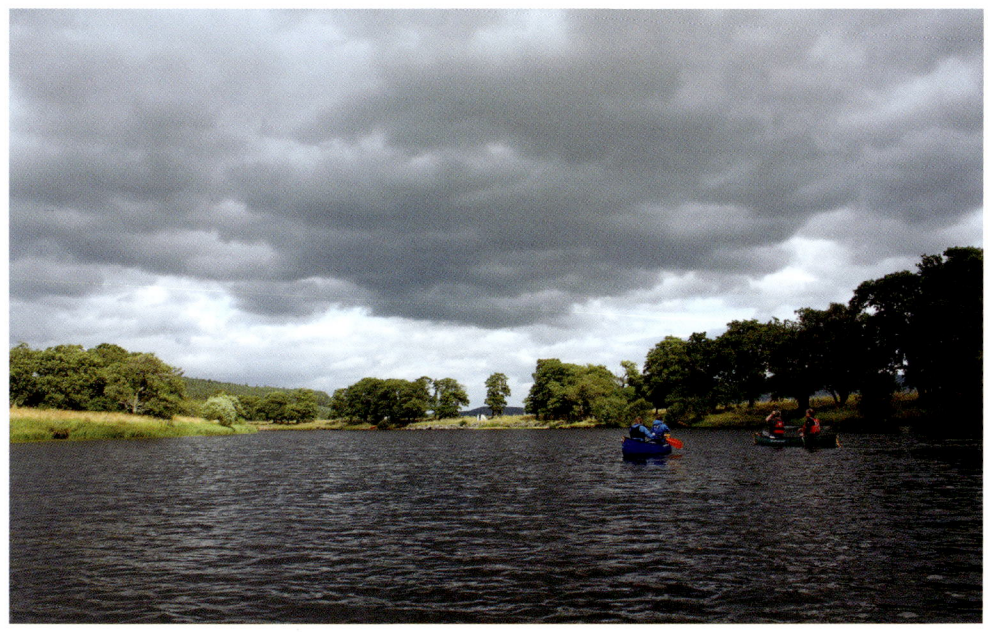

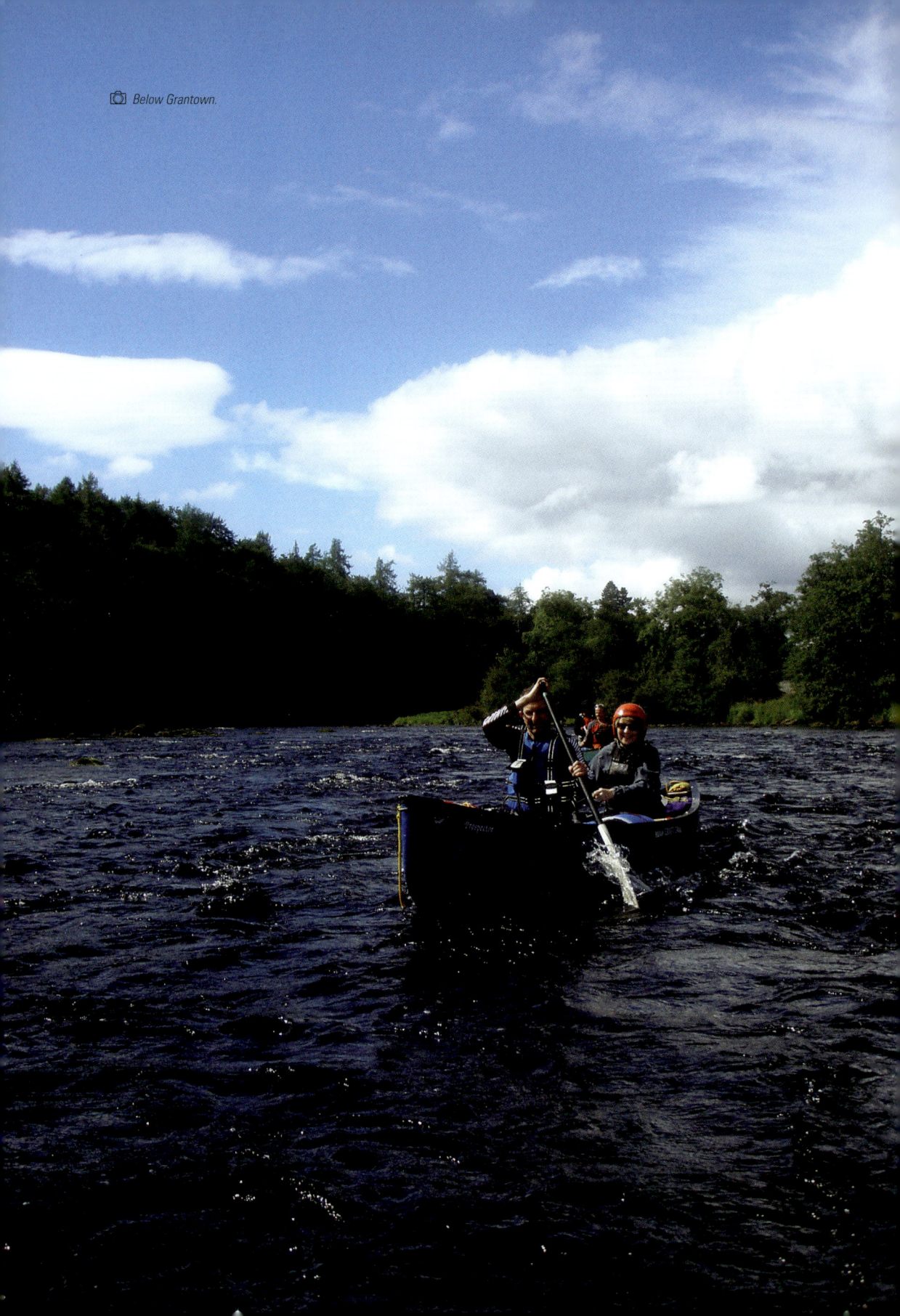
📷 Below Grantown.

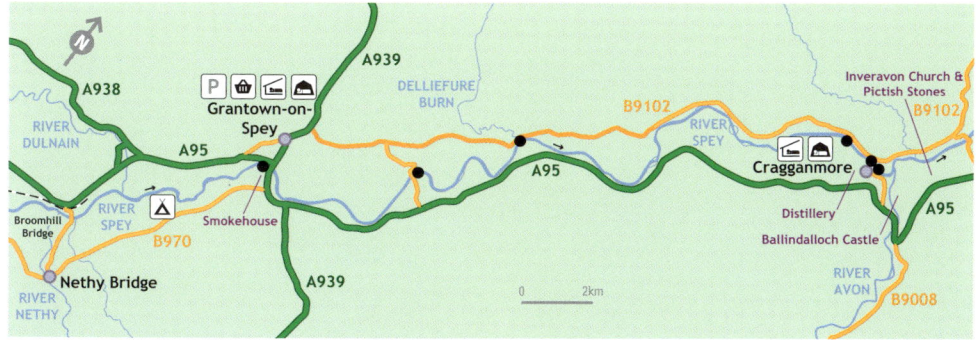

Section 4

Boat of Balliefurth to Cragganmore

Distance 26.5km
Start Grantown-on-Spey, NJ 028 266
Finish Cragganmore Bridge, NJ 169 368
Difficulty Grade 1 and grade 2 rapids

Agreed access points

Grantown-on-Spey, NJ 028 266 – parking spot just off the A95 about 500m above the main road bridge.

Cromdale Church, NJ 066 289 – parking just off the road on the downstream side of the bridge. Access to the river via the track below the bridge.

Delliefure Burn on the left of river, NJ 085 316 – limited parking by the track leading to the fishing hut upstream; be very careful not to block access.

Advie Bridge, NJ 120 354 – left-hand side access via the five-bar gate, parking on verge being careful not to block road.

March Pool, Ballindalloch, NJ 158 369 – left-hand side of river; difficult parking here due to boulders on the side of the road.

Ballindalloch, NJ 167 368 – limited parking on the side of the road. Access is walking via a gate and down a track to the river.

Delnapot/Cragganmore Bridge, NJ 169 368 – just below the bridge on the left-hand side. You can get access to the Speyside Way here which will take you to the camping spot at Cragganmore village.

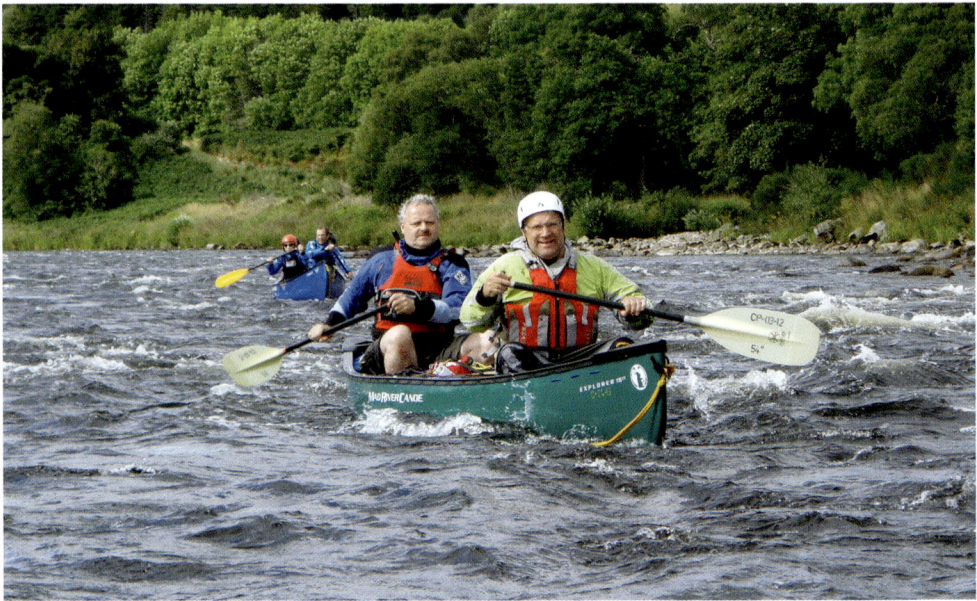
Enjoying the river.

Nearby attractions

The following attractions are on or just off your route: Grantown-on-Spey village; Anagach Woods; Spey Valley Smoke House, Grantown; Revack Estate; Grantown Museum; Ballindalloch Castle and Gardens; Cragganmore Distillery; Inveravon Pictish Stones.

Accommodation

The following campsites and hostels are within easy walking distance of the river: Ardenbeg Bunkhouse, Grantown; Grantown-on-Spey Caravan and Camping Park; Cromdale Outdoor Centre; Ballindalloch Station Bunkhouse; Ballindalloch Station Campsite at Cragganmore. B&B and hotel information for Grantown to Cragganmore can be found through the tourist information centre in Grantown on 01479 872242 or Dufftown on 01340 820541.

Description

Continuing down the river you start to notice the speed of the river picking up a bit and there are a few easy grade 1 rapids before you get to Grantown. Fishing here is controlled by the Grantown Fishing Association and permits can be bought for different beats in the village of Grantown-on-Spey from Mortimer's shop. This is on the High Street next to the post office.

Marking the edge of Grantown is the old graveyard seen on the left-hand side of the river. There is a small but lovely sandy beach just further down on the left, which gives easy access if you are planning to take out or put in here. From the beach you can see the top of the first of the bigger, longer rapids (around grade 1+ depending on water levels) on the Spey that takes you under the road bridge and down to Grantown Old Bridge. From the top of this rapid just under the road bridge you can see a route down the right-hand side moving left towards a concrete fishing pier. From the fishing pier the river continues straight down and then takes a sharp left-hand bend under the old bridge. In bigger water conditions this rapid may reach grade 2. This is a good fishing spot, and you often get a few fisher folks in this area.

Leaving Grantown Old Bridge you immediately notice that the river has picked up speed and is now going from rapid to rapid. The scenery around you has rounded off and the dominating mass of the Cairngorms on the right-hand side has been replaced by the rolling Cromdale hills. To the left of the river you are passing through Anagach Woods, a beautiful section of Scots pine and carefully managed forest, which is run by the Anagach Woods Trust. If you are lucky you may see crossbills, capercaillie and the elusive pine marten, amongst other rare woodland species.

The rapids from here to Cromdale feel a little more remote than before although the main trunk road, the A95 from Grantown to Elgin, runs close by. The rapids in this section are generally straightforward and are around grade 1(+) depending on water level. Many of the rapids are fairly long as you are travelling down them, and if you are in a group you might need to suggest specific meeting places on the river to regroup. You are also into an area where people pay more for their fishing and you will often see ghillies out with their clients. Some of these may be in the traditional green rowing boats. Make your approach known to people by whistling or a shout of "good day", and ask which way they

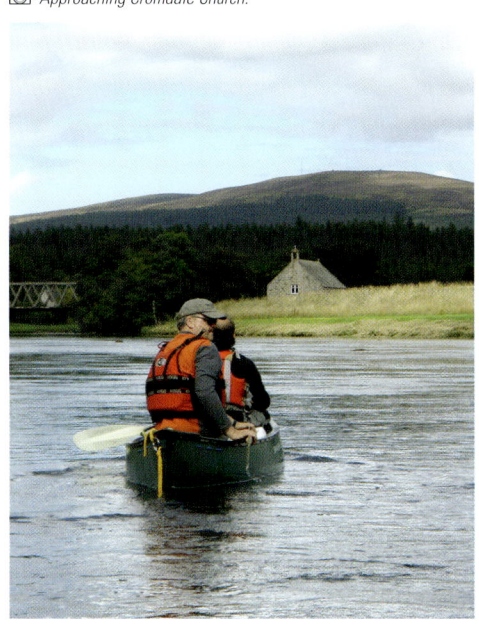
Approaching Cromdale Church.

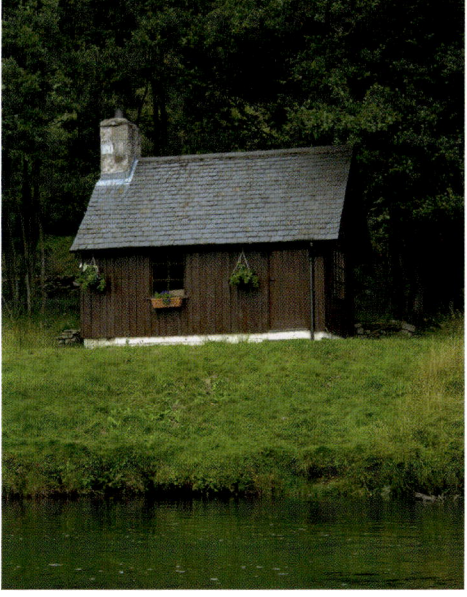
King's Hut.

would like you to pass them. Normally they will ask you to paddle behind them if possible. Most are very pleasant, but if you are the tenth group of paddlers that has passed in the last hour then you can perhaps understand any frustrations shown.

Paddling towards Cromdale Bridge and church you will see a manicured lawn on the right-hand side just in front of the church. This is an agreed access and egress point and a lovely place to stop for a break. The first bridge here at Cromdale was a suspension footbridge built in 1881, and the current road bridge was built in the 1920s. Before this there was a ferry crossing over the river which gave the name Boat of Cromdale, now one of the house names near the river.

Cromdale itself is about 1km up the road on the church side of the river. It is a very small village with big Scottish historic claims to fame. The Battle of Cromdale was fought in this area in 1689, ending one of the Jacobite rebellions, and the Scottish folk song 'The Haughs of Cromdale', supposedly penned after this event, is a very popular tune still.

In low water you might see the remnants of a bird's lunch on the shore in the form of freshwater mussel shells. These are one of the rare sightings found on the River Spey; freshwater pearls were almost fished to extinction and are now a protected species. If you see large quantities of shells in one area, or see people walking in the river with a glass-bottomed bucket, you should report this to the police. See the SCA website for current advice.

Leaving Cromdale Bridge you are again into a section of grade 1(+) water where the flow gently leads you downstream. The river meanders between the busier A95 and the very quiet B9102, neither of which really intrude on your journey. From Dalriach to the farm at Mains of Dalvey there are a few fishing huts. One of the more interesting looking is the King's Hut on the left-hand side of the river. It is a small stone and wood-built hut with antlers adorning it, so called because King Edward VII and various other royalty used to fish here often.

There is a small bridge on the main A95 road over a tributary burn near the farm at Mains of Dalvey which has a set of traffic lights so that only one vehicle can travel at any one time. If you have not been paying attention to the map, this is a good relocation point for you.

After the traffic lights there is a set of islands opposite Culfoichbeg with some fun rapids around them; sometimes these rapids can get a little bigger than grade 1. Following this there is a nice run of gentle rapids down to Advie Bridge.

At Advie Bridge in higher water it is possible to go down the right-hand channel which takes you straight through the bridge, but in lower water levels the main flow tends to go round the left-hand side of the island, which is all fine until you round the last corner just before the bridge. At this point, just before reaching the new bridge on the river left, there are some old submerged bridge pillars that can easily trip a boat up before reaching the eddy line under the bridge. The flow of the current here also takes you towards the new bridge pillars, so this is an area to be aware of. It is worth aiming for the middle gap to avoid the hazards. Once over the excitement of Advie Bridge you can relax and enjoy the river for a while. You are now getting into the area of one of the most paddled sections of the river down to the Knockando rapids. If you lift your eyes from the water you should be now be starting to see the Corbett, Ben Rinnes with granite tors at its summit. The hills to the left of the river are much smaller, and are now home to a wind farm, although the turbines are generally hidden from view here. Between the bridge at Advie and the old railway bridge at Cragganmore there are a number of grade 1+ rapids, which are great to give you a warm-up for the slightly bigger ones still to come. After Advie Bridge you pass a few more grade 1+ rapids before you reach the main access point for this section at the Ballindalloch Pools. There is a second access point in this area. This leads you down a track towards the river and an open field with Cragganmore Bridge below it. At Cragganmore Bridge you can get access to the Speyside Way Campsite, which has basic facilities. Stop just under the bridge on the left-hand side and walk up onto the path on the disused railway. Walk south-west along the railway footpath and you will get to the campsite (approx. 250m). If you have any energy left here you can always go for a walk and discover one of the local distilleries at Cragganmore, go for a quick game of golf up at Ballindalloch Castle Golf Course, walk around the castle grounds, or visit the standing stones at Inveravon.

Approaching Cragganmore Bridge.

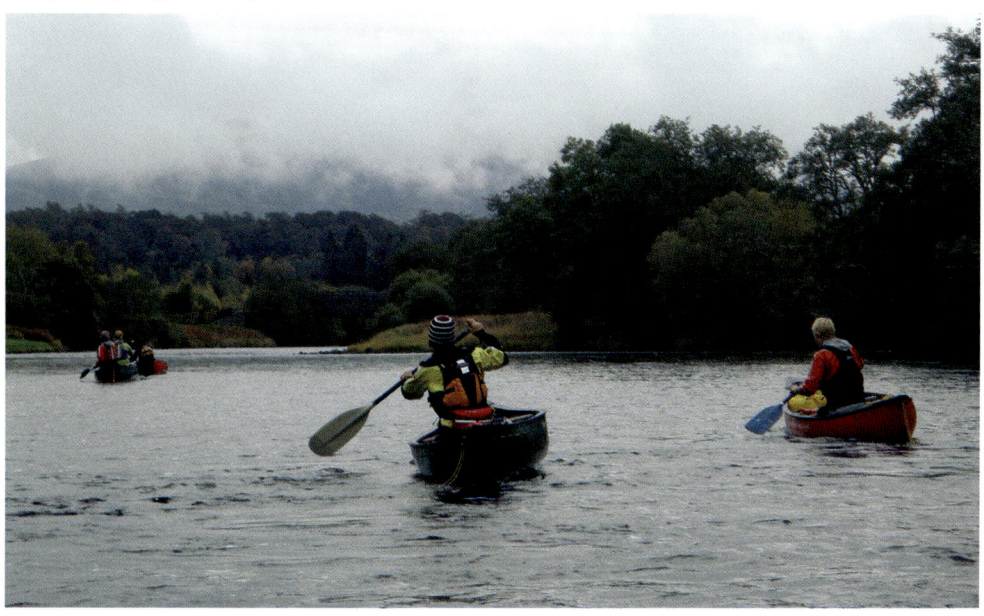

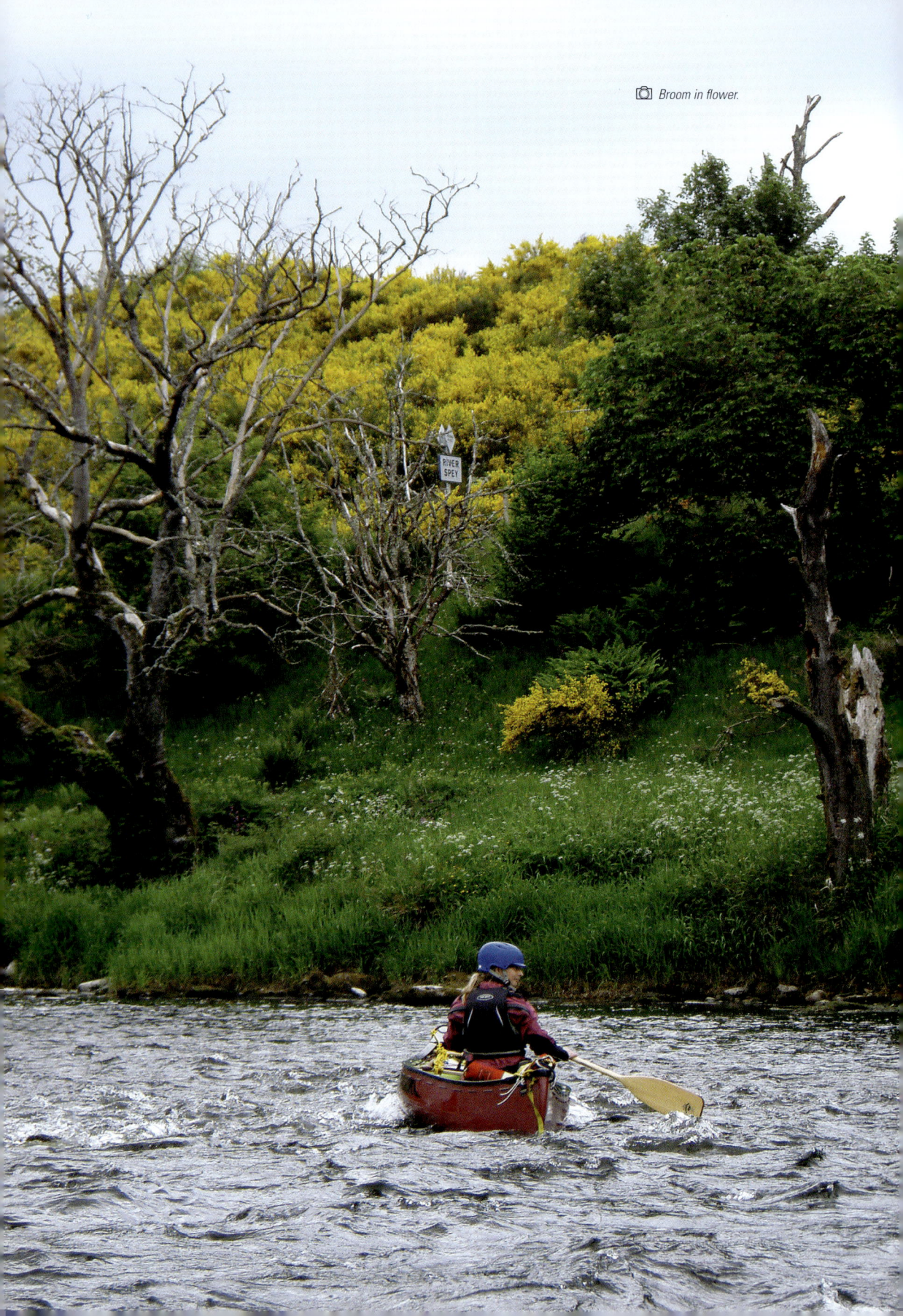
📷 Broom in flower.

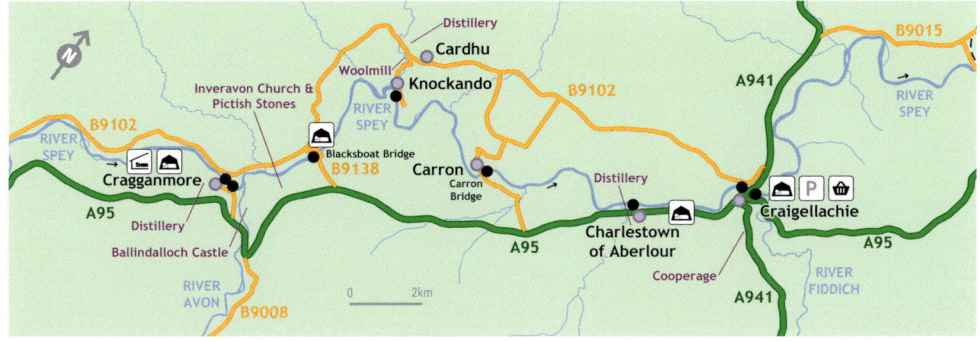

Section 5

Cragganmore to Craigellachie

Distance 21.5km
Start Cragganmore Bridge, NJ 169 368
Finish Craigellachie, NJ 290 452
Difficulty Grade 1 and grade 2 rapids

Agreed access points

Delnapot/Cragganmore Bridge, NJ 169 368 – river left below the railway bridge. If you are starting at the campsite there is possibly parking there.

Cragganmore village, NJ 171 367 – river right, immediately before the houses that are signposted Cragganmore village from the A95. Lay-by on the south side of the B9137. There is a footpath opposite leading to the riverside.

Blacksboat Bridge, NJ 184 389 – river left, just upstream of the bridge.

Knockando, NJ 190 416 – river left below the Tamdhu Distillery. There is parking in the old railway station, and access to the river by the path at the upstream end of the railway platform, passing composting toilets and changing rooms.

Carron Bridge, NJ 225 411 – river left at the bridge. For loading and unloading boats you can use the passing place at the bridge, but please park in the car park in Carron village if leaving the vehicle.

Aberlour, NJ 262 428 – river right on the grassy bank upstream of the Victoria footbridge.

Craigellachie, NJ 285 452 – river right on the sandy beach just below the Thomas Telford bridge. Small car park just next to the beach.

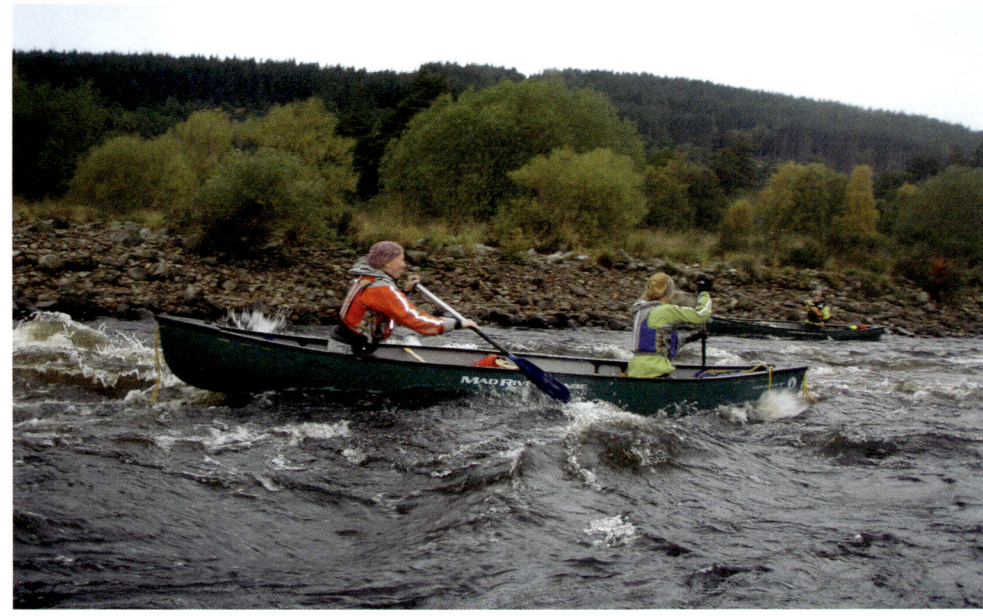
Running the Washing Machine.

Craigellachie, NJ 290 452 – river right near a fishing hut, there is an L-shaped boat park to tie boats to and a quick walk upstream to the Speyside Way. Then turn left on the path and follow it to Fiddich Park where there is good car parking as well as the camp site.

Nearby attractions

The following attractions are on or just off your route: Cardhu Distillery, Knockando Woolmill, Aberlour Distillery, Walkers Shortbread Factory, Speyside Cooperage in Craigellachie.

Accommodation

The following campsites are within easy walking distance of the river: Blacksboat Station camping area, Aberlour Gardens Caravan and Camping Park, Boat o' Fiddich camping area, Craigellachie. For B&B or hotel information contact the tourist information centre in Dufftown on 01340 820541.

Description

This section of the river contains the most regularly paddled water in the guidebook, from Cragganmore to Knockando. The Knockando rapids themselves have an agreed whitewater training section on them. This is agreed with the Knockando Estate in conjunction with the SCA. Due to the high usage, a composting toilet and changing room facility has been built at the Knockando rapids take-out point.

Starting down the river from Cragganmore Bridge, you turn the corner to the left and the river starts to flow more northerly until you reach the confluence of the River Avon (locally pronounced A'an).

In big water conditions the River Avon is one of the main tributaries of the Spey and is one of the reasons why the Spey does not behave like a traditional river, where the closer to the sea you get, the easier the paddle. The Spey picks up pace as it continues downriver, assisted by the water it gains from the Avon and other lower tributaries. The catchment for the Avon is far up in the Cairngorm Mountains. Starting high on the plateau near Ben Macdui, many smaller burns flow into Loch Avon high on the hills. These then drain into the River Avon, which flows remotely through the mountains all the way past Tomintoul and down to the point you are at just now. For more adventurous and skilled paddlers the River Avon from the Tomintoul area down is a great grade 3+ run, and the whole river has in the past been paddled by kayak from Loch Avon down. Getting to Loch Avon and the start of the River Avon involves an epic portage up and over Cairngorm Mountain.

Just after the mouth of the River Avon you get a bigger rapid (grade 2) which turns the corner to the right and leads into another bigger wavetrain. Don't worry if you take on a bit of water here, as there is a calm section and a small beach on the left at which to bail. This is a prime fishing spot, so if there is fishing going on here it is usually best not to linger in the area. If there is no fishing going on it is a lovely rapid at which to practise skills.

After this, another long grade 2 rapid follows the river around a gentle right-hand bend at the top and bounces you down a long straight.

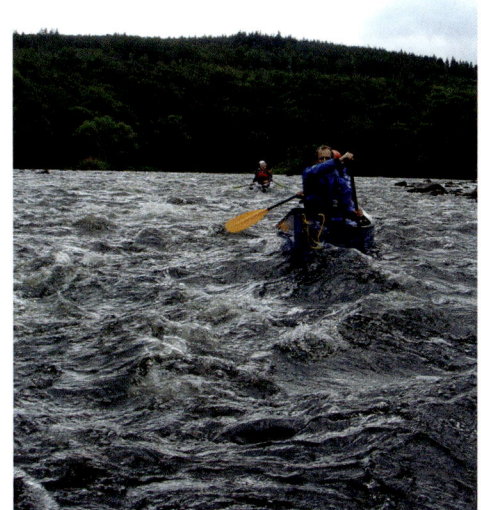

Enjoying the rapids.

There are a number of stone-built fishing piers in this area. At the bottom of the rapid there is an eddy behind a fishing pier on the right-hand side and this is a good stopping point to catch your breath.

The biggest rapid so far is just about to appear. You can usually hear it and it sounds worse than it is. However, it is worth getting out to inspect it if you are concerned. To get out and look it is usually easiest on the river right. The river narrows at the rapid and turns slightly left. In normal water conditions you can't quite see the bottom of the rapid. There is a big, bouncy wavetrain that takes you through the Washing Machine grade 2 (sometimes known as Blacksboat rapid). Following the main part of the rapid, the river stays narrow with a shingle beach for a couple of hundred metres. This channels the water

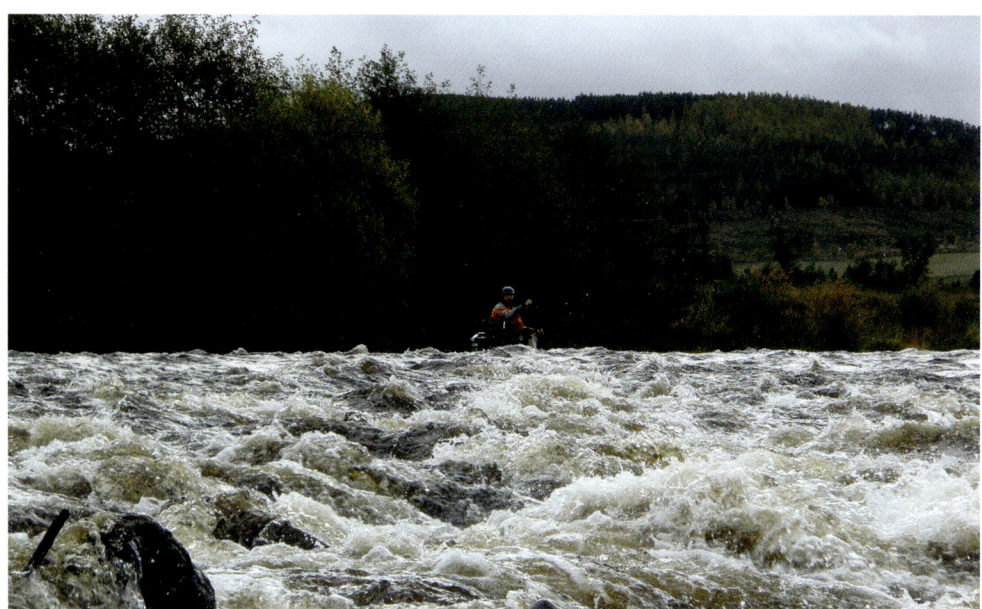
Top of the Washing Machine.

through quickly, which means that you need to plan your break-out and be very active in your paddling to make it. In low water the rapid is actually steeper than in high water, when it fills in and widens out below, over the shingle bank. You will often need to bail your boat after the Washing Machine. This is easily done on the shingle bank river right at the bottom of the rapid.

Following this, the river takes you into a gentle rapid with a lovely playspot on the right, and continues down towards Blacksboat Bridge where there is access just above the bridge on the left. You can walk from here to the campsite at Blacksboat camping area. There are no facilities here other than running, cold water. Walkers and bikers on the Speyside Way use this camping spot as well.

There is a lovely fishing hut just underneath the bridge and the anglers are keen that you pull in at the access point on the upstream side of the bridge if you need to do so, rather than in front of their hut. Please phone the estate on 01807 500205 to let them know that you will be leaving boats on the river bank.

Blacksboat Bridge (originally the site of another ferry) is followed by Craigroy Island which is normally taken by following the line on the left-hand side with a lovely grade 1+ rapid. At NJ 181 410 you will see an estate sign on the right-hand bank requesting that paddlers stay to the right-hand side; this is a very popular fishing pool.

Round the corner from here you get to another island. In higher water levels you can paddle either side of this, but in lower water, it gets very shallow on the right, although it is usually possible to paddle. The left-hand channel has some tight moves around a tree and boulder at the top of the rapid, and then flows into a pleasant, bouncy wavetrain. There is a sign on the left-hand side of the river asking you to stay on the right-hand side of the river. This is part of a local river users' agreement with the landowners.

You are now at the top of the Knockando rapids, grade 2, which are probably the most well-known rapids on the river. Here, river levels depending, you have a choice of routes. In higher water you can shoot either side of the next island, but in lower water, or if you are wanting the more technical route down in high water, you should go down the left-hand side of the main islands round the outside of the bend.

At the top of the rapid at Knockando on the right-hand side you will see there is a white post on the bank. This marks the top of the whitewater training area, and there is a similar post opposite the put-in point at the bottom of the rapid. Knockando Estate agreed to this designation, and you can train and paddle between these posts between 10am and 10pm. There is a portage trail on the right-hand bank of the river (opposite side to the car parking and toilet). On the left-hand side on the riverbank there is good parking, a composting toilet, and basic male and female changing rooms. Coming down to the river from the car parking area there are some steep steps that go down passing the toilet; paddlers are requested to use these rather than the older steps slightly further down the rapid. When using the composting toilet you are requested to put a handful of sawdust down the hole after, but nothing else as other items do not compost down. Note that nobody is employed to clean the changing rooms and toilets, however, the local RAF centre and Glenmore Lodge do a good job of raking the compost below and replenishing the sawdust in the bin above. Please leave the toilets and changing area as clean as possible.

Leaving Knockando rapids you are again into a series of longer grade 1+ to 2 rapids, you will normally go down the right-hand side of Roary Island, and this leads you round to the next major rapid on a right-hand bend at NJ 210 420. It is another rapid where you have to get quite close to the top to actually see down. It is big and bouncy grade 2 with a large wavetrain at most water levels. At low water you

Composting toilets at Knockando.

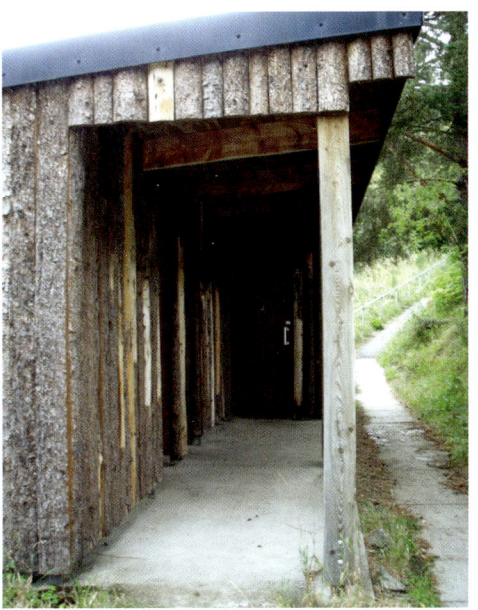

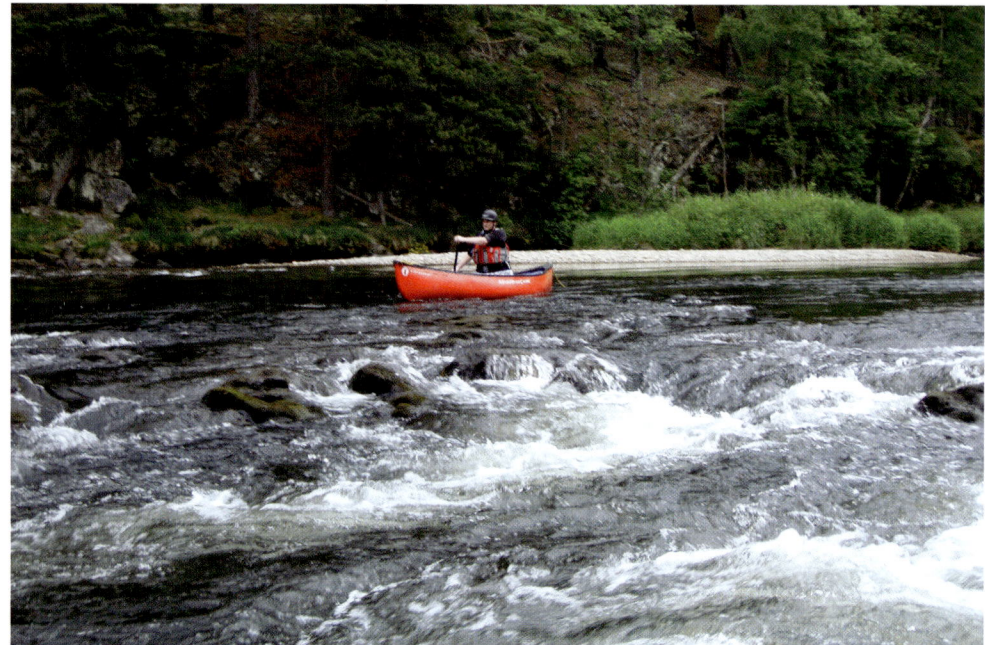

Top of the Knockando rapid in low water.

normally have to start the rapid on the left and move right through the flow. From here you have some lovely scenery and pass through a few more easy-to-read rapids. Soon you will start seeing the chimneys of the derelict Imperial Distillery on the left-hand side. There is a sharp left-hand bend in the river and this leads you round and under the majestic arches of the bridge at Carron.

From Carron Bridge to Victoria Bridge in Charlestown of Aberlour there are some great grade 1 and 2 rapids. Keep your eyes open for one that has a bit more oomph to it at NJ 243 426. It is a long grade 2 rapid with a large wave near the top. Depending on water levels you can usually skirt around it to the right or left, but if you go through it can easily swamp a boat. At the bottom of the first section of rapids there is a second rapid that flows around a left-hand corner. From this point the rapids become a bit easier again taking you down towards Aberlour.

The Victoria Bridge at Aberlour is a footbridge that crosses the River Spey and is locally known as the Penny Bridge after the toll that was once charged to cross it.

Aberlour was originally famous for its orphanage which closed in 1967, but is now mostly famous for its two main industries which are whisky and shortbread. Walkers have had a shortbread factory there for over 100 years and you often get a lovely smell wafting over the river as you paddle past. There are about 50 whisky distilleries within a 15 mile radius of Aberlour, some of which you have already paddled past.

From Aberlour to Craigellachie there is a section of grade 1+ rapids keeping things moving along. By now you will be so used to them that you probably are not noticing them quite so much. As you approach Craigellachie, you get a superb view of the Thomas Telford designed bridge, completed in 1815. Its iron arch spans the river and is still open to pedestrians and cyclists although not to vehicles; a new road bridge was built slightly downstream. You can get access to the river just below the bridge on the right where there is a lovely sandy beach with a small car park. If you are planning to camp here then you should continue down the river under the new road bridge, and about 500m further on the right-hand side there is a small, black fishing hut just above the confluence of the Fiddich Water (NJ 289 452). Pull in below here and you will see an L-shaped boat rack where you can lock up your boats overnight. To get to the campsite, walk towards the fishing hut and you will see some steps which lead you up to the main Speyside Way. Turn left (downstream) on this path, go through a gate and walk under a stone-arched road bridge until you reach Fiddich Park car park, where you will find a basic toilet block and water pipe. The camping area here (free) is just beyond the car park and is signposted on the left-hand side. It is a lovely flat area behind a raised, grassy earth bank. Although Craigellachie is a small village, there are a few hotels with a superb selection of Speyside whiskies in them; it is worth sampling a few of them during an evening here.

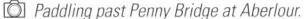
Paddling past Penny Bridge at Aberlour.

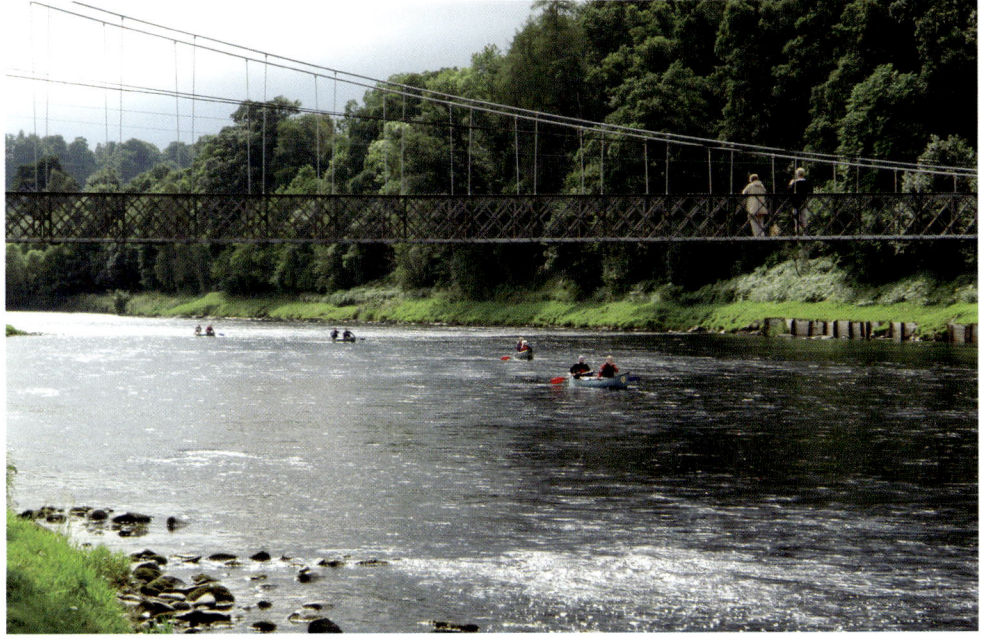

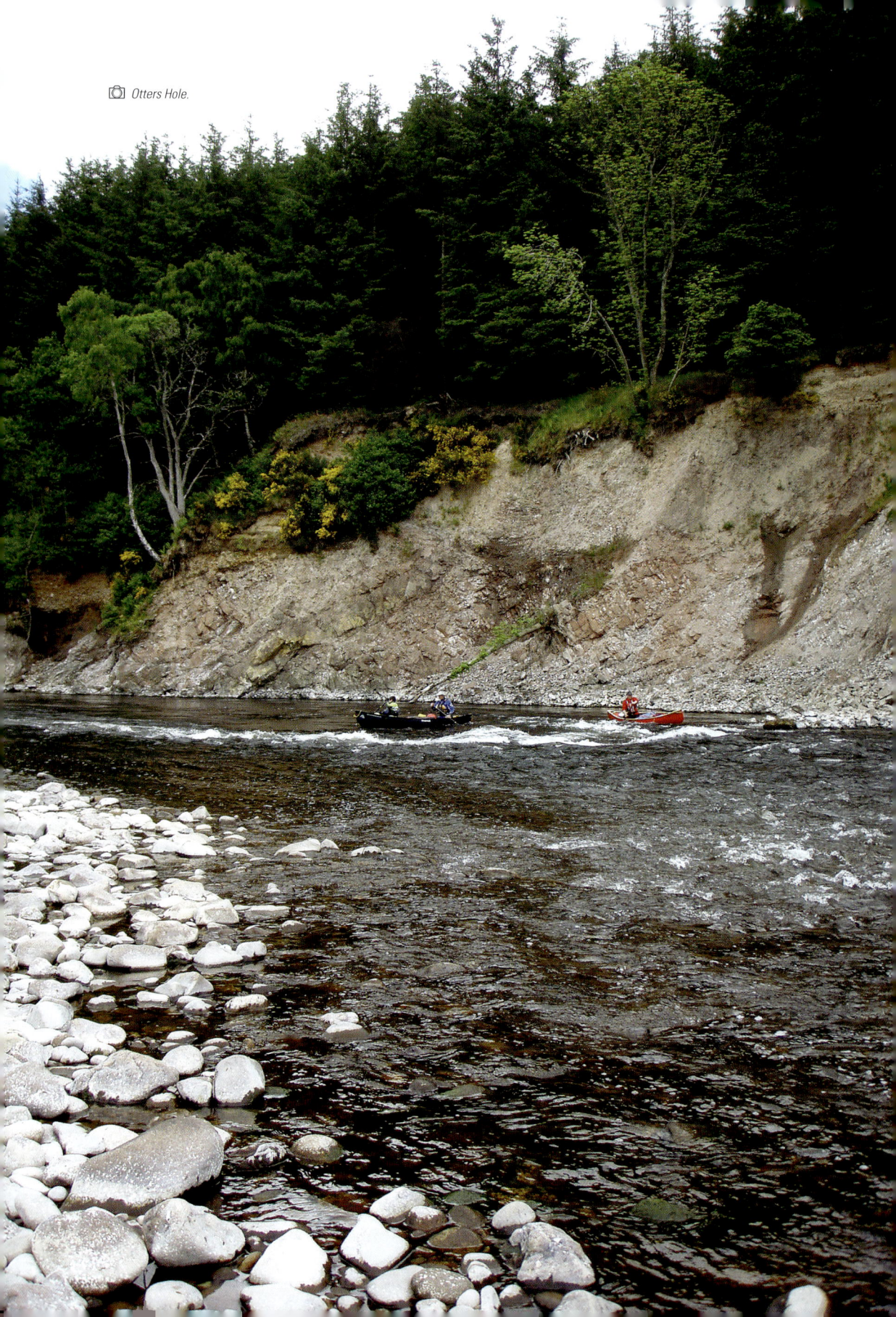
Otters Hole.

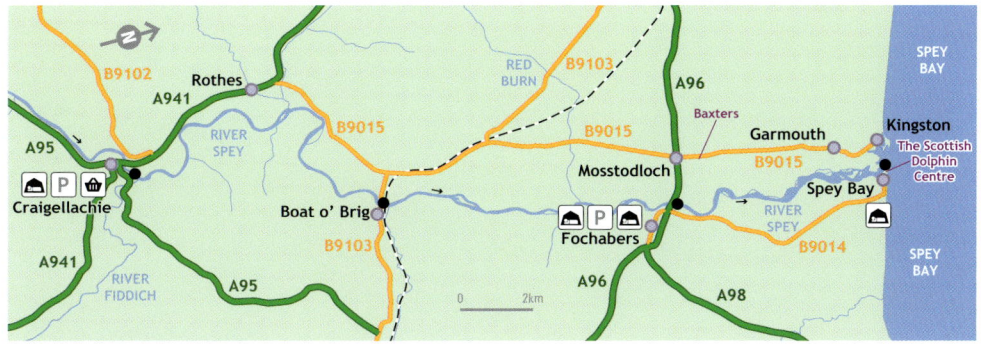

Section 6

Craigellachie to Spey Bay

Distance 28km
Start Craigellachie, NJ 290 452
Finish Spey Bay, NJ 348 654
Difficulty Grade 1 and grade 2 rapids

Agreed access points

Craigellachie, NJ 290 452 – river right near a fishing hut, there is an L-shaped boat park to tie boats to and a quick walk upstream to the Speyside Way. Then turn left on the path and follow it to Fiddich Park where there is good car parking as well as the camp site.

Boat o' Brig, NJ 318 517 – river left at the bridge, access via the track leading past the water board building. There is a small car park between the bridges.

Fochabers, NJ 341 595 – river right, below the road bridge. The parking lay by is situated on the Spey Bay road (B9104) giving access to a track to the river.

Spey Bay, NJ 348 654 – river right next to the buildings and car park, marked as Tugnet on the map.

Nearby attractions

Baxters, Fochabers, The Scottish Dolphin Centre, Spey Bay.

Accommodation

The following campsites are within easy walking distance of the river: Burnside Caravan Park, Fochabers. Spey Bay Golf Club and Caravan Site. For B&B and hotel accommodation contact Elgin Tourist Information Centre on 01343 562608.

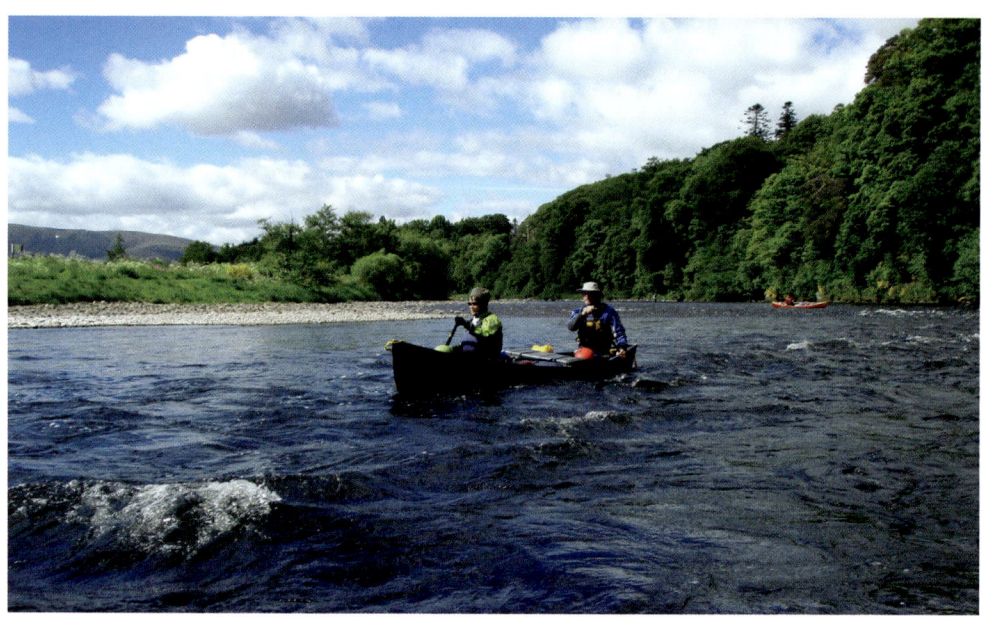
Near Craigellachie Bridge.

Description

As you leaving the riverbank at Craigellachie, stay on the right-hand side, if possible, until you are at the next rapid. Enjoy the last day of paddling. You are gong to pass through some superb scenery and beautifully manicured lawns of fishing estates and huts. The river continues dropping downhill at a great rate and continues offering you rapids of grade 1 to 2 throughout the day.

At the island opposite Rothes (NJ 286 498) there is often a tree (or tree debris) which overhangs the main low water channel on the left-hand side. This means that this is an area to be very aware of, particularly in low water where you are channelled very close to the edge of the island. From here down you continue meandering along the river from rapid to rapid (all grade 1 to 2, but very easy to read).

Just before you arrive at Boat o' Brig, there is a rapid at NJ 312 506. This has a nasty boulder in the middle of the river which should be avoided; it has been the scene of many upsets in a canoe. The river then continues from one easy rapid to the next until you get to the road and rail bridges at Boat o' Brig.

Haugh Island is your next decision, you can go down either side, but again be aware of tree debris that can collect in this area. Just below here you have some stunning crags along the right riverbank, and another good rapid where the river funnels through a smaller gap. Then the land opens out again until you reach the Orton earth pillars (sometimes known as the Seven Pillars of Hercules) which are red, clay pillars sticking out into the river. There is a small recirculating eddy near one of them that can have you going around for a wee while in high water. You can also sometimes get some strong gusts of wind around the cliffs in this area. When you see the huge power lines crossing above the river you have 3km to go until you reach Fochabers.

The run into Fochabers has a few interesting rapids on it with two to note. Just after the huge sandstone cliffs at NJ 339 575 (again look out for the sand martin colonies that inhabit here), there are two large rock dykes in the water on the right-hand side, these are a major hazard to a paddler. Make sure you give them a wide berth on their left-hand side. There is then another right-hand bend rapid, and then after a few more rapids you turn another sharp corner to the left coming towards Fochabers. Here, particularly in low water, you have to be active in your paddling to avoid the wall and the trees. You then follow the river into the final section to the bridges at Fochabers. You can get access onto the river just below the bridge here. At this point you can often smell what is cooking in the Baxters' factory. The factory shop has a good cake stop and is just a short walk from here.

Between Fochabers and Spey Bay the river changes on a regular basis, with tree debris getting washed down and the gravel banks changing the river flow each flood. The rapids are still mostly around grade 1 to 2 depending on the water level, and in high water this section can be quite exciting and dangerous due to the debris.

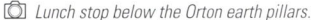
Lunch stop below the Orton earth pillars.

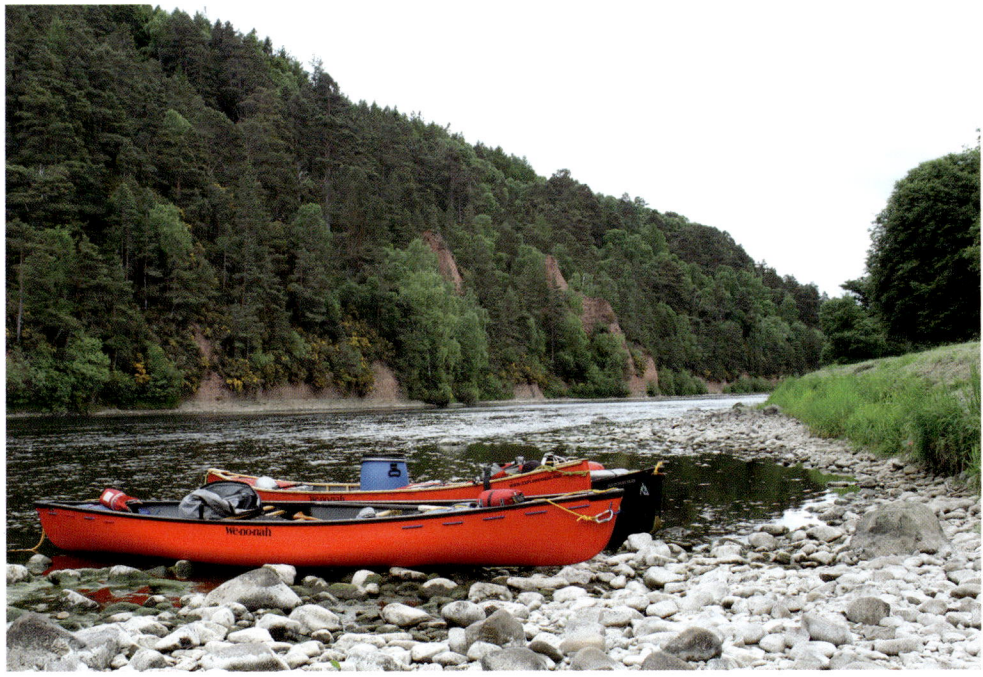

The old railway bridge near Garmouth is a really convenient marker that gives you a 1km warning until you reach Spey Bay. There is often tree debris caught on the bridge pillars, so care is required here. This is now used as part of the Moray Coastal Path and you can sometimes see walkers and cyclists travelling across it. If you have chosen to do your shuttle by public transport you will walk across the bridge to get to the village of Garmouth.

This last section of the Spey generally has a lot of fishing going on and it sometimes feels like a slalom course, working out which is the best line down through all of the islands and avoiding the folks fishing. Occasionally if you get the wrong line in low water you may end up having to jump out and portage across to a different channel; don't worry, all of the flowing channels will lead you towards the sea, some go a bit more directly or more easily than others. Often you can see ospreys flying and fishing in the area, which is a real treat at the end of the trip.

When you get to the point that you can see the buildings at Tugnet and further onto the open sea, you know you have completed a really special journey. Far away on the left-hand side of the river you can see Kingston and Garmouth. These were once the major shipping ports that took all of the logs that came from further up the river, off down south. Originally Garmouth was the port, then over the years the river moved away and the port changed to Kingston. Kingston was also a popular ship building port in the late 1700s to late 1800s.

As you reach the lagoons near the sea you start to feel the effect of the tide on your journey, and if you dip your hand into the water at certain points of the tide it is starting to taste salty.

Check the tides for your planned day of arrival at Spey Bay; if the tide is going out when you arrive then be aware of this as you paddle down the last section. Tidal flow and river water make a strong current flowing out of the lagoons and it can be difficult to get back into the shore, especially if there is an offshore wind blowing. If you have tide and river flowing out with an onshore wind (northerly), you can get a line of breaking waves to go through which can be quite daunting as well. When the tide is coming in, and is pushing against the flow of the river, you can again get a line of breaking waves near the mouth of the river. At slack tide and low winds it can be absolutely lovely to get out into the sea and have a short paddle out there to complete your journey. As you return to shore, the river flow often creates an eddy for you to cross when you come back into the lagoon area.

Even if you decide not to go out onto the sea there is a lovely feel to the area at Tugnet and Spey Bay. The shingle banks are beautiful to look at and wander across. On the shingle banks of the shore here there are many remnants of the tree debris that has floated down the river. Most of the logs are bleached by the sunshine and weather. You get frequent sightings of seals, dolphins and occasionally whales in the area.

The buildings at Tugnet started off life as part of the fishing station, including a domed ice-house to preserve the salmon caught when they used to net the river and catch everything that was going up. Some of these buildings have now been converted into the Moray Firth Wildlife Centre, which is part of the Whale and Dolphin Conservation Society. They also house a great café for well-earned tea and cakes at the end of your journey. If you want to stay at the seaside for your final night, a campsite has recently opened at the Spey Bay Golf Course near the old Spey Bay Hotel. The journey down the River Spey is a magical paddle, coming from the high mountains through the long Strathspey with majestic scenery surrounding you, travelling through villages and towns, taking in the history as you go, the mountains gradually shrinking and disappearing as you reach the sea. It is a journey to savour and enjoy throughout. I hope you have as much fun on the river as I do.

Paddling across the lagoons.

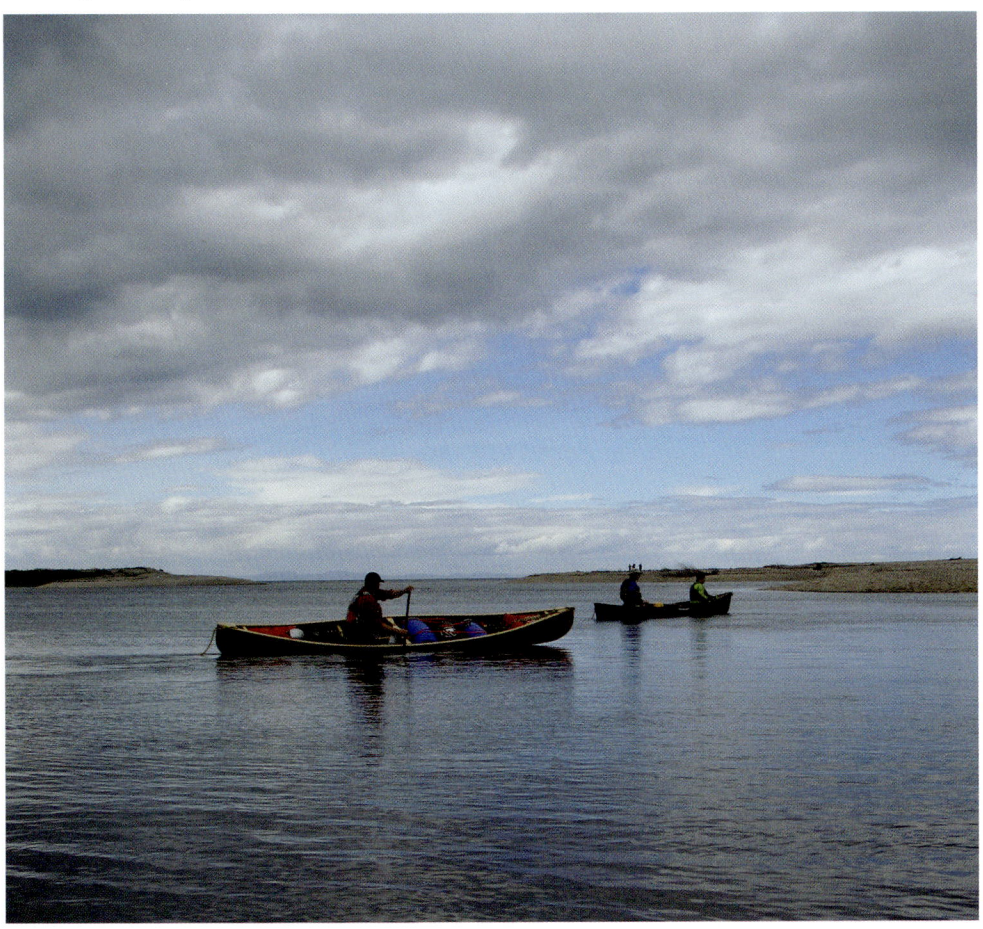

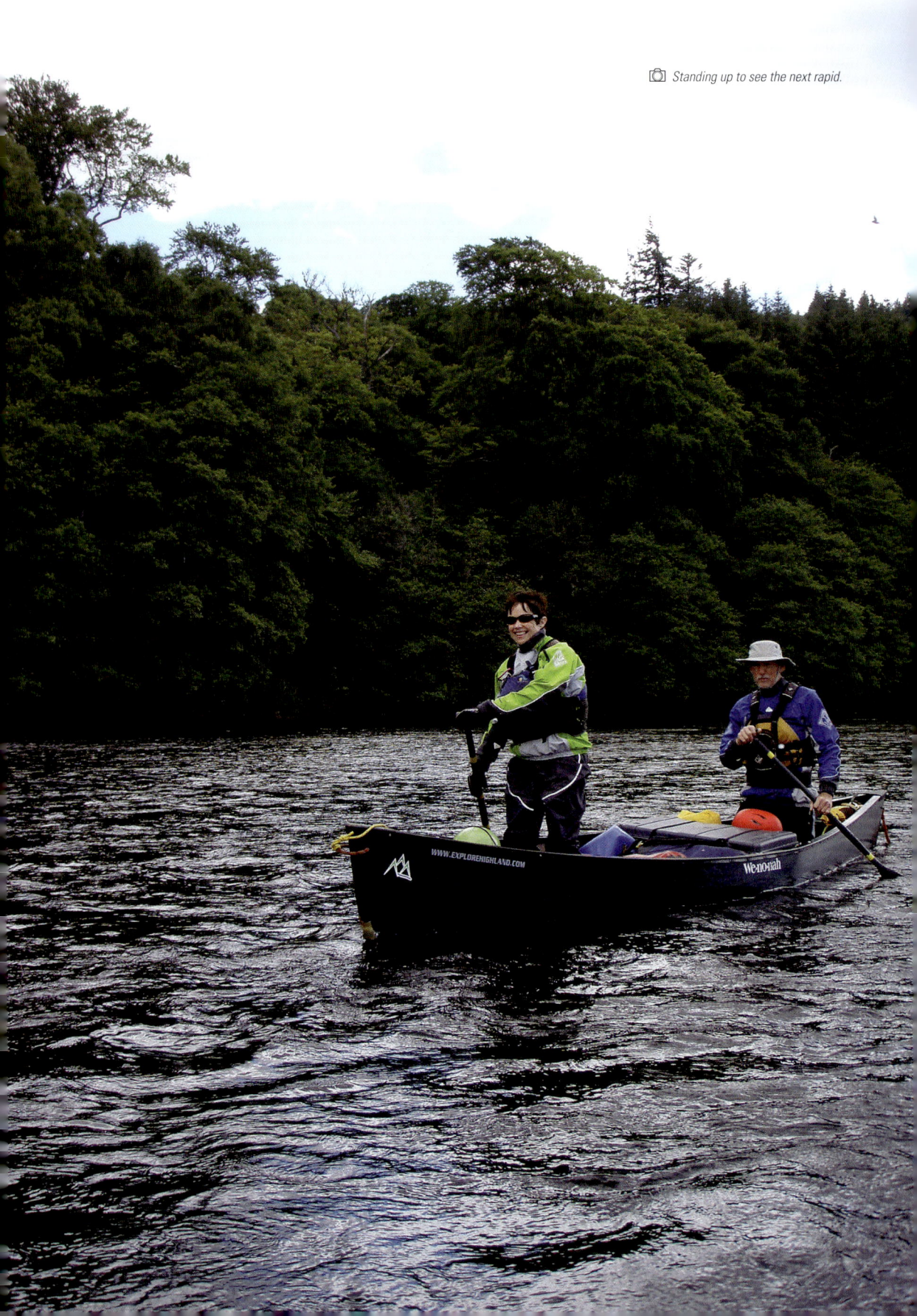
Standing up to see the next rapid.

Safety and Rescue

Being able to look after yourself, and the other boats and people that you are travelling down the river with, is a really important skill. There are many good books and DVDs on the subject, so I will just highlight a few things.

- Wear appropriate safety kit including a buoyancy aid and helmet, and carry a river knife and safety gear.

- Make sure you have you boat kitted out with buoyancy bags, swim lines (open canoe), and have a spare throw bag.

- Inspect rapids if you are unfamiliar with them before going down them, either by standing up in the boat and having a look, or by walking down the bank to check them out.

- Learn to read a rapid before you go down it so that you can choose to take the dry line or safe route, therefore reducing the chance of capsizing or swamping your boat.

- Learn how to use a throw bag and to rescue a canoe (or your chosen craft) before you go, so if it does all go wrong you have practised it beforehand.

Try reading

White Water Safety and Rescue by Franco Ferrero
BCU Canoe and Kayak Handbook which has a chapter on safety and rescue

Try watching

White Water Safety DVD by Bruce Jolliffe and Dougie Shannon

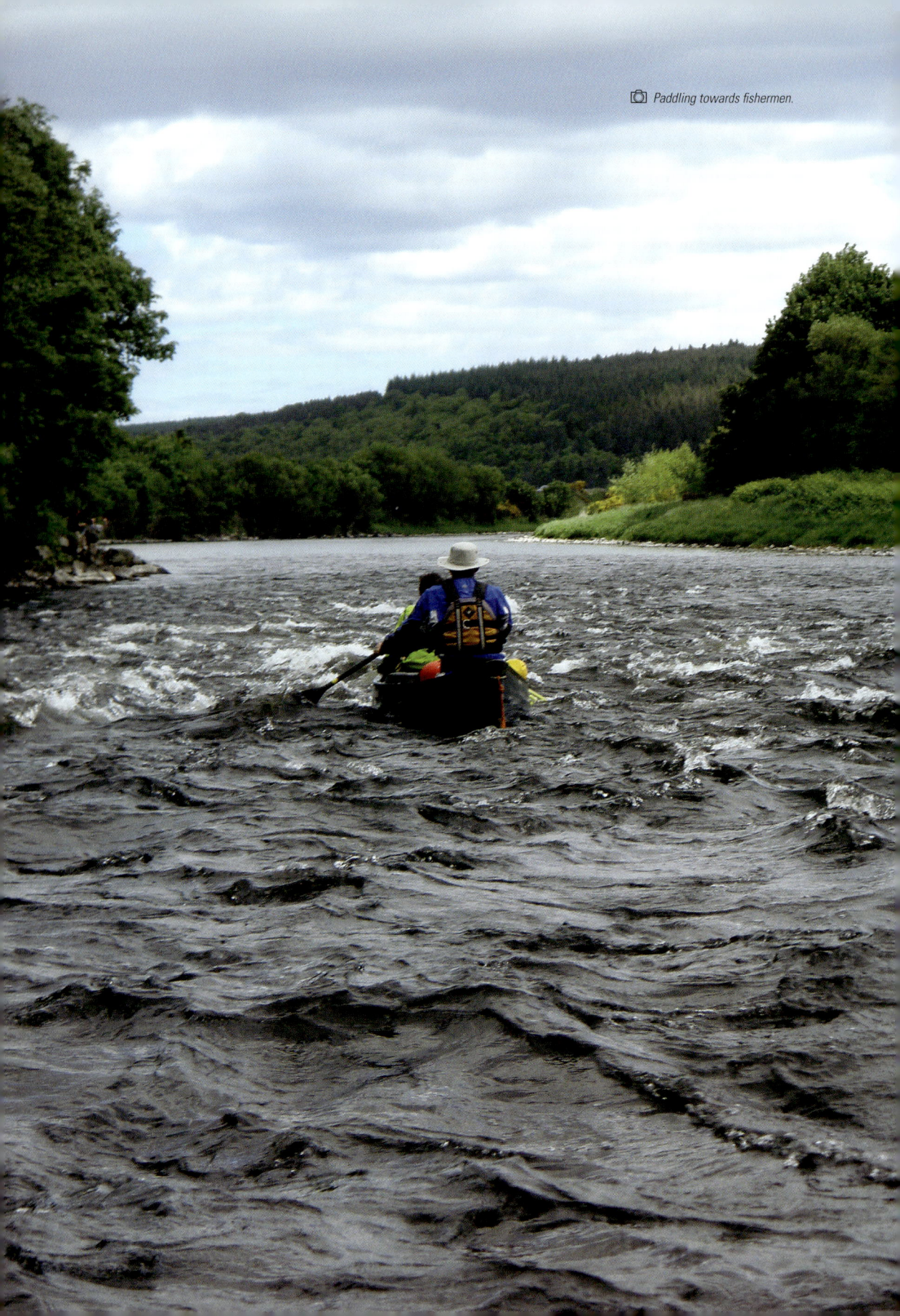
Paddling towards fishermen.

Access, Wild Camping and Fishing

In Scotland we have The Scottish Outdoor Access Code. This code gives us a good explanation of our rights to accessing the countryside, but also states that with those rights comes responsibility and we need to recognise this when we are paddling or getting to the river. You can find more information at www.outdooraccess-scotland.com.

The three key principles of the code are: take responsibility for your own actions, respect the interests of others, and care for the environment. One of the main other river user groups on the River Spey is anglers, and a good rapport has been built up between the angling community and regular river users over the years. Dave Craig, the current SCA River Adviser for the Spey, has been a key player in forming and maintaining the Spey Users Group, which meets on a regular basis to address any issues that have arisen on the water or on the riverbanks. He is a good contact to chat to about any updates on and off the river. Dave can be contacted on 01540 673826 and davecraig1@btinternet.com.

Wild camping

Although in this guide I have suggested routes that start from recognised campsites, there are many beautiful wild camp spots on the Spey, particularly on some of the islands and riverbanks close beside the river. To stay within the framework of the Scottish Access Code you should keep your group small, camp away from houses or roads, ensure adequate toilet facilities are used (this may be a trowel), and you should aim to leave your campsite with no trace of you being there. There is a paddlers' wild camping guide on the Scottish Canoe Association (SCA) website which contains very useful information.

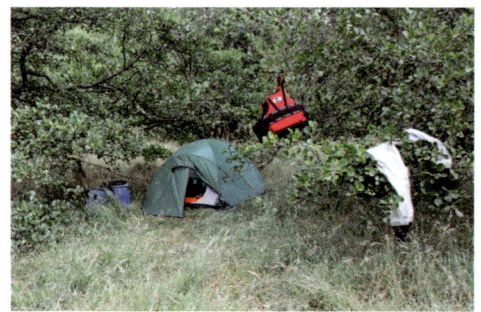
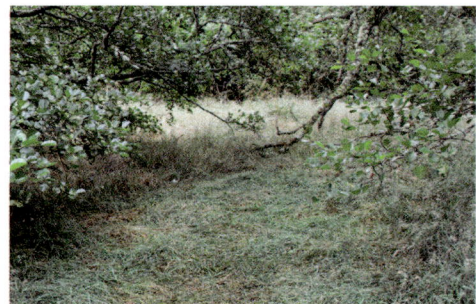

Leaving no trace.

Toileting

If you are going to the toilet out of doors there are some basic guidelines that should be followed. Go to the toilet a minimum of 30m away from the river, with care and consideration for others and the environment. This means burying or taking out any waste. If burying faeces please do so a minimum of 15cm below the soil level to allow proper decomposition. Please do not leave any visible evidence of your visit; toilet paper especially dries in warm weather and can then blow about and get into the river. Any sanitary products should be taken out, as they do not biodegrade. I have a toilet kit that I take with me on camping journeys which is in an identified dry bag and contains a trowel, toilet paper, zip lock bags for toilet paper and sanitary items, and gel hand wash.

Campfires

Campfires can be lit in suitable sites (away from any vegetation or trees) making sure that you leave no evidence of your fire. A firebox is ideal to use, or have your fire on a shingle beach or sandbank where you will be able grind up any left over ash so it will disperse more easily. If this is not possible, then lifting a turf and then replacing it afterwards is an alternative.

For more ideas on minimising our impact as we travel down the river try contacting the 'Leave No Trace' organisation on www.lnt.org. The above sections on toileting and campfires are two of the seven principles of their leave no trace policy.

Responsible camping kelly kettle.
Photo | Donald Macpherson.

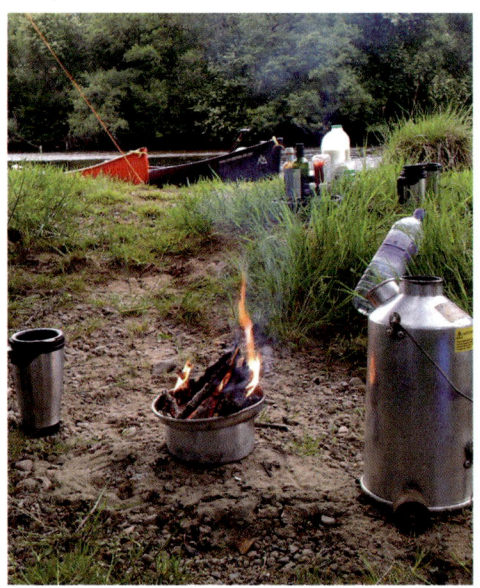

Fishing

The River Spey is one of Scotland's top salmon fishing rivers as well as being a must for paddlers. The fishing season is between 11th February and 30th September which covers the prime paddling time. With this in mind the SCA and the Spey Fishery Board issued a Spey Anglers Guidance for when kayaks and canoes approach.

The SCA also has a leaflet detailing a Paddlers' Access Code, which asks us to keep an eye out for anglers. The key principles are as follows. If you see someone fishing think about how it is best to pass them with the least disturbance. Where possible it is best to stop upstream and attract the angler's attention before passing, this is best done with a whistle. If they have a line in the water, wait for a signal to proceed and then follow the route that they indicate, if safe and practical to do so. An angler should point to the side they want you to pass by on. Many anglers wading in the water will want you to paddle behind them. It is also asked that

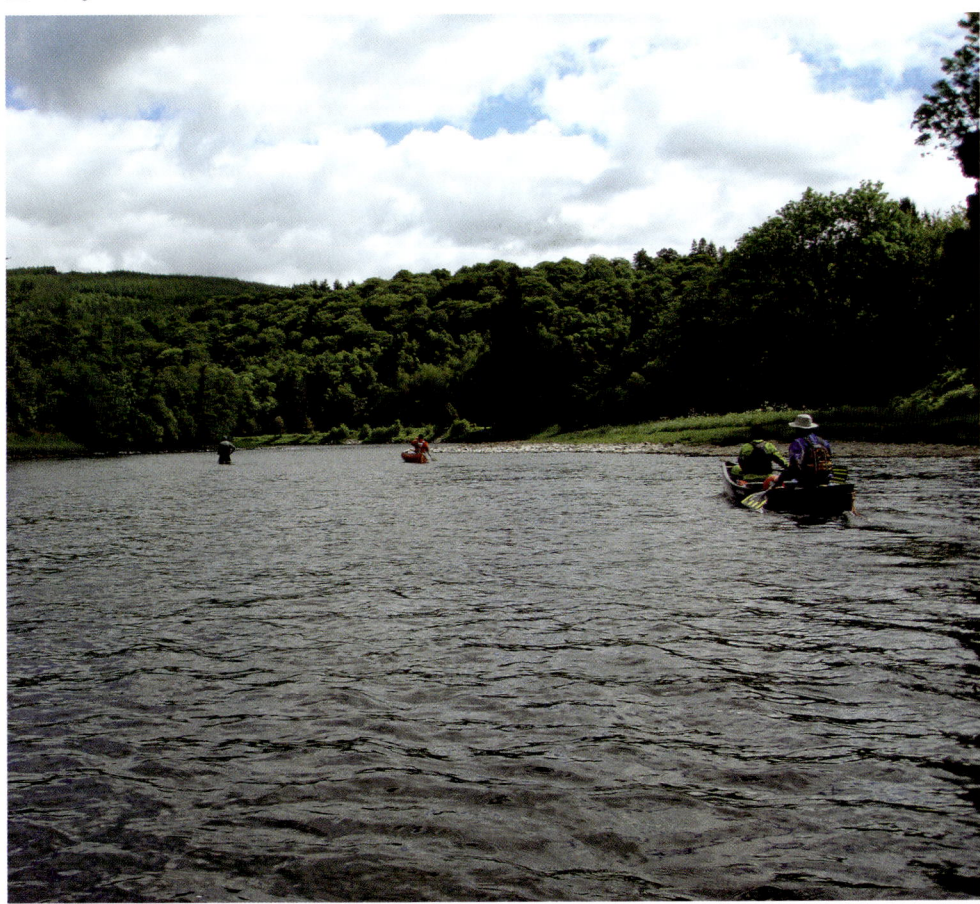
Passing behind a fisherman.

you identify yourself to anglers or landowners if requested; anglers should reciprocate if asked by you.

There are an increasing number of boats paddling on the river, and ideally the fishing and paddling community can continue the positive dialogue that has been happening over the past number of years. For this to continue it needs both anglers and paddlers to be aware of the others' needs, and to try to accommodate them as best as possible. So as a paddler, be aware that although you may have been having an amazing wilderness experience, the angler that you pass may have already seen several groups of boats passing them throughout the day, which may detract from their overall experience on the river. A cheery smile, a wave and a "hello" often go a long way to help the situation.

If you do have a problem there are a number of ways of reporting it. For a serious problem contact the police. The SCA have an online form that is used for reporting incidents, and you can also contact the local access officer for the area. From Laggan to Dellifure Burn contact the Cairngorm National Park Outdoor Access Team on **01479 873535**. For the Tulchan Estate contact the Highland Council Access Officer, Stuart Easthaugh on **01463 255287**, and from Ballindalloch to Spey Bay contact the Moray Council Local Access Officer, Ian Douglas **01343 557049**.

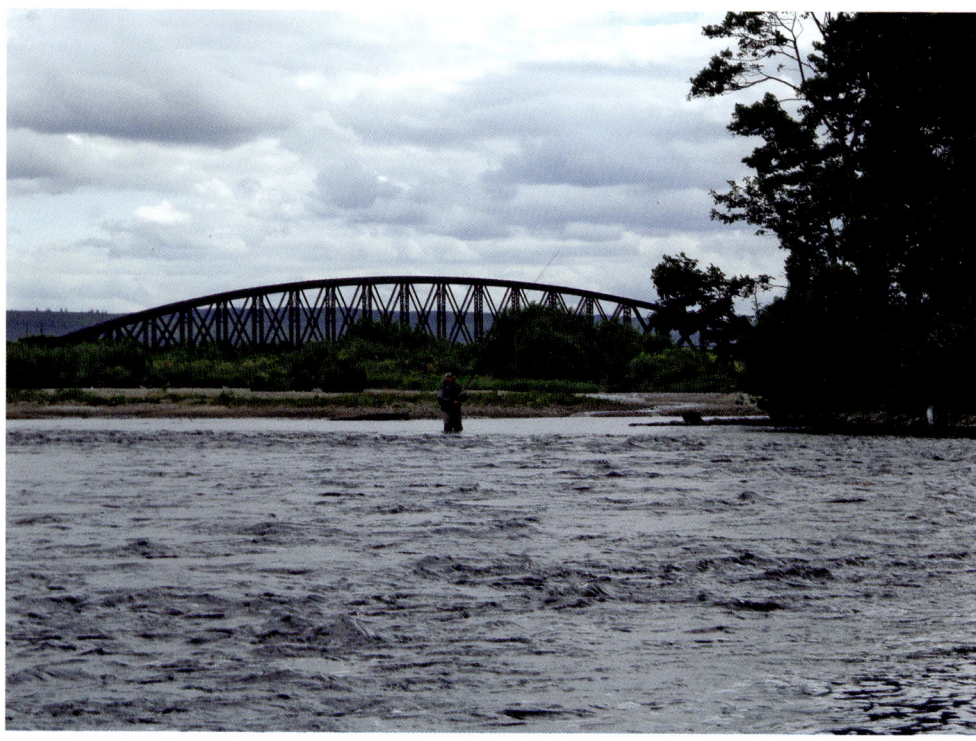
Fishing on the lower stretches of the Spey.

Spey Anglers Guidance

Anglers can reasonably expect:
- The leader of the paddling group will endeavour to ensure the angler is aware of their presence by either shouting or ideally blowing a whistle (most likely to be heard over water noise).
- Once contact is established the leader will seek information on the angler's preferred line of passage for the group.
- Paddlers will wish to cause minimum disturbance to the angler's direction of casting and, water depth/obstructions allowing, paddlers will move in the direction indicated. Where the angler is standing on the bank, direction indicated may include towards the angler, even under the rod, or towards the opposite bank. If the angler is wading, canoeists will be very happy, where possible, to pass behind, i.e. between the angler and the bank.
- Leaders will endeavour to have their group pass in fairly close formation, with a reasonable, safe distance between each boat, thus minimising the time taken to pass.
- If an angler is playing a fish, paddlers normally wait upstream until the fish is landed or until there is indication from the angler or ghillie that it is safe to pass towards the direction indicated.
- In the event of inadvertent capsize, paddlers will do utmost to affect efficient rescue and refloat upturned canoe as soon as possible. Currents can catch out even the most experienced paddlers!
- Once past, the party will continue on their way downstream. Paddlers will not loiter unnecessarily or play in a pool where someone is actually fishing.

Anglers are requested to:
- Acknowledge they are aware of the presence of paddlers.
- Carefully consider which line is most practical for both angler and paddler.
- Give clear direction as to the preferred side for the craft to pass.
- Not always necessary to take in line. However, refrain from casting while boats pass by.
- As soon as the boats have safely passed, the angler may very soon resume fishing.

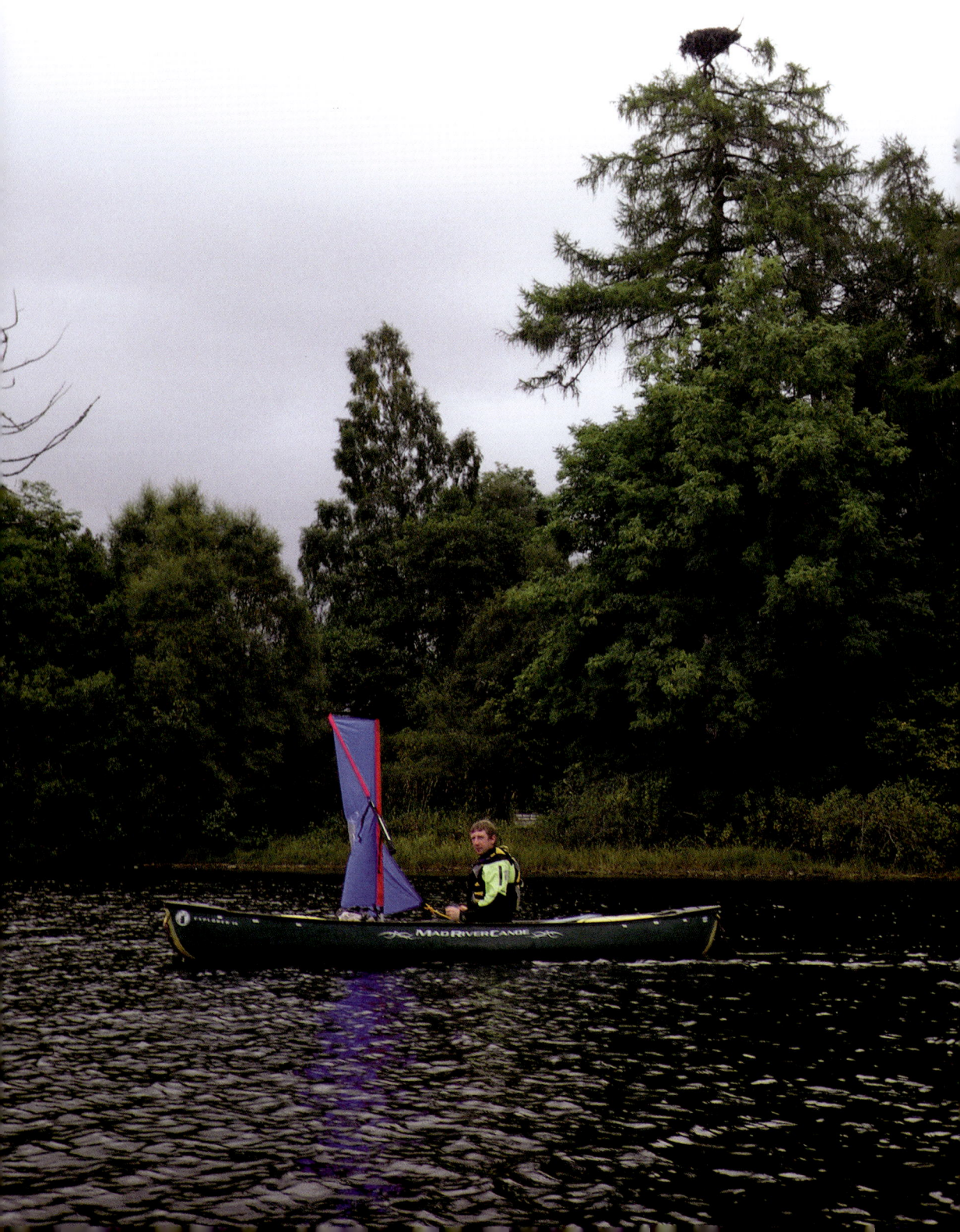

Sailing past an osprey nest on Loch Insh.

Wildlife

For me, a huge part of the joy of travelling down the River Spey is what I see when I am passing by. There are numerous creatures that live in the river and on the riverbanks and they, alongside the wildflowers and trees, help to characterise the river as being a great wilderness journey. Some of the most regularly spotted creatures you might see are:

In the water

Salmon

Salmon are regularly seen leaping when you are paddling the River Spey, and they are the reason that most of the anglers are standing on the side of the river. Salmon spawn and hatch in gravel banks in fresh water. Once large enough (they will stay up to 3 years where they were hatched) they migrate down to the sea, and then return to the River Spey between one to four years later to complete the cycle and spawn themselves. Salmon are a member of the trout family. Other species that you might also find in the River Spey are brown trout and sea trout. Salmon regularly leap out of the water and you may be lucky enough to see this at close quarters. A once-in-a-lifetime experience is to have a salmon jump over your boat, or as happened to one client on the river, have one jump out of the water and hit your buoyancy aid. We all turned round wondering what the huge shout and clatter was – it had knocked him off his seat before bouncing back into the water!

Bottlenose dolphins

The Moray Firth is the home of a group of bottlenose dolphins that travel around the East Coast. They are grey in colour with a darker back and dorsal fin and are up to 4m long. Dolphins usually travel round in schools or pods, so you are likely to see a few at a time. They are often sighted at Spey Bay, but for a more guaranteed sighting pop along to

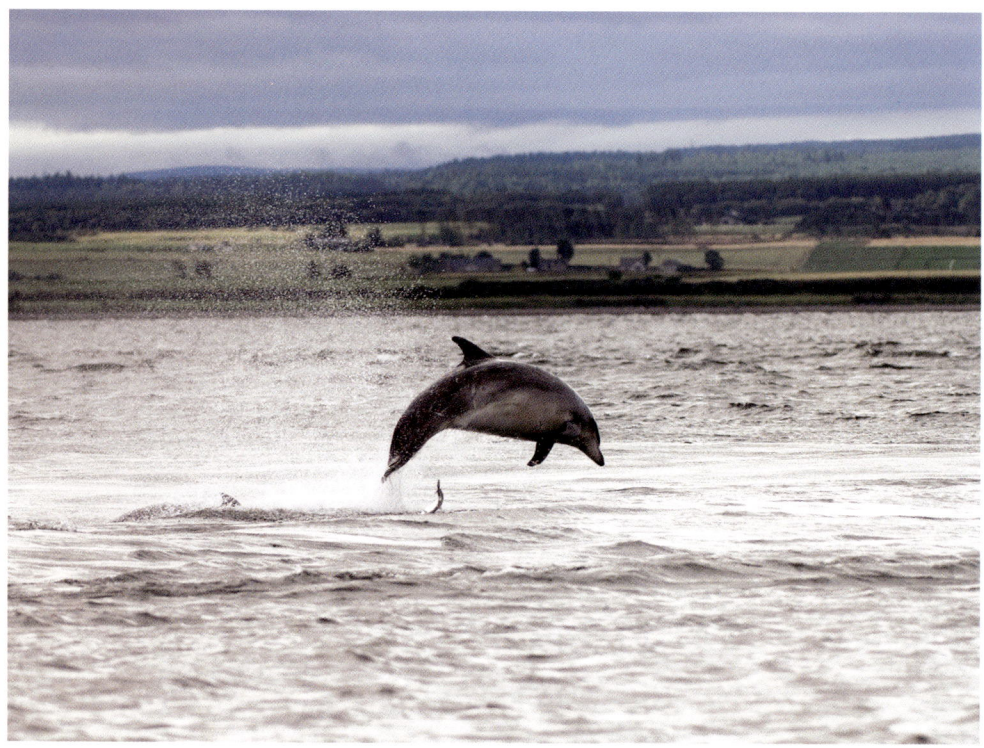
Dolphin at Chanonry Point. Photo | istockphoto.com.

Chanonry Point as they go there to feed. The Scottish Dolphin Centre is at Spey Bay and they will help you spot dolphins and other coastal wildlife.

Seals

Both common and grey seals are spotted in the Moray Firth and they fish around the mouth of the River Spey. Common seals are slightly smaller than the grey seals, they tend to have a darker coat with a longer nose, and it is often said they look a bit like a dog. The grey seals are the largest UK seal, and can be told apart by their distinctive roman-style nose, and their coat which is often blotchy grey, brown and black.

Minke whales

Minke whales are a small whale which are occasionally seen on the coast around the mouth of the River Spey. Their body is usually dark on the top with a lighter belly, they are around 7m to 11m in length, and their dorsal fin is quite tall, being positioned about two-thirds of the way along their back. They have a very graceful slow, deep dive.

On the land

Red squirrels

The red squirrel is native to Britain and is a fairly common sighting in and around the woodlands surrounding the River Spey. They are often seen in the trees on the riverbank and have a red-brown coat with a white tummy and little tufts of fur coming out of their ears. You can sometimes hear them shouting at you with a distinctive 'chuk chuk' noise and perhaps a bit of foot stomping. I think perhaps one of the most wonderful sightings that I have had of squirrels on the River Spey was when I watched them swimming across the river using their tail as a rudder. It took a while to recognise what the animal was, as I had not expected to see them doing that.

Otters

Otters are elusive creatures but are seen regularly in the early morning or late evening on the River Spey. They are territorial and like to live in areas of undisturbed undergrowth on the riverbank. They mark their territory with their droppings, which you may come across if you are exploring the riverbank thoroughly. You might also find a worn patch on the riverbank where an otter has been regularly getting in and out. The Spey has a healthy population of otters. This is thought to be a reflection of the good habitat for them, such as reed beds, islands, and a plentiful food supply.

Wild cat

Known as the 'Tiger of the Highlands' you will be very lucky to catch a glimpse of a true wild cat. There are many sightings that prove to be the offspring of feral cats who have at some point mated with a wild cat. It is estimated that there are around 100 genuine wild cats left in the area. Their coat is black with brown stripes, with a very muscular body, and a thick tail with

Red squirrel. Photo | istockphoto.com.

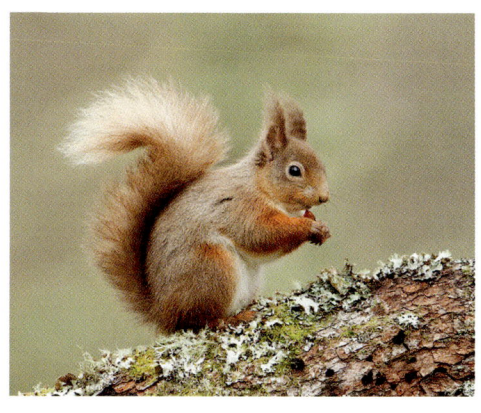

Otter. Photo | istockphoto.com.

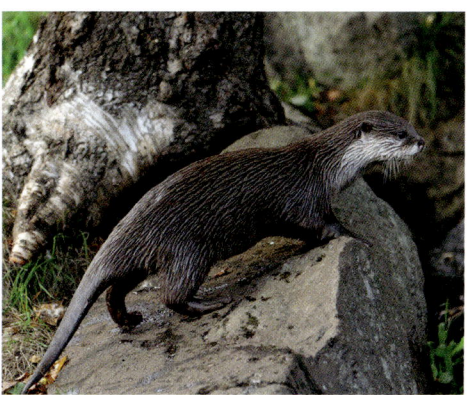

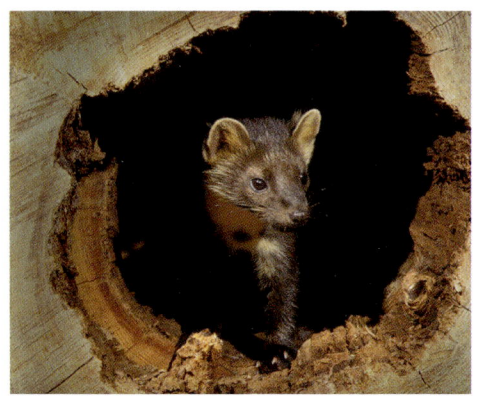
Pine marten. Photo | istockphoto.com.

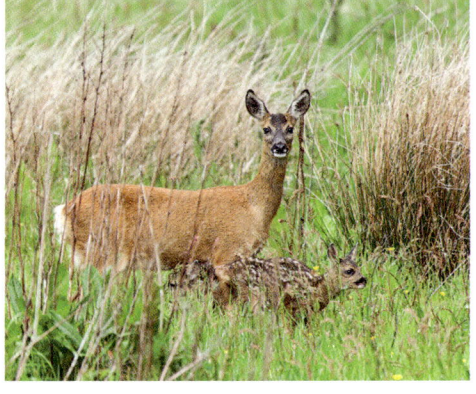
Roe deer. Photo | istockphoto.com.

a blunt black tip. If you want to guarantee a sighting, go the Highland Wildlife Park where they are helping with a breeding programme.

Pine marten

Pine martens are becoming a more common sighting around the Badenoch and Strathspey area. They are of similar size to a cat, with dark brown fur and a white throat. They are members of the weasel family and are a protected species. You will often see them in wooded areas where they eat other small mammals, fruits and berries. In areas where they are frequent sightings many people attract them into their gardens by feeding them; they seem to have a fondness for jam and peanut butter.

Red and roe deer

Higher up the river there are some herds of red deer that roam around. They are common sightings around Loch Spey and down to Laggan. Red deer have the typical stag heads that you see adorning an estate house wall. They have a reddish-brown to brown coloured coat which will turn more greyish in the winter. They are around 110cm to 120cm at the shoulder on average. The stags have large antlers with many branches, the older they get the bigger the antlers. They have been recorded living up to 18 years old.

There are also many roe deer in the area and you will often find them in forested areas. They have a lighter, reddish-brown coat, which turns pale brown in the winter. They are very much smaller than red deer, being about 60cm to 75cm at the shoulder.

Badgers

Seldom seen in daylight, the badger is an easily recognisable animal with its dark grey body and black and white striped head. They are social animals and live in networks of tunnels called setts. They have a fierce reputation, however their favourite food is earthworms. They have short, powerful legs for digging out their setts and foraging for food. They are around 90cm in length and are commonly known in Scotland by the name 'Brock'.

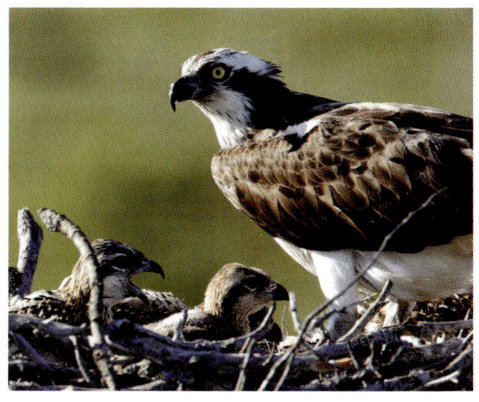
Osprey. Photo | istockphoto.com.

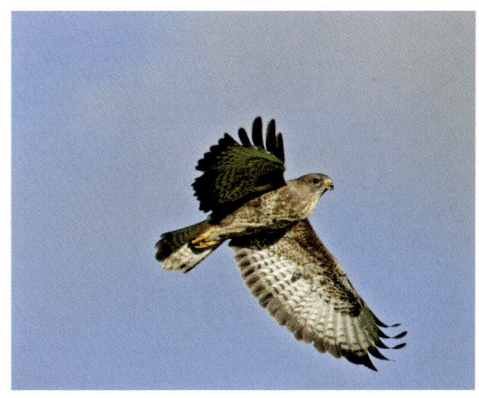
Buzzard. Photo | istockphoto.com.

In the air

Osprey

Seen from below the osprey has a white breast. It has long graceful wings with a black elbow joint and wing tips. The osprey has a wing shape similar to a gull and is often mistaken for one, however it is a much larger bird and once closer is easy to distinguish. It is an amazing sight to see one swooping down to grab a fish and then fly off with it grasped firmly in its talons. You can see ospreys at any point along the River Spey, but good places to regularly see them are; Rothiemurchus Fishery, Loch Insh where there is a nest on the island (do not land there between April and October), Loch Garten where there is a camera trained in on an osprey nest, and the last section of the river at Spey Bay.

Buzzard

Buzzards are commonly found all along the banks of the River Spey. It is a large bird having broad, rounded wings with 'fingers' on the ends of their wing tips. They have a large fan-like tail. Their back is brown, and seen from below they have a lighter coloured breast with a dark leading edge of the wings. You will often spot them when you are doing the shuttle as well as when you are on the river, as they like to sit on fence posts and survey the land around them.

Sand martin

Sand martins are very small birds, wintering in Africa and making the flight back over to Scotland and the River Spey in spring each year. They have dark brown upper bodies, and dark under their wings with very white tummies. They are very agile fliers catching insects over the water. They create their homes in the sandy riverbanks, and you will often see a collection of holes high in the sand cliffs which you will see on your journey down the river. They flit in and out of these with insects for their young.

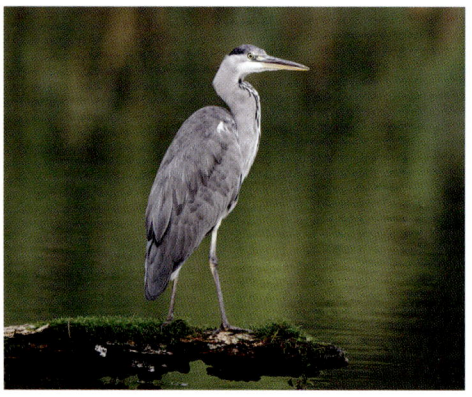
Heron. Photo | istockphoto.com.

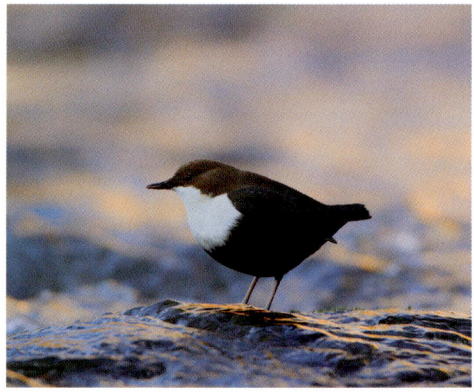
Dipper. Photo | istockphoto.com.

Goldeneye duck

These are a medium-sized diving duck with a distinctive yellow eye. The males are black and white with a green head, and the females are smaller with a grey-brown head. They nest in trees, or in specially constructed boxes, and the young, once ready, jump down and into the water. When you see the height that the nest boxes are placed it seems a daunting prospect to jump and land safely. They however do it, and seem to be making a success of it, as there appears to be an increasing number of them on the River Spey.

Mallard

The mallard is one of the most common ducks found on the River Spey. They are a relatively large duck. The male is stunning with his green head, yellow bill and dark body with a little curl to his tail. The female is less bright with her feathers being flecked brown and having a more brown-coloured beak. You will often see lines of chicks following their mothers around in the spring and summer months.

There are not so many brightly coloured males in the summer, they moult and start looking a similar colour to the female for part of the summer until they get back into their breeding plumage.

Grey herons

Grey herons are one of the most commonly seen birds on the river. They are very tall with long legs, a long beak and are predominantly grey in colour with some black and white feathers as well. They often look prehistoric when they take off and can remind people of a pterodactyl with long, slow flaps of their huge wings. Herons nest in trees and hunt in the River Spey, with fish and frogs being some of their favourites. They tend to harpoon their prey with their long beak and may walk very slowly, or be absolutely still, when hunting.

Dippers

Dippers are beautiful, small, plump birds with a black or dark body and a white chest. They

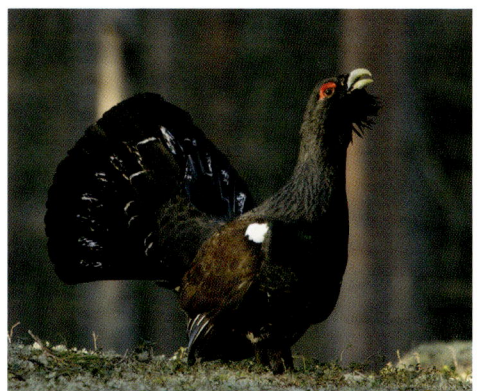
Capercaillie. Photo | istockphoto.com.

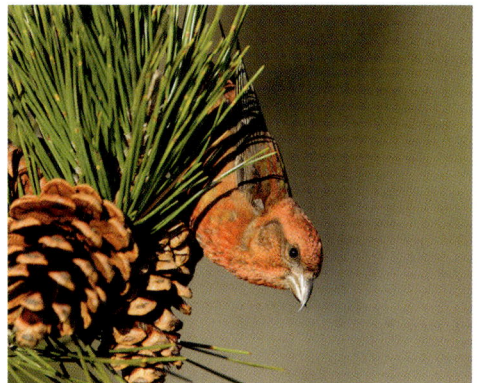
Crossbill. Photo | istockphoto.com.

have a very distinctive bobbing motion. You will often see them sitting on rocks in the middle of the River Spey. Occasionally, if you are really lucky, you might see them walking into the water or swimming underwater to feed. They feed on insects found in the water, and may also eat fish eggs or small fish.

Capercaillie

A huge grouse-like bird with a spectacular tail in the breeding season. Commonly spotted in the forests surrounding the River Spey above and below Aviemore. If you want to watch the lek (mating display) in its full glory, the Loch Garten Nature Reserve run a Capercaillie watch in April and May. They are quite rare in the UK, so a treat to watch.

Goosander

These birds have a serrated bill (sawbill family) making them look like they have teeth which they use to catch and eat fish. They are a handsome bird with black and white plumage, a green head and a red-coloured beak. You will often see them racing along the riverside running on the water. In the late spring and early summer you will see whole families hiding underneath the foliage on the riverbanks.

Red-breasted merganser

These are another of the sawbill family with the goosander. Another fish-eating duck. The males are black and white with a green tufted head and a browny-red chest, the female is grey with a browny-red tufted head, and both have a red beak.

Crossbill

These are sometimes seen in the scots pine woodlands in the Badenoch and Strathspey area. They are a large finch that often flock together eating seeds from pine cones as they go. Males are a distinctive red-orange colour and females are more yellow-green with grey-brown. Their bill has a distinctive curve to allow them to get the pine seeds out.

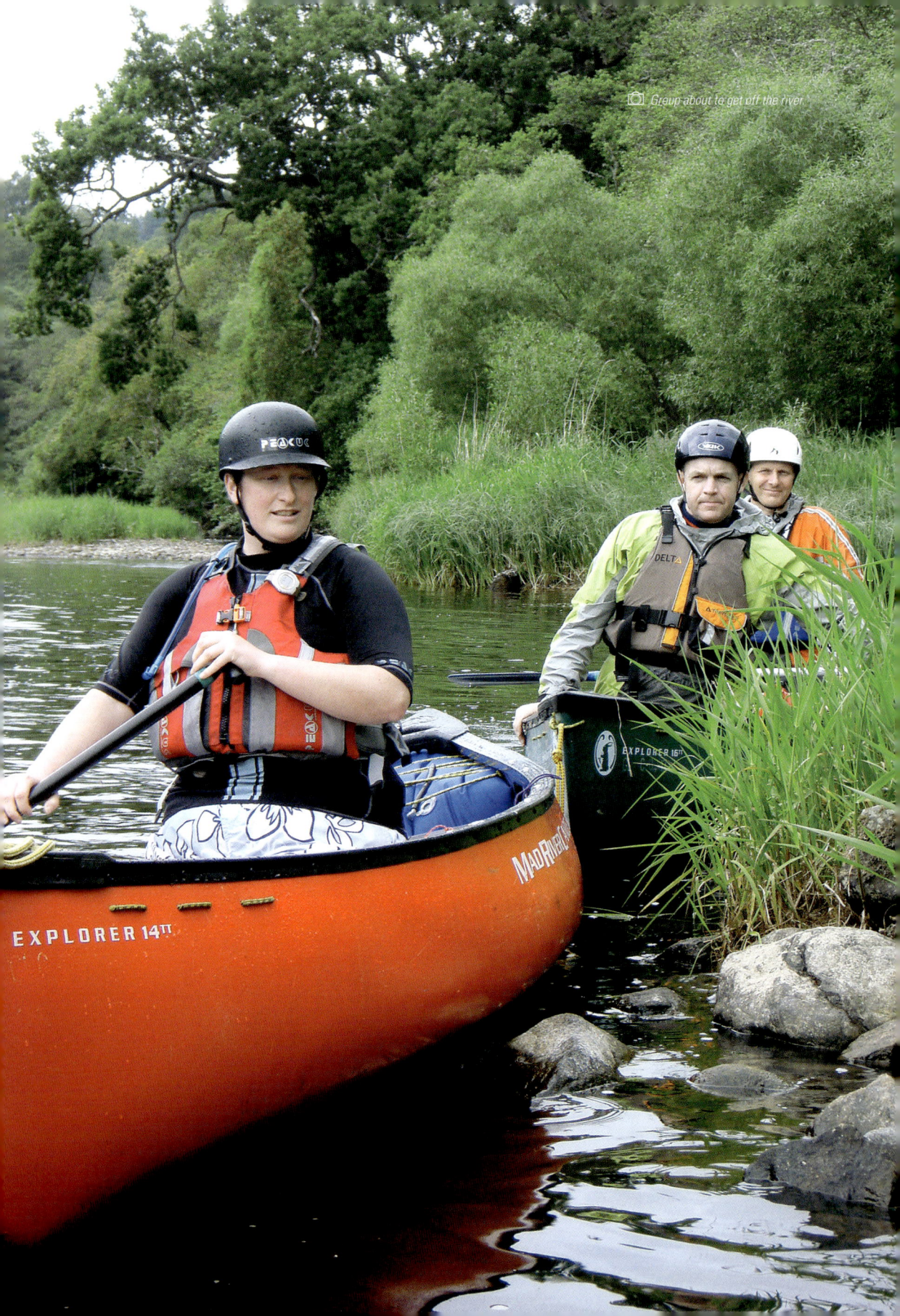
Group about to get off the river.

Environmental Issues

There are a number of environmental issues that are starting to become more prevalent. At each of the agreed access points you will find a sign that has been put up highlighting *Gyrodactylus salaris* and signal crayfish. These ask you to ensure that if you have been paddling, fishing, or in the water in another river or country, then to make sure that your boat, equipment and personal kit has been thoroughly washed.

Gyrodactylus salaris is a salmon parasite, which is found at present in large quantities in Scandinavia, it is also found in other European salmon rivers. It is vitally important to river ecology and economy that this parasite is not brought into the UK as it could have a devastating effect on rivers.

Signal crayfish are from North America and have established themselves in the UK. At present they are just found in England and the south of Scotland. They eat a wide range of species and have a particular fondness for fish eggs, which again could have a huge impact on the fish stocks and other areas of the ecology of the River Spey.

Freshwater mussels are a protected species, which have a recovering population in the River Spey. At one point they were almost fished to extinction for the freshwater pearls that they contain. If you see anybody acting suspiciously, for example walking in the water with a glass-bottomed bucket, or come across large quantities of the shells, you should report it to the police and the National Wildlife Crime Unit; use the number 101 to report it, or 999 in an emergency case.

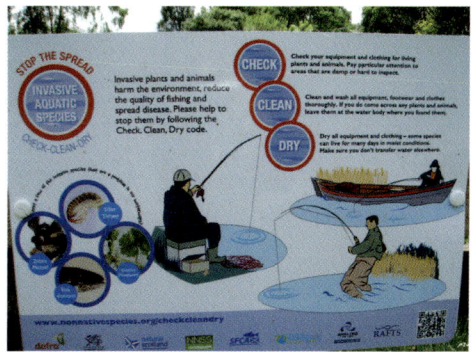

Sign on the river.

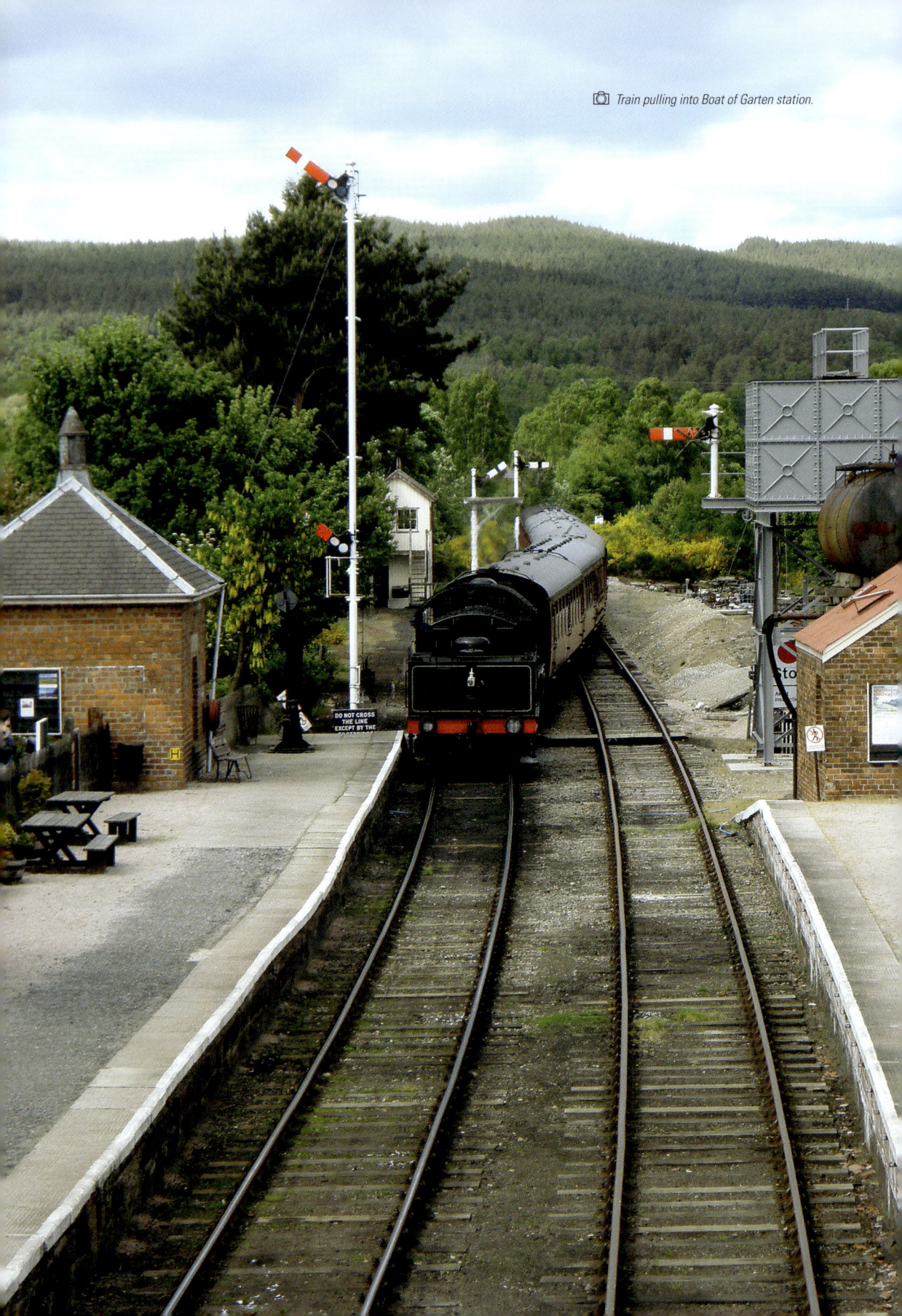
Train pulling into Boat of Garten station.

History of the River Spey

The River Spey has a long history of people working, travelling down it, and living along its shores, from the Pictish settlements evidenced by their standing stones, all the way through to our more recent recreational uses of the River Spey for canoeing and kayaking. In the 1970s Clive Freshwater from Loch Insh Watersports Centre won navigation rights for paddlers down the river, which has benefited us all greatly. More recently the River Spey has been designated a Core Path in the Cairngorms National Park Authority. I have added in a few bits of information here, but there are many more interesting stories to be found in other publications. I have certainly enjoyed researching them.

Logging

In the 1700s there were a number of logging businesses on and around the River Spey. Timber was cut in the forests of Nethy Bridge, Glenmore and Rothiemurcus and transported to the nearest running water source where they built small dams. You can still find remains of some of these dams in the Glenmore Forest area. When there was a suitable amount of logs in the burn, the men would open the dams and send them down to the Spey where they were caught and stored until made into a raft and floated to the sea. They were originally stopped at the port of Garmouth, but later on the port changed to Kingston as the river changed direction. There was much ship building on the coast, and the logs were loaded onto the ships and transported to many towns in the south of Scotland and England, particularly London.

At the mouth of the River Druie, one of the Spey tributaries that floated the logs down from Rothiemurcus and Glenmore, there was a basic bothy which was specifically for the logging men. Most of the men were from the coastal areas and had no other accommodation in the area. The men all knew the river well, and would wait in the bothy until they had enough logs to create their rafts and send them downstream. They would then return to it after they had walked or ridden back to Aviemore to start making the next one. There are no remains of the bothy now.

Originally men in currachs (large coracles) would guide the logs and rafts down river; there are records of this from the Rothiemurcus Estate dating back to the 1500s. In the 1700s the style of rafting the logs changed to building a larger raft that had planks on top, allowing two men to steer it. The river was 'improved' to allow rafts to flow down it more easily. This involved removing obstacles such as boulders. In the late 1700s there was a court case in Edinburgh where it was claimed that the log rafts were damaging fishing on the river. The court upheld the use of the rafts and they were allowed to continue.

There were also a number of sawmills and boring mills in the area. There is still a house called the Boring Mill in the Rothiemurcus area. This was used to drill holes in very straight logs for water pipes. Many of these went down to London to help with sanitation issues there. Logging and rafting like this had largely stopped by the early 1800s. There is a lovely description of the logging trade in 'Memoirs of a Highland Lady' by Elizabeth Grant.

Whisky and distilleries

A huge number of whiskies are distilled in the area surrounding the River Spey, and it is one of the industries that has stood the test of time. Up until 1820 there were no legal distilleries in the area, although there was apparently no shortage of whisky either. It is suggested that there were up to 200 illegal distilleries in the area. After the Excise Act in 1823, distilleries in the area became recognised, although there are records that the excise men still managed to uncover illicit stills every now and then. Whisky has gone from strength to strength in the area, each one praising the water that it uses to make its Uisgebaugh (water of life). There are a number of very good distillery tours in the area for those wanting to know more and to sample some of the unique flavours produced in the area.

Railways

It is not unusual to see a steam train puffing along the tracks when you are travelling from Aviemore to Broomhill Bridge; the best views from the river are usually between Boat of Garten and Broomhill Bridge, where you often get a friendly wave from the train driver and passengers.

There were two train lines in the area. The train from Perth and further south originally came up over Drumochter, onto Dalwhinnie, and through the villages to Aviemore, Boat of Garten, Broomhill, Grantown-on-Spey, Dava and up to Forres where it joined up with the line going to Inverness. It was originally known as the Highland Line. It is now known as the Strathspey Steam Railway.

At Boat of Garten there was a second line built and this was the Strathspey Line. It ran parallel to the Highland Railway and then went over the river to Nethy Bridge (you can still see the bridge pillars on the river), and from there follows what is now the Speyside Way up towards Craigellachie where it met the Keith to Dufftown lines and Elgin to Lossiemouth lines. It was opened in 1863 and became a tourist trip for many folks taking a day out, as well as transporting whisky, sheep, cattle, and other freight. It passed through many of the stations that are now camp spots or recognised access and egress points for us as paddlers. You will see many bikers and walkers following the long distance route that is the Speyside Way mostly following the railway line from Buckie, through Spey Bay and up to Aviemore. You may even meet a few of them in the Speyside Way campsites if you use them.

Farming and droving

Crofting in the Badenoch and Strathspey area has had a long history. The Highland Folk Museum in Newtonmore gives a very good picture of life in Badenoch and Strathspey, with croft houses and other industries in the area set up to show life through the past. It was a hard and basic lifestyle with most folks being tenant farmers. In the times of the clearances many people were driven off the land in favour of sheep, although not all moved away from the area. The villages grew bigger as people relocated down to them and worked locally.

Many of the traditional drove roads from further up in the Highlands came through the Badenoch and Strathspey area, and were used by people taking cattle to the markets or trysts in Crieff and Falkirk, and possibly even further south. There were good pastures in the area which encouraged the drovers to stop for a break here allowing the animals to rest before taking the journey over Drumochter further south. The book 'The Drove Roads of Scotland' gives a very good account of some of these meetings in the area.

Salmon fishing at Spey Bay

Until the 1940s salmon fishing at Spey Bay was a commercial activity employing over 100 people at its height. The salmon were caught in large nets which were rowed upstream and across the estuary, left for a while, and then brought in by hand. The fish were then dispatched by the fishermen onshore and taken off to the ice-houses for storage, before being transported to market, often in London.

At Tugnet you can see the three domes of the ice-houses, where the salmon, once caught, were stored. In the winter, the ice from the river was stored in the insulated ice-houses and used to preserve the fish for transportation. In winter and spring it was possible to send fish all the way to London before they became spoiled. Later on in the summer, when the ice had melted, they used a different method of preserving the salmon. The salmon were boiled in vinegar and then salted, and this kept them good in the heat of the summer. You can see the boilers and read more about the history of the ice-houses at the Dolphin Centre.

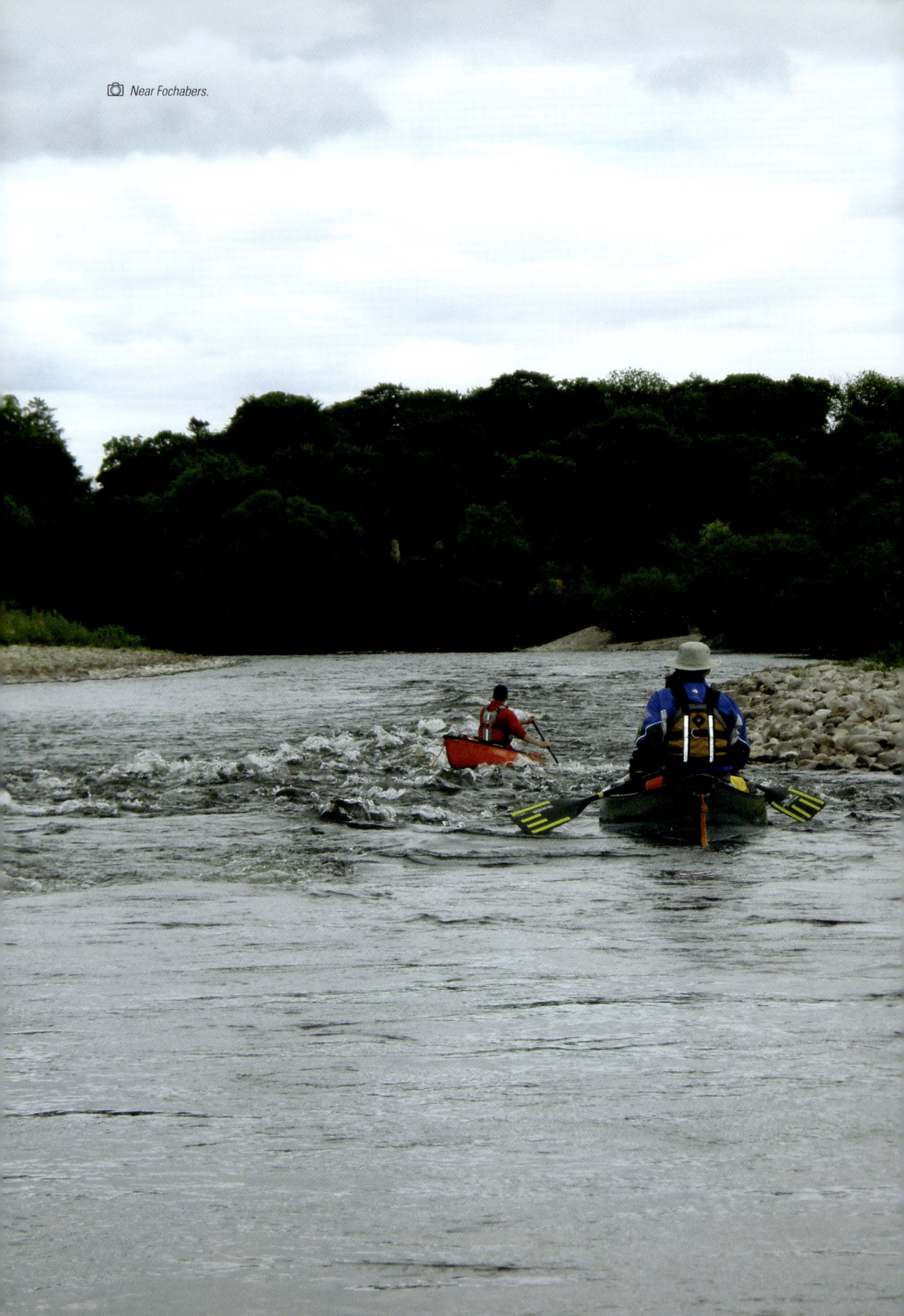
Near Fochabers.

Navigation Skills for the River

Navigation and map reading skills are really useful to have when you are paddling down a river. They will help you find the put-in and take-out points and, if you need to identify where you are for any reason, relocation skills will help you with that. A GPS is a fantastic addition to your kit to do this, however it is also very useful to be able to read a map just in case the batteries run out. As an alternative to a GPS unit, many smartphones have useful GPS or mapping apps on them.

Grid references

When you know where you are on a map you can give an accurate position. This is called a grid reference. In the UK we have a great mapping system which splits the country down into 100km blocks. Each block is given a unique double letter, which are found on the map. If you are printing off a map from any computer based mapping programme, make sure that you print off the double letters. If you ever have to contact the emergency services, you will be asked for them.

These 100km blocks are then split down into 1km grid squares that we see on a map. The grid lines mark out each of these 1km blocks and each grid line has a number.

From this you can easily identify where you are by giving the double letter (which is the 100km identification) and the relevant numbers.

For example, on the map below, if you want to identify the square that shows Carron Bridge, you start with the letters NJ (on OS sheet 28 Elgin & Dufftown).

The double letter identification on a map - NJ.

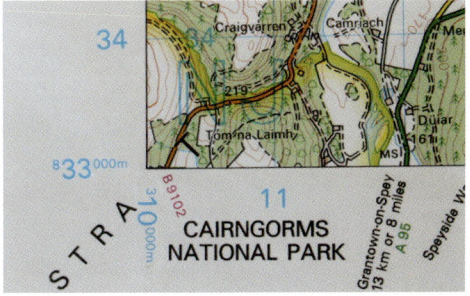

Now you take the number of the grid line along the western edge of the square, found along the bottom of the map sheet (22), and then the number of the grid line along the southern edge of the square, seen at the side of the map (41), and that will give you a 4-figure grid reference, NJ 2241.

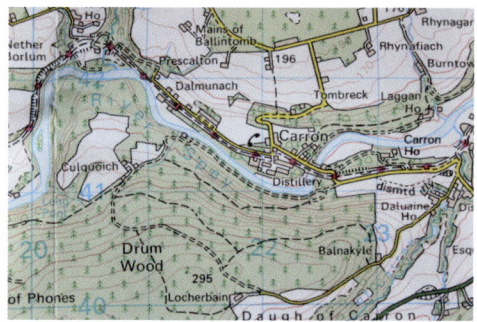
The 4-figure grid reference for Carron Bridge - NJ 2241.

To make the grid reference even more accurate you can split the 1km square down into 10 equal squares across the bottom of the square and 10 up the side of the square. This now gives you a 100m square. So the 6-figure grid reference at Carron Bridge would be NJ 225 412.

If you use a GPS it will normally come up with an 8-figure grid reference, which being within a 10m square is even more accurate again. It may also have a location position on a map if you are using a GPS with maps loaded into it.

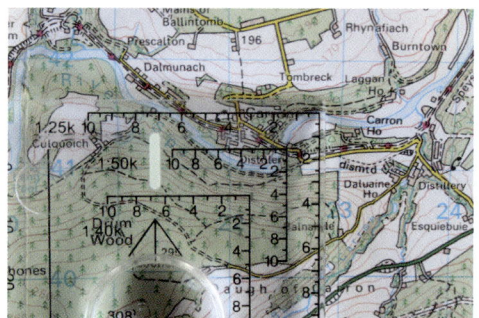
Using the scale on a compass to get a 6-figure grid reference for Carron Bridge - NJ225 412.

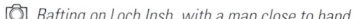
Rafting on Loch Insh, with a map close to hand.

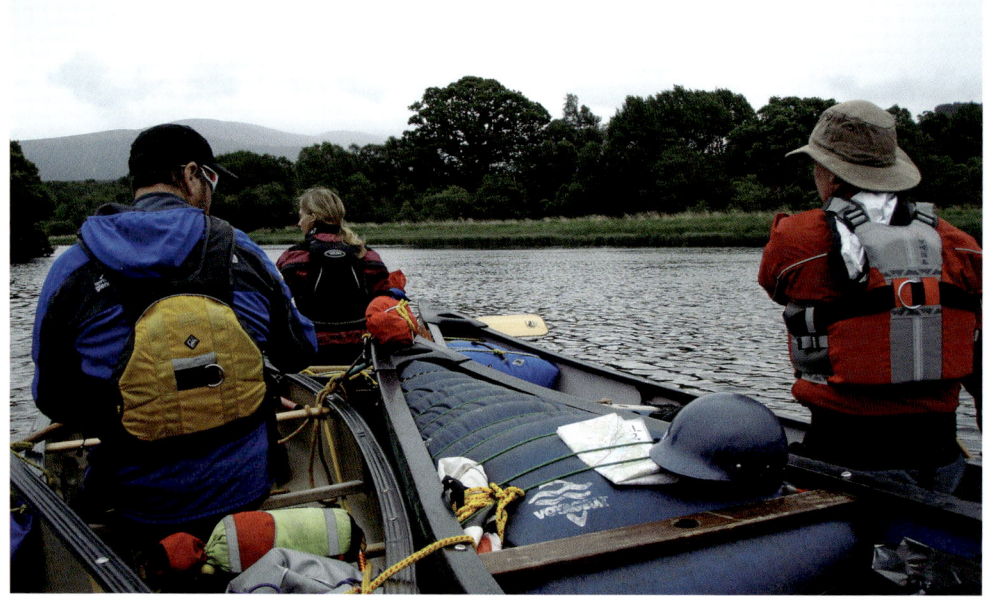

Using features to identify where you are

To help make sure you know where you are when on the river, here are some top tips.

- Have your map folded to the correct area, waterproof it and attach it to the boat or to you so you can see it during the day.
- At the start of the day, pick out any features that you will definitely see when you are travelling down the river, and tick them off in your head as you are journeying past. For example the section from Cragganmore to Craigellachie, "I am going to pass the confluence of the River Avon, Blacksboat Bridge, the islands at Knockando with some tight bends on the river, Carron Bridge, the bridge at Charleston of Aberlour and the two bridges at Craigellachie. Ben Rinnes should go from being in front of me, to be at the side of me, and then behind me, and then possibly out of sight."
- Time how fast you are paddling on different flows of water and this can help you estimate how long a section will take. Between 4km to 6 km per hour is a good estimate if travelling continuously. This obviously depends on the flow of the river.

Relocation skills

If you do not know where you are, some basic relocation skills for use on the river are helpful.

- Take your last known point and estimate how long you have paddled from there.
- Are there any easily identifiable features beside the river, for example: bends in the river, bridges, buildings, tops of hills, etc. You may have to go ashore to find this.
- You can take a bearing down the river and see which direction it is going in. To do this you need to point your compass downstream and line up your compass with the edge of the river. Keep the compass flat and away from any metal in your boat or in your buoyancy aid. Turn the dial round until the floating red needle is hovering above the hatched red arrow on your compass and then add on any variation (currently around 3.5 degrees on sheet 28). Then you can put the compass onto the map and without moving the dial, line up the grid lines with the north/south lines on the compass.
- You should find that in some places on the map the edge of the river should match the direction that the compass is pointing. This limits the number of places where you can be, and using the other skills you can narrow it down further.
- Ideally if you keep an eye on the map throughout the day you should be able to continually see where you are and it should be easy to identify your location.

Index

A

Aberlour 53, 58, 59
Aberlour Distillery 54
Access 69
Accommodation 32, 37, 41, 48, 54, 61
Advie Bridge 47, 50
Anagach Woods 48, 49
Anagach Woods Trust 49
Aviemore 37, 39, 41
Avon, River 54, 55

B

Badgers 42, 78
Ballindalloch 47
Ballindalloch Castle 48
Ballindalloch Castle Golf Course 51
Ballindalloch Pools 51
Battle of Cromdale 50
Baxters 61, 63
Blacksboat Bridge 53, 56
Blacksboat Rapid 55
Boat o' Brig 61, 62
Boat of Balliefurth 41, 47
Boat of Balliefurth Campsite 45
Boat of Cromdale 50
Boat of Garten 41, 43
Broomhill 44
Broomhill Bridge 41, 44
Buzzard 79

C

Campfires 70
Capercaillie 49, 81
Cardhu Distillery 54
Carron Bridge 53, 58
Cragganmore 47, 53
Cragganmore Bridge 47, 51, 53, 54
Cragganmore Distillery 48
Craigellachie 53, 59, 61, 62
Craigroy Island 56
Crayfish 83
Creag Dhubh 25, 31, 32
Cromdale 50
Cromdale Bridge 50
Cromdale Church 47, 50
Crossbill 49, 81
Culfoichbeg 50

D

Dalfaber golf course 42
Dalriach 50
Deer 78
Dippers 80
Distances 29
Distilleries 86
Dolphins 64, 75
Droving 87
Duke of Gordon's Monument 39

E

Environmental issues 83
Equipment 15
Equipment list 18

F

Farming 87
Fiddich Park 54, 59
Fiddich Water 59
Fishing 49, 64, 69, 71, 72, 87
Fochabers 61, 63
Freshwater mussel 50, 83

G

Garmouth 64
Garva Bridge 23
Goldeneye duck 80
Goosander 81
Grantown Fishing Association 48
Grantown Museum 48
Grantown Old Bridge 49
Grantown-on-Spey 47, 48
Grid references 89
Group paddling 13
Gyrodactylus salaris 83

H

Haugh Island 62
Heron 80
Highland Badgers 43
Highland Folk Museum 32, 87
Highland Line 86
Highland Wildlife Park 32, 37, 78
History of the River Spey 85

I

Imperial Distillery 58
Insh Marshes National Nature Reserve 32, 34
Inveravon Pictish Stones 48
Invertruim House 32
Itineraries 27

K

Kinchurdy Farm 43
Kincraig Church 31, 35, 37, 38
King's Hut 50
Kingston 64
Kingussie 31, 34
Kinrara House 39
Knockando 53
Knockando rapids 51, 54, 57, 58
Knockando Woolmill 54

L

Laggan 24
Laggan Bridge 24
Lagoons 64
Lochain Uvie 23, 25, 31
Loch Avon 55
Loch Garten Osprey Centre 41
Loch Insh 31, 35, 37
Loch Insh Water Sports Centre 31, 32, 35, 37
Loch Spey 23
Logging 85

M

Mains of Dalvey 50
Mallard 80
Monadhliath Mountains 23
Moray Firth Wildlife Centre 65

N

Navigation skills 89
Nethybridge 41
Newtonmore 31, 32, 33

O

Old Bridge Inn, Aviemore 37, 39, 41, 42
Orton earth pillars 62
Osprey 38, 79
Osprey Centre, Loch Garten 41
Otter 77

P

Packing a canoe/kayak 15
Paddlers Access Code 71
Parasite (salmon) 83
Penny Bridge 58, 59
Pine marten 49, 78
Planning 13, 27

R

Railways 86
Red-breasted merganser 81
Rescue 67
Revack Estate 48
River Avon 54, 55
River levels 19, 20
River Spey, Upper 23
Roary Island 57
Rothes 62
Rothiemurchus 39
Rothiemurchus Estate 37
Ruthven Barracks 31, 32, 34

S

Safety and rescue 67
Salmon 75
Salmon parasite 83
Sand martin 42, 63, 79
Scottish Dolphin Centre 61, 76
Scottish Outdoor Access Code 69
Seals 64, 76
Seven Pillars of Hercules 62
Shuttles 14
Signal crayfish 83
Spey Anglers Guidance 71, 73
Spey Bay Golf Course 65
Spey Bay (Tugnet) 61, 64
Spey Bridge 31, 33
Spey Bridge Campsite 31
Spey Dam 24
Speyside Cooperage 54
Speyside Way campsite 51
Speyside Wildlife 41
Spey Valley Smoke House 48
Squirrels 77
Strathspey Steam Railway 41, 44, 86

T

Tamdhu Distillery 53
The Haughs of Cromdale 50
Toileting 70
Tomintoul 55
Tom Nan Carragh 45
Tugnet 61, 64, 65

U

Upper River Spey 23

V

Victoria Bridge 58

W

Walkers Shortbread Factory 54
Washing Machine Rapid 56
Weather 19
Whale and Dolphin Conservation Society 65
Whales 64, 76
Whisky 86
Wild camping 69
Wild cats 77
Wildlife 75

Spirit of the Spey

OPEN CANOE JOURNEYS
With Spey Specialist
Dave Craig

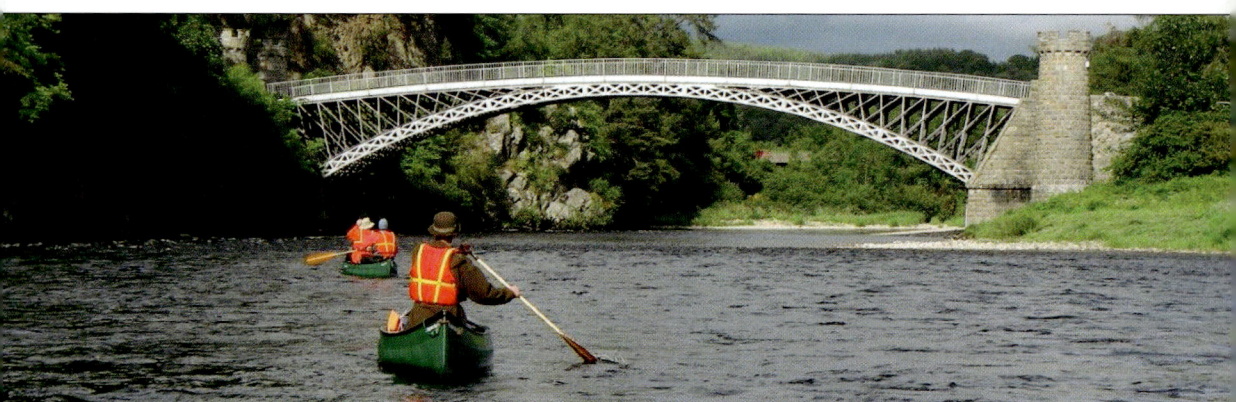

Canoe Journeys ~ Whisky Tours ~ Coaching Sessions
01540 673 826 • 0787 033 8110
www.spiritofthespey.co.uk

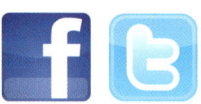 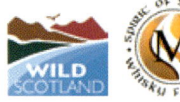 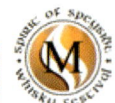

beyond ADVENTURE

Guided River Spey canoe trips
Shuttles & canoe/kayak transport
Canoe hire & outfitting service

t: 01887 829202
e: email@beyondadventure.co.uk
w: beyondadventure.co.uk

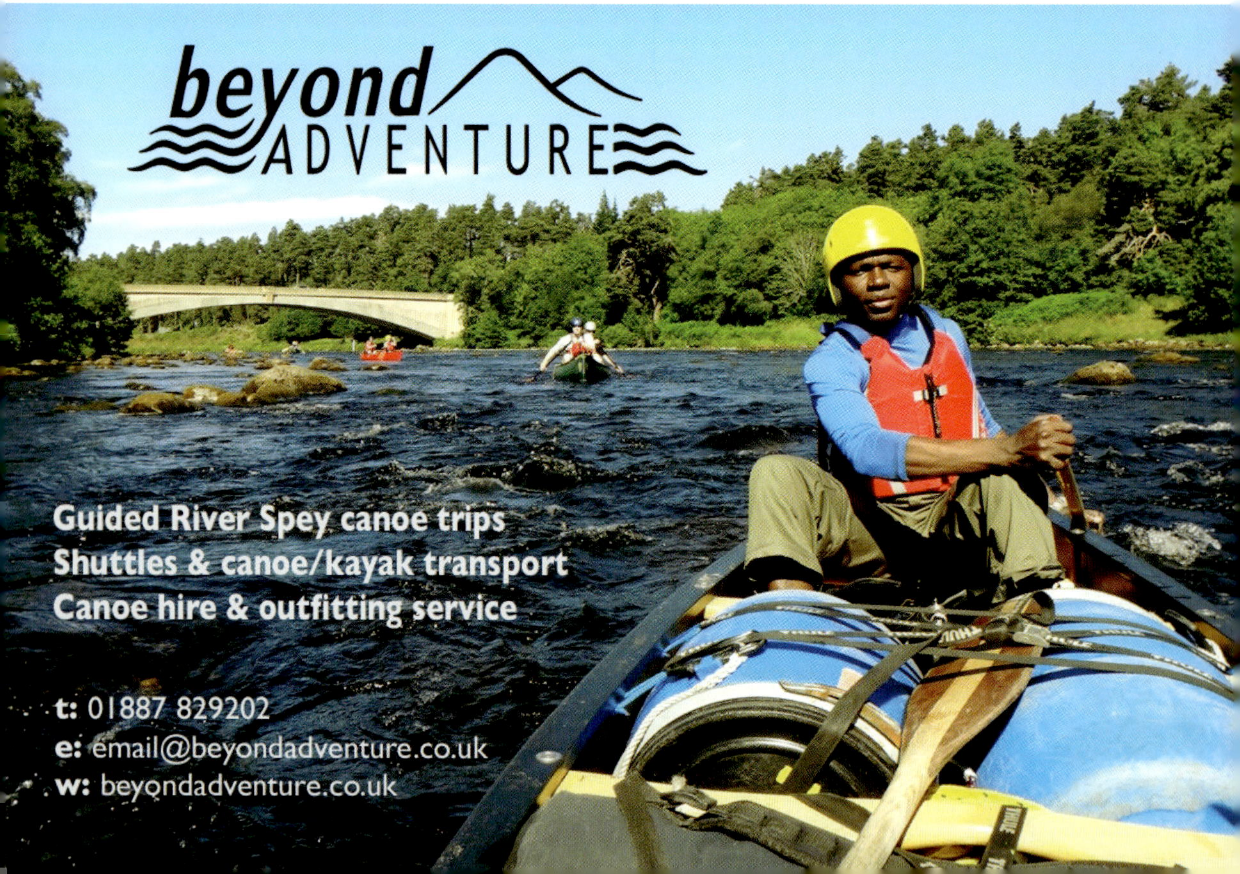